Medial Mandibular Ramus

Ontogenetic, idiosyncratic, and geographic variation in recent *Homo*, great apes, and fossil hominids

Gary D. Richards
Laboratory for Human Evolutionary Studies, Department of Anthropology,
University of California, Berkeley, CA 94720

Department of Anatomy, University of the Pacific,
School of Dentistry, San Francisco, CA 94115

Rebecca S. Jabbour
Ph.D Program in Anthropology, City University of New York and NYCEP,
New York, NY 10036

John Y. Anderson
Department of Anthropology, University of New Mexico,
Albuquerque, NM 87131

BAR International Series 1138
2003

Published in 2019 by
BAR Publishing, Oxford

BAR International Series 1138

Medial Mandibular Ramus

© The authors individually and the Publisher 2003

The authors' moral rights under the 1988 UK Copyright,
Designs and Patents Act are hereby expressly asserted.

All rights reserved. No part of this work may be copied, reproduced, stored,
sold, distributed, scanned, saved in any form of digital format or transmitted
in any form digitally, without the written permission of the Publisher.

ISBN 9781841713335 paperback
ISBN 9781407325385 e-book

DOI https://doi.org/10.30861/9781841713335

A catalogue record for this book is available from the British Library

This book is available at www.barpublishing.com

BAR Publishing is the trading name of British Archaeological Reports (Oxford) Ltd.
British Archaeological Reports was first incorporated in 1974 to publish the BAR
Series, International and British. In 1992 Hadrian Books Ltd became part of the BAR
group. This volume was originally published by John and Erica Hedges in conjunction
with British Archaeological Reports (Oxford) Ltd / Hadrian Books Ltd, the Series
principal publisher, in 2003. This present volume is published by BAR Publishing,
2019.

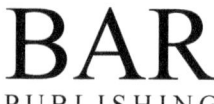

BAR titles are available from:

BAR Publishing
122 Banbury Rd, Oxford, OX2 7BP, UK
EMAIL info@barpublishing.com
PHONE +44 (0)1865 310431
FAX   +44 (0)1865 316916
www.barpublishing.com

ACKNOWLEDGMENTS

We thank Drs. Tim D. White and F. Clark Howell; Henry Gilbert and Faysal Bibi; and three anonymous reviewers for their comments and suggestions on an earlier version of the manuscript. We also thank Drs. Nuria Garcia and J. L. Arsuaga for information regarding specimens in their care and Dr. Erik Trinkaus for information on trait scoring criteria. For access to specimens and collections, we thank Drs. F. Clark Howell and Tim D. White, LHES, UCB; Dr. Dorothy Burk, Department of Anatomy and Dr. Dorothy Dechant, The Institute of Dental History and Craniofacial Study, UOP; Dr. Erik Trinkaus, Department of Anthropology, Washington University; and Drs. Ian Tattersall and Kenneth Mowbray, Department of Anthropology, American Museum of Natural History. For help in translation of various publications, we thank Bettina Behrens, Dr. K. Polosukhina, Marta and Michael Thoene, and Dr. Yohannes Zeleke.

Table of Contents

Acknowledgments
Abstract

INTRODUCTION 1

MATERIALS AND METHODS

I. Comparative anatomical collections 3
    1. Recent *Homo sapiens* and great ape osteological samples 4
    2. Fossil hominid sample 4
    3. Recent *Homo sapiens* soft tissue sample 4

II. Methods 8
    1. Methodology for developmental age determinations 8
    2. Criteria used in assessing medial pterygoid tubercle occurrence rates 8
    3. Procedures for collecting hard and soft tissue data 8
    4. Terminological issues and definitions 10
    5. Statistical procedures 11

RESULTS OF OBSERVATIONS AND DESCRIPTION OF MEDIAL RAMAL BONY AND SOFT TISSUE ANATOMY IN MODERN AND FOSSIL HOMINOIDS

I. Assessment of the medial pterygoid tubercle character state, as defined, in recent *Homo sapiens* 14
    1. Introduction 14
    2. Percentage occurrence of the character state by age group 14
    3. Geographic distribution of the character state 14

II. Description of bony medial ramus anatomy in an ontogenetic series of recent *Homo sapiens* and related soft tissues in adults 16
    1. Introduction 16
    2. Observations on ligaments and fascia of the medial ramus region 16
    3. Observations on neurovascular and related soft tissues of the medial ramus region ... 18
    4. Overview of hard and soft tissue relationships in the recent *Homo sapiens* series 20

III. Description of bony medial ramus anatomy and related soft tissues in ontogenetic samples of great apes 26
    1. Introduction 26
    2. Overview of hard and soft tissue relationships in ontogenetic samples of great apes ... 26

IV. Description of bony medial ramus anatomy in ontogenetic samples of Plio-Pleistocene hominids 29
    1. Introduction 29

2. Description of the bony medial ramus in fossil hominids 29
   2.1. *Australopithecus afarensis* 29
   2.2. *Australopithecus africanus* 31
   2.3. *Australopithecus robustus* 31
   2.4. *Australopithecus boisei* 33
   2.5. *Homo habilis* (*sensu lato*) 33
   2.6. *Homo erectus* (*sensu lato*) 33
   2.7. Archaic *Homo sapiens* 36
   2.8. Neanderthals 36
      2.8.1. Subadult Neanderthals 36
      2.8.2. Adult Neanderthals 38
      2.8.3. Morphology of the superior aspect of the medial pterygoid tubercle 41
      2.8.4. Morphology of the medial aspect of the medial pterygoid tubercle 41
   2.9. Anatomically modern *Homo sapiens* 42
   2.10. *Homo sapiens* ssp. indet. 44
   2.11. Bilateral occurrence of medial ramal features and limitations of the fossil record 44

DISCUSSION OF THE ONTOGENY OF MEDIAL RAMAL BONY AND SOFT TISSUE ANATOMY IN MODERN AND FOSSIL HOMINOIDS

I. The medial pterygoid tubercle in recent *Homo sapiens* and an introduction to the necessity for a broader assessment 45
   1. Assessment of the recent *Homo sapiens* data 45
   2. Rationale for the need of a broader assessment of medial ramal anatomy 45

II. Overview of the ontogeny of recent *Homo sapiens* medial ramus morphology 47
   1. Overview of the development of medial ramal morphology 47
   2. Factors influencing tubercle area and projection 49
   3. The role of ligaments in producing and maintaining medial ramal morphology 50
   4. Summary 51

III. Ontogeny of medial ramal anatomy in great apes and issues in character homology 53
   1. Overview of great ape medial ramal anatomy 53
   2. Discussion of medial ramal tubercle homology in great apes and recent *Homo sapiens* 54
   3. Summary 55

IV. Ontogeny of medial ramal anatomy in fossil hominids 56
   1. Medial ramus morphology of australopithecines 56
      1.1. *Australopithecus afarensis* 56
      1.2. *Australopithecus africanus* and *Australopithecus robustus* 57
      1.3. *Australopithecus boisei* 57
   2. Medial ramus morphology of *Homo* 58
      2.1. *Homo habilis* (*sensu lato*) 58
      2.2. *Homo erectus* (*sensu lato*) 58
      2.3. Archaic *Homo sapiens* 59
         2.3.1. Morphology of the medial pterygoid region 59
         2.3.2. Population level variation in the medial pterygoid insertion 60
         2.3.3. Subadult morphology 60
      2.4. Neanderthals 60

  2.4.1. Lingular and mylohyoid groove bridging 60
  2.4.2. Morphology of the medial pterygoid region 65
  2.4.3. Population level variation in the medial pterygoid attachment 65
  2.4.4. Shape characteristics of medial pterygoid related insertion tubercles 66
 2.5. Anatomically modern *Homo sapiens* 66
 2.6. *Homo sapiens* ssp. indet. 66
3. Bilateral development of medial ramal features and the value of anomalous
development for understanding observed medial ramus morphology 67

SUMMARY OF MORPHOLOGICAL DIFFERENCES AND EVOLUTIONARY CHANGE IN THE MEDIAL RAMUS FROM *AUSTRALOPITHECUS* TO RECENT *HOMO SAPIENS*

I. Derivation of Australopithecine medial ramal morphology 68
 1. Evolutionary change and revision of mandibular skeletal units 68
 2. Change in medial ramal morphology from the presumed ancestral condition 68

II. The Australopithecine - *Homo* transition and medial ramus evolution in *Homo* 70
 1. Stasis and change in early *Homo* 70
 2. Early *Homo* to *Homo erectus* (*sensu lato*) 70
 3. *Homo erectus* (*sensu lato*) to Archaic *Homo sapiens* 71
 4. Archaic *Homo sapiens* and Neanderthals 71
 5. Neanderthals and anatomically modern *Homo sapiens* 73
 6. Anatomically modern *Homo sapiens* to recent *Homo sapiens* 74

III. Summary 75

ROLE OF TENDONS, LIGAMENTS, AND MUSCLES IN CRANIOFACIAL GROWTH

I. Tendon and ligament development and function 76
 1. Introduction 76
 2. Tendon and ligament development and mechanics in craniofacial growth 76
 3. Correlation of primary and literature-derived data 79

II. Muscle physiology and architecture and their effects on medial ramal morphology 82
 1. Muscle structure and physiology 82
 2. Impact of cultural behaviors on masticatory muscles 83
 3. Gross structure and function of masticatory muscles 84
 4. Summary 85

MUSCULAR FUNCTION, CRANIOFACIAL ONTOGENY, AND MODELING MANDIBULAR GROWTH

I. Muscular function and craniofacial morphology 87
 1. Introduction 87
 2. Mandibulofacial development in relation to the ontogeny of masticatory function 87
 3. Masticatory muscles and craniofacial shape 89
 4. Summary 89

II. Impact of current work on model of mandibular growth 91
   1. Migration of musculotendinous attachments 91
   2. Suggested revision to mandibular growth model 92

ONTOGENY AND VARIATION IN SYSTEMATICS

I. Ontogenetic and phylogenetic issues related to the medial pterygoid tubercle 93

II. Morphological variation and systematics 94

CONCLUSIONS 95

BIBLIOGRAPHY 97

ABSTRACT

The study of human evolutionary systematics rests on a foundation comprising observations of gross morphology. Even in recent cases where discussion of the taxonomic status and phylogenetic position of fossilized remains of human ancestors has revolved around analysis of mitochondrial DNA, the analyzed fossils required prior taxonomic assignment. Species determinations for these fossils relies, in large part, on the analysis of features and character states of the osseous craniofacial complex; however, generally-accepted guidelines for establishing feature and character state validity are not available and, resultantly, criteria used in species recognition are not consistently applied in paleoanthropology. Whereas it is beyond the scope of this work to propose a complete set of such guidelines, this study illustrates the importance of considering interactions between soft and hard (bone) tissues throughout ontogeny and the variation produced by these interactions in defining features and character states.

Numerous osseous indicators have been proposed and employed in assessing generic, specific, and subspecific affinities of modern humans and their ancestors. In this work we focus on the morphology of the medial mandibular ramus as its topography reflects changing relationships within the Hominoidea between the midface, mandible, cranial base, and neck. Specifically, we focus on a mandibular ramus character state, the 'medial pterygoid tubercle' (MPT), as its usage raises broad issues related to interpreting osseous morphology in ontogenetic, taxonomic, and phylogenetic contexts. This character state is also of historic interest as its position coincides with a previously defined feature, the *tuberculum pterygoideum inferius* (*tpi*). The *tpi* and the MPT are also positionally related to other medial ramus features and character states which are employed in taxonomic and phylogenetic studies. Further, knowledge of how bony topography arises and is maintained throughout ontogeny has direct relevance to all analyses of skeletal remains.

To evaluate the MPT character state we employ two approaches. First, we address the validity of the autapomorphic status of the character by assessing it as an isolated feature of the medial ramus. Second, because features of bone do not arise in isolation we examine the character as part of a developing system.

To assess the ontogeny and evolution of the medial ramus and address issues of character homology, we examine both dry bone and soft tissue samples. We examine ontogenetic series of recent *Homo sapiens*, great ape, and fossil hominid (*Australopithecus* through anatomically modern *Homo sapiens*) mandibles. We supplement these dry bone assessments with observations of soft tissues deriving from both human cadaver dissections and literature descriptions.

In our first assessment, we conclude that the MPT character state is not autapomorphic for Neanderthals, as it occurs at a high frequency in recent *Homo sapiens*. We also conclude that this character state is insufficiently defined for use in taxonomic assessments and that it should, therefore, no longer be employed. In our second assessment we detail medial ramus ontogeny and variation in recent *Homo sapiens*, great apes, and fossil hominids and the evolutionary trajectories of medial ramal structures in the Hominidae. Note that our observations are limited to expanding our understanding of the development of the *musculus pterygoideus medialis* insertion site and not directly to the ontogeny and evolution of each of the following structures. On this basis, we document variation present throughout ontogeny in the: (1) *crista endocondyloidea*; (2) *sulcus colli*; (3) *lingula mandibulae*; (4) *foramen mandibulae-canalis mandibulae*; (5) mylohyoid groove (*sulcus mylohyoideus mandibulae*); and (6) *m. pterygoideus medialis* insertion site. By incorporating these dry bone data with those gained from cadaver dissections, we also delineate: (1) bony insertion morphology relative to *m. pterygoideus medialis* septa; (2) the soft tissue construction and insertion sites of the *ligamentum sphenomandibulare*, *ligamentum stylomandibulare*, and deep cervical fascia; and (3) the relationship of these and associated neurovascular structures to the development of medial ramal morphology.

From our recent human data we specifically demonstrate that a combination of genetic, epigenetic, and idiosyncratic factors are involved in the production and maintenance of *m. pterygoideus medialis* insertion morphology, in bridging of the mylohyoid groove and *l. mandibulae*, and in extension of the *l. mandibulae*. We also document how the insertion sites of the *m. pterygoideus medialis* and *l. sphenomandibulare* are impacted by ontogenetic events related to this muscle's maturation and by the changing relationships of associated functional matrices of the medial ramus. From these data we suggest a range of factors involved in producing and maintaining medial ramus bony topography.

Using our assessment of modern great ape and hominid fossil morphology we clarify issues surrounding the homology of *m. pterygoideus medialis* insertion tubercles between great apes and hominids. We also document a range of differences between these groups and suggest pathways for shape change in the medial ramus associated with a significant shift in locomotion and behavior. Further, we document how these changes in craniofacial relationships result in significant soft tissue repackaging and modified functional requirements and how these impact the insertion of muscles and ligaments of the medial ramus. Specifically, we document changes in positioning of *m. pterygoideus medialis* insertion tubercles and follow a general series of changes in this attachment throughout the hominid lineage. We also document the relationship between presumed changes in the structure and insertion relationships of the *l. sphenomandibulare* and the origin and evolutionary development of the *l. mandibulae*. Given these results and observations on the evolutionary and ontogenetic trajectories of other medial ramal structures, we discuss how muscles, ligaments, neurovascular structures, and related tissues interact to form the bony topography of the medial ramus. These data demonstrate clearly that expression of *m. pterygoideus medialis* insertion tubercles (cf. MPT, *tpi*), aspects of the horizontal-oval foramen character state, and features of the *crista intermedia* are partially linked and heavily impacted by changing relationships and functions throughout ontogeny.

By employing our observational data, we document significant shape change of the osseous medial ramus both during ontogeny and throughout evolution. These data, however, do not allow us to fully address the question of how these features of bone develop. To better understand factors involved in producing variation in the osseous phenotype we review the literature covering: (1) muscle, tendon, and ligament architecture and physiology; (2) the importance of these to understanding the musculotendinous-bone interface; (3) the relationships of these soft tissues to development of medial ramus morphology; and (4) the general relationship between developing craniofacial functional matrices and medial ramal anatomy. By combining this review with data obtained from our dry bone observations and cadaver dissections we document some of the complexities of the relationship between soft and hard tissues. Within this context we establish a framework from which we resolve some of the issues related to the production of medial ramal topography. We also indicate numerous areas where available data is insufficient to resolve current questions. We conclude that resolution of these issues in conjunction with a more developed understanding of how osseous structures develop and change throughout ontogeny will provide a more firm basis for the delineation of useful features and character states. It is our belief that an expanded emphasis on understanding ontogeny and variation throughout growth will provide an improved basis for the taxonomic study and significantly expanded understanding of the phylogenetic history of hominids.

INTRODUCTION

Discussion of the specific status of modern humans and Neanderthals has historically relied on anatomical description and metric and non-metric assessments of the craniofacial complex. Recent discussion has, however, emphasized results from analysis of mitochondrial (mtDNA) and nuclear DNA extracted from fossilized remains (fDNA: Krings et al., 1997; Golovanova et al., 1999; Höss, 2000; Krings et al., 2000; Ovchinnikov et al., 2000; Scholz et al., 2000; Caramelli et al., 2003). Evidence available from mtDNA and fDNA, although seen by some as confirming the taxonomic status of Neanderthals as a separate species (Krings et al., 1997; Golovanova et al., 1999; Höss, 2000; Ovchinnikov et al., 2000; Scholz et al., 2000) or as relegating morphological analyses to a supporting role in such assessments (Lieberman, 1999), is not conclusive. Significant questions arise in the phylogenetic meaning of differences observed and in the relationship of mtDNA to nuclear DNA in species recognition (Eckhardt, 1989; Nordborg, 1998; Fay and Wu, 1999; Hey, 1999; Relethford, 1999, 2001; Wolpoff and Caspari, 1999; Hawks and Wolpoff, 2001; Templeton, 2002). Further, a recent mtDNA study of the Mezmaiskaya Cave (Layer 3) infant purports to confirm the findings of Krings et al. (1997), who found Neanderthals to be a separate species; however, the Mezmaiskaya Cave study relies on a taxonomic assessment based on phenotypic characters of the fetal-infant craniofacial region (Golovanova, 1994; Golovanova and Romanova, 1995; Golovanova et al., 1999; Höss, 2000; Ovchinnikov et al., 2000). Given our current methodological paradigm, difficulties encountered in determining the phylogenetic status of subadult remains from discrete and continuous characters expressed in the phenotype are well known (Weidenreich, 1945; Heim, 1982; Tillier, 1982, 1988, 1989, 1992, 1995, 1998; Madre-Dupouy, 1991; Lieberman, 1995, 2000; Rak and Kimbel, 1995; Trinkaus, 1995b; Creed-Miles et al., 1996; Schwartz and Tattersall, 1996a; Mann and Vandermeersch, 1997). These problems notwithstanding, the morphological assessment of the Mezmaiskaya Cave infant which resulted in its designation as *Homo neanderthalensis* (Golovanova, 1994; Golovanova and Romanova, 1995; Golovanova et al., 1999) is also a clear example of a typological approach (see Mayr, 1974:108) to taxonomy. The mtDNA analysis of this individual (Ovchinnikov et al., 2000) currently provides no confirmatory evidence regarding the specific status of Neanderthals nor can it be said to increase the available sample of Neanderthal mtDNA (contra Krings et al., 2000). Resultant problems created from the specific assignment of the Mezmaiskaya Cave infant remains serve, however, to underscore the need for ontogenetic analyses which: (1) employ appropriate samples and sample sizes; (2) fully detail the observed range(s) of phenotypic variation; (3) employ data which allow for the interpretation of skeletal units through their associated functional matrices; and (4) recognize that few adult character states occur in subadults (see Straus, 1962; Mann et al., 1990; Winkler, 1991; Tillier, 1995, 1998). It is within this context, and by examining a purported medial ramal character state as an example, that we provide description and review of the ontogeny of soft and hard tissues of the medial ramus region in hominoids. Given these data we attempt to delineate how specific bony features arise on the medial ramus and how an increased emphasis on understanding the ontogeny of soft and hard tissues can provide features and character states of greater value to systematics.

Features and character states of the craniofacial region constitute most of the basis for our understanding of relationships between Middle-to-Upper Pleistocene hominids (Minugh-Purvis, 1988, 1998; Trinkaus, 1990, 1993; Rosas et al., 1991; Tillier, 1992, 1998; Akazawa et al., 1995a, b; Franciscus and Trinkaus, 1995; Lieberman, 1995, 2000; Rak et al., 1994; Rosas, 1995, 1997; Schwartz and Tattersall, 1995, 1996a, b; Hovers et al., 1996; Laitman et al., 1996; Arensburg and Belfer-Cohen, 1998; Dodo et al., 1998; Hublin, 1998; Rak, 1998b; Stefan and Trinkaus, 1998a, b; Coqueugniot, 1999; Franciscus, 1999; Sanchez, 1999; Schwartz et al., 1999; Smith et al., 1999; Churchill and Smith, 2000; Rosas, 2000, 2001; Lebel et al., 2001; Rosas et al., 2002). Controversy exists, however, regarding interpretations derived from these analyses (Trinkaus, 1993, 1995b; Antón, 1994b, 1995, 1996; Rak et al., 1996; Franciscus and Trinkaus, 1995; Hovers et al., 1995, 1996; Lieberman, 1995; Richards and Plourde, 1995; Rightmire, 1995; Creed-Miles et al., 1996; Rhoads and Franciscus, 1996; Schwartz and Tattersall, 1996a, b; Arensburg and Belfer-Cohen, 1998; Hublin, 1998; Jabbour and Richards, 1998; Quam and Smith,1998; Rak, 1998a, b; Stefan and Trinkaus, 1998a, b; Tillier, 1998; Tyrrell and Chamberlain, 1998; Coqueugniot, 1999; Franciscus, 1999; Jabbour et al., 2002). A subset of the latter works (see below) focuses on mandibular morphology with important re-assessments and discussions of phenotypic features traditionally utilized to distinguish Neanderthals from recent and anatomically modern humans (AmHs) at the specific or subspecific level. In addition to the traditionally utilized features of the medial mandibular ramus (i.e., gonial angle shape and its mediolateral orientation, the presence or absence of a preangular notch, the general topography of the *musculus pterygoideus medialis* insertion site, basic configuration of the *sulcus colli*, and the presence or absence of mylohyoid groove (= *sulcus mylohyoideus mandibulae*) and *lingula mandibulae* bridging: McCown and Keith, 1939; Smith, 1976; Billy and Vallois, 1977; Wolpoff et al., 1981; Trinkaus, 1983; Rosas, 1987, 1995, 2001; Tillier et al., 1989; Rosas et al., 1991; Tillier, 1991; Arensburg and Belfer-Cohen, 1998; Coqueugniot, 1999; Churchill and Smith, 2000; Jidoi et al., 2000; Lebel et al., 2001; and citations below), a new character state has been proposed, the so-called 'medial pterygoid tubercle' (MPT: Rak et al., 1994, 1996).

Prior to definition of the MPT character state (Rak et al., 1994), the insertion region of the *m. pterygoideus medialis* had received only cursory attention in descriptions of fossil hominids (Schoetensack, 1908; Boule, 1911-1913; Martin, 1923; Buxton, 1928; Weidenreich, 1936; Boule and Vallois, 1957; Patte, 1958; Arambourg, 1963; Piveteau, 1963-1966; Ferembach, 1969, 1970; Suzuki, 1970; Heim, 1974, 1976; Sausse, 1975; Smith, 1976; Vandermeersch and Tillier, 1977; de Lumley et al., 1982; Johanson et al., 1982; Tillier, 1982, 1983b, 1984, 1989, 1991, 1998; Tillier et al., 1989; Madre-Dupouy, 1991; Tobias, 1991; Wood, 1991; Faerman et al., 1994). In Neanderthal adults the attachment site had been described as rugose with well developed crests and tubercles (Boule, 1911-1913; Boule and Vallois, 1957; Patte, 1958; Heim, 1974, 1976; Trinkaus, 1983; Tillier et al., 1989), whereas in subadult Neanderthals it was only noted as vast (Patte, 1958) or strongly developed (Tillier, 1983b). The generally strong degree of bony development of the *m. pterygoideus medialis* insertion in this group was variously considered as: (1) a Neanderthal trait (Tillier et al., 1989; Tillier, 1991); (2) a primitive retention (Le Double, 1906; Billy and Vallois, 1977); or (3) similar in both modern and Pleistocene *Homo* (Boule, 1911-1913). Morphology of the attachment site in AmHs was less well delineated but noted as: (1) presenting with strong muscle associated crests in Qafzeh 9 and 11 (Vandermeersch and Tillier, 1977; Tillier, 1984) and, thereby, being similar to Skhul V (Vandermeersch, 1981); and (2) being a strongly developed, archaic feature in the similarly aged subadults Skhul 1, Roc de Marsal 1, and Barakai (Tillier, 1998).

Combining portions of this history with their analysis of the region, Rak et al. (1994) and Hovers et al. (1995) state that the following individuals or taxa share a generalized (symplesiomorphic) morphology of the insertion site for *m. pterygoideus medialis* with modern *Homo sapiens*: (1) *Gorilla*; (2) *Pan troglodytes*; (3) *Australopithecus robustus* (SK 23); *A. boisei* (KNM-ER 729, Peninj); *Homo erectus* (*sensu lato* (s.l.): Zhoukoudian, Ternifine); and archaic *H. sapiens* (s.l.: Arago). On the other hand, the nature of this muscle's insertion site, as denoted by the MPT character state, is considered to be autapomorphic for Neanderthals by Rak et al. (1994, 1996), Rak and Kimbel (1995), Creed-Miles et al. (1996), and Rak (1998a). The character's importance derives from being considered to be under direct genetic control, as opposed to a character which results from either epigenetic (*sensu* Atchley, 1993) or nonheritable idiosyncratic variation. Evidence for a genetic basis for the trait derives from analysis of the 10-month-old Amud 7 infant. The character's presence in such an early growth stage, well prior to the initiation of its perceived adult function, is considered by Rak et al. (1994) as direct confirmation of a genetic underpinning. By presenting in early developmental stages the MPT character state could be considered as similar to features such as positioning, but not necessarily number, of *foramina mentale*. Positioning of this foramen is associated with the course and distribution of the third branch of the *nervus trigeminalis* and is currently considered to reflect craniomandibular relationships established in the earliest stages of development (Merida-Velasco et al., 1993; Trinkaus, 1993; Anderson, 2000; Moore et al., 2003). Further, since the MPT character is suggested to be directly related to *m. pterygoideus medialis* hypertrophy it is considered to have little or no function in its pre-adult state (Rak et al., 1994; Hovers et al., 1996).

Discussion of the *m. pterygoideus medialis* insertion site and the MPT character state are of anatomical, taxonomic, and phylogenetic interest. Recognition of a MPT in the Amud 7 infant, in conjunction with other 'character states', has provided support for a taxonomic assessment of this specimen as *H. neanderthalensis*. Given this taxonomic designation, the presence of the character state in Amud 7 is seen to confirm the presence of Neanderthals in the Middle East. It also has cultural implications as it provides supporting evidence for both intentional burials by Neanderthals and the first evidence in the Levant of the possible association of grave goods with a Neanderthal burial (Rak et al., 1994; Hovers et al., 1996).

Given the above, recognition of the MPT character state carries with it broad ontogenetic, functional, taxonomic, and phylogenetic implications and impacts reconstructions of Pleistocene cultures. For these reasons, Richards and Plourde (1995) presented results which demonstrated that the MPT character state did not allow differentiation of recent *H. sapiens* from Neanderthals. This result was independently confirmed by Antón (1995) in conjunction with her suggestion that the functional argument accounting for the character state was incorrect. Subsequently, Creed-Miles et al. (1996) concluded that the MPT character: (1) could not yet be considered as autapomorphic in immature Neanderthals due to problems in defining such traits in early postnatal stages; (2) is ubiquitous and autapomorphic in adult Neanderthals; and (3) is the same structure for which Weidenreich (1936) employs the term '*tuberculum pterygoideum inferius*' (*tpi*). They also noted that further consideration of growth changes of the medial mandibular ramus would be required in order to homologize this structure between juvenile and adult specimens (Creed-Miles et al., 1996). In a simultaneously published response, Rak et al. (1996) disputed the claims of Creed-Miles et al. (1996) regarding the identification of the MPT as a *tpi* and referred instead to a second tubercle superior to the MPT as the *tpi*. On this basis, Hovers et al. (1995) and Rak et al. (1996) rejected the differing conclusions of Creed-Miles et al. (1996) and, thereby, reinforced: (1) the validity of the MPT character state; (2) their naming of muscle related tubercles in the superior *m. pterygoideus medialis* attachment site; (3) the homology of the latter tubercles in great apes and hominids; (4) the taxonomic assignment of the Amud 7 infant and cultural implications drawn therefrom; and (5) the validity of the taxon *H. neanderthalensis*. Subsequently, Antón (1996) provided a metric analysis of MPT projection, concluding that, on average, Neanderthals have MPTs which are slightly more projecting than those of recent humans. Recently, Quam and Smith (1998) observed that the MPT is variably expressed but clearly present in 70% of Neanderthals. These authors further suggest that the MPTs presence on the Tabun C2 mandible (= non-Neanderthal,

Quam and Smith, 1998) may indicate a possible Neanderthal contribution to this individual's ancestry, if the assessment of Rak *et al.* (1994, 1996) is correct. Tillier's (1998) assessment results in the conclusion that the insertion site morphology in Neanderthals is plesiomorphic. Coqueugniot (1999) not only concludes that, the character state is not autapomorphic for Neanderthals but also strongly questions the validity of a divison of the insertion site into two distinct characters, the *tpi* and MPT. Most recently, Lebel *et al.* (2001) state that this character state, or a similar one, is variably expressed on Neanderthal and other Middle Pleistocene mandibles but that the higher frequency of occurrence in later Neanderthal samples appears distinctive.

Description and discussion of the *m. pterygoideus medialis* insertion site and MPT character state by Rak *et al.* (1994) raises several issues in the: (1) anatomical relations and range of soft tissues involved in producing and maintaining bony ramal morphology; (2) role(s) of muscle, tendon, and ligament function in producing and maintaining bony ramal morphology; (3) functional role(s) of morphological features of the bony medial ramus during ontogeny; (4) interpretation of osseous morphology in taxonomic and phylogenetic contexts; and (5) role of ontogeny in phylogenetic reconstructions. To address some of these issues, we initially evaluated the MPT character state as an isolated feature of the *m. pterygoideus medialis* attachment site in recent *H. sapiens* and Neanderthals (Richards and Plourde, 1995). We include the complete results of that work here. As outlined above, subsequent discussion of the character state by Antón (1994a, 1995, 1996), Creed-Miles *et al.* (1996), Hovers *et al.* (1996), and Rak *et al.* (1996) have expanded the breadth and complexity of issues pertaining to the character state while providing little resolution of the problems. The extensive assessment of the character state by Coqueugniot (1999) provides important new observations and conclusions regarding the ontogeny of the insertion site, but does not resolve numerous important issues. The current situation is further complicated by the continued use of this, or a similar, character state in taxonomic and phylogenetic assessments of Pleistocene *Homo* (Hublin, 1998; Quam and Smith, 1998; Smith *et al.*, 1999; Schwartz and Tattersall, 2000; Churchill and Smith, 2000; Jidoi *et al.*, 2000; Lebel *et al.*, 2001; Rosas *et al.*, 2002). For these reasons, and because features of bone do not arise in isolation, we expanded our analysis to include structures of the medial mandibular ramus inclusive of and inferior to the *crista endocondyloidea*. The sample has also been expanded to include all hominid taxa with preserved ramal regions and representatives of three great ape genera. Further, dissections of adult human cadavers were carried out to evaluate soft tissue structures of the medial ramus. Our data and those derived from a broad review of the anatomical and paleontological literature are employed here to: (1) provide a basic outline of the ontogeny of the medial ramus in recent humans, great apes, and fossil hominids; (2) relate hominid to ape morphology to resolve issues in tubercle homology; (3) delineate the evolutionary trajectory of medial ramal structures in hominids; (4) clarify the role(s) of soft tissues and ontogeny in producing and maintaining observed bony morphology of the medial ramus; and (5) clarify the anatomy and developmental origin(s) of variously related features and character states of the medial ramus and their applicability to hominid systematics. It is important to note that this expanded analysis is not confined to an assessment of the MPT character state. Features and character states of the medial ramus that are in some way linked to the development of the *m. pterygoideus medialis* are also examined. Further, in this work we do not attempt to divide morphological variation into discrete 'types' or character states. Our intent is to provide, by way of a sample character state (MPT), some insight into the processes by which ontogeny and function interact to produce phenotypic variations, the foundations of evolutionary change.

MATERIALS AND METHODS

I. COMPARATIVE ANATOMICAL COLLECTIONS

1. Recent *Homo sapiens* and great ape osteological samples

To evaluate aspects of medial mandibular ramus morphology we both examined dry bone specimens and carried out dissections of adult human cadavers. We compiled a large ($N = 728$) and geographically diverse sample of recent *H. sapiens* mandibles, retaining 689 of these for analysis. The osteological sample population ranges in developmental age from newborn to adult (> 20.6 years). Mandibles used in the examination of dry bone features derive from: (1) Phoebe Hearst Museum of Anthropology (PHMA), University of California, Berkeley (UCB), CA; and (2) The Institute for Dental History and Craniofacial Study, University of the Pacific, School of Dentistry, San Francisco, CA (UOP). Individuals in the PHMA collections derive from archaeological contexts in Alaska ($N = 1$), Nevada ($N = 1$), and California ($N = 288$). The California subsample derives from 87 localities in 25 counties, the majority of which are from Central California. Dates of occupation for localities included in this subsample fall within the time range of between ~ 4,500-100 BP, with the vast majority deriving from localities younger than ~ 500 BP. Individuals from these sites can be considered as representative of a hunter-gatherer mode of subsistence. The UOP sample ($N = 399$) comprises individuals from modern, non-archaeological contexts. The geographic ranges and sample sizes for this subsample include: (1) Mexico and South America ($N = 50$); (2) India ($N = 23$); (3) Europe and China ($N = 9$); and (4) geographic origin unknown ($N = 317$). We believe the majority of individuals in the latter category derive from the Indo-Pakistan region and Mexico. The subsistence pattern for the UOP individuals is unknown. Individuals with hemifacial microsomia ($N = 3$) derive from the UOP collection. We also evaluated bony anatomy of the medial ramus in great apes ($N = 48$) including: (1) *Pan troglodytes* ($N = 9$ adult, 8 subadult); (2) *Pan paniscus* ($N = 7$, 0); (3) *Pongo pygmaeus* ($N = 4$, 5); and (4) *Gorilla gorilla* ($N = 13$, 2). Originals and casts of great apes are housed in the Laboratory for Human Evolutionary Studies (LHES), UCB and UOP (Table 1).

2. Fossil hominid sample

Observations and discussions of subadult and adult fossil *Australopithecus* and *Homo* mandibular morphology are based on direct observation of original specimens and casts ($N = 74$: Table 1). Totals for the groups examined are: *A. afarensis* ($N = 10$); *A. africanus* ($N = 4$); *A. boisei* ($N = 2$); *A. robustus* ($N = 4$); *H. habilis* (*s.l.*, $N = 1$); *H. erectus* (*s.l.*, $N = 13$); archaic *H. sapiens* (ArHs: $N = 6$); Neanderthal ($N = 20$); anatomically modern *H. sapiens* (AmHs: $N = 13$); and *H. sapiens* ssp. indet. ($N = 1$). Original fossil specimens examined are housed at the Ethiopian National Museum, Addis Ababa, Ethiopia. Fossil casts examined are housed in the LHES; the Department of Anthropology, American Museum of Natural History, New York, NY; and the laboratory of Dr. Erik Trinkaus, Department of Anthropology, Washington University, St. Louis, MO. We recognize that the use of original specimens is preferable to the use of casts, as no cast duplicates the intricate detail of the original specimen. We are confident, however, that our use of casts has no negative impact on our observations. Prior to data collection: (1) all casts were evaluated against multiple literature descriptions, plates, and figures so as to eliminate any cast in which poor resolution of anatomical detail, mold part lines, or other casting artifacts might obscure scoring criteria or bony landmarks; and (2) all observations were carried out under a binocular microscope (10-30x) to ensure that observable morphology was not artifactual. Further, we both note throughout the text instances in which cast quality precludes accurate assessment of the morphology and maintain a level of anatomical description appropriate to the use of casts (i.e., determination of the more general configuration versus a focus on minute detail). Specimens examined, their taxonomic attributions, and individual age assessments are detailed in Table 1.

3. Recent *Homo sapiens* soft tissue sample

Two of us (GDR, RSJ) also evaluated adult bony and soft tissue anatomy of the medial mandibular ramus in a mixed-sex sample of 62 human cadavers. Chronological ages for the human cadavers range from between approximately 50.0 and 100.0 years of age. There is a slight female bias in this sample (~ 60% female) but it comprises individuals which sample a wide range of size and robusticity. Specimens derive from undissected portions of cadavers which remained at the termination of the UOP gross anatomy course. The level of dissection carried out prior to our work included the superficial face, brain removal, and midline bisection of the head. Structures deep to the superficial face or superficial to the sagittal plane remained intact.

Table 1: Taxonomic designations and developmental ages for fossil hominid and modern pongid mandibles examined

Taxon[1]	Specimen[2]	Age in years[3]	Taxon[1]	Specimen[2]	Age in years[3]
A. afarensis	AL 288-1	Adult	H. erectus (s. l)	Zhoukoudian F1 (c)	8.0 - 9.0
	AL 333-43b	~2.0 – 3.0		Zhoukoudian G1 (c)	Adult
	AL 333-100	Adult		Zhoukoudian H1 (c)	Adult
	AL 333-108	Adult			
	AL 333w-1e	Adult	ArHs	Arago II (c)	40.0 - 55.0
	AL 333w-16	Adult		Arago XIII (c)	~18.0 – 20.0
	AL 333w-52	Adult		Ehringsdorf F (c)	Adult
	Mak VP-1/2	Adult		Ehringsdorf G[4] (c)	11.0 – 12.0
	Mak VP-1/12	Adult		Mauer (c)	Adult
	Mak VP-1/83	Adult		Montmaurin 1 (c)	Adult
A. africanus	MLD 40 (c)	Adult	Neanderthal	Amud 1 (c)	Adult
	Sts 36 (c)	Adult		Circeo III (Guattari III) (c)	18.0 – 20.0
	Sts 52b (c)	Adult		Gibraltar 2 (Devil's Tower) (c)	4.0 – 4.5
	Stw 498 (c)	Adult		Kebara 2 (c)	Adult
				Krapina 53 (mand. C)[5] (c)	10.0 – 11.0
A. boisei	KNM-ER 729 (c)	Adult		Krapina 59 (mand. J) (c)	> 20.0
	Peninj (c)	Adult		Krapina 63 (ramus 1) (c)	> 20.0
				La Chapelle-aux-Saints (c)	Adult
A. robustus	SK 12 (c)	Adult		La Ferrassie 1 (c)	Adult
	SK 23 (c)	Adult		La Quina H5 (c)	Adult
	SK 64 (c)	~5.0 – 6.0		Pech de l'Azé (c)	2.0
	SKW 5 (c)	Adult		Régourdou 1 (c)	Adult
				Roc de Marsal 1 (c)	2.0 - 3.0
H. habilis (s. l)	OH 13 (c)	Adult		Saint Césaire (c)	Adult
				Shanidar 1 (c)	Adult
H. erectus (s. l)	KNM-BK 67 (c)	Adult		Tabun C1 (c)	Adult
	KNM-ER 820[1] (c)	5.3 – 6.5		Tabun C2[6] (c)	Adult
	KNM-ER 992 (c)	Adult		Teshik Tash (c)	8.0 – 11.0
	KNM-WT 15000 (c)	10.5		Vindija 207 (c)	Adult
	OH 22[1] (c)	Adult		Zafarraya (c)	Adult
	SK-15 (c)	Adult			
	Thomas Quarry 1 (c)	Adult	AmHs	Border Cave 2 (c)	Adult
	Ternifine (Tighennif) II (c)	Adult		Border Cave 4 (c)	Adult
	Ternifine (Tighennif) III (c)	Adult		Dar es Soltan 5[7] (c)	Adult
	Zhoukoudian B1 (c)	8.0 – 9.0		Ein Gev I (c)	30.0 – 40.0

Table 1 (continued): Taxonomic designations and developmental ages for fossil hominid and modern pongid mandibles examined

Taxon[1]	Specimen[2]	Age in years[3]	Taxon[1]	Specimen[2]	Age in years[3]
AmHs	Fish Hoek (c)	~30.0	P. paniscus	RG 24060	Adult
	Haua Fteah I (c)	>18.0 <25.0		RG 27012	Adult
	Haua Fteah II (c)	12.0 -14.0		RG 29047	Adult
	Omo-Kibish 1 (c)	Adult	P. troglodytes	LHES 1	Adult
	Qafzeh IX (c)	Young adult		LHES 2	Adult
	Qafzeh XI (c)	12.0 - 13.0		LHES 3	Adult
	Skhul 4 (c)	Adult		LHES 4	Adult
	Skhul 5 (c)	Adult		LHES 5	Adult
	Zhoukoudian 101 (c)	Adult		LHES 6	Adult
H. sapiens ssp. indet.	Amud 7 (c)	~ 0.83		LHES 7	Adult
Gorilla gorilla	LHES 1	Adult		LHES 8	Adult
	LHES 2	Adult		LHES 9	Adult
	LHES 3	Adult		LHES 10	9.0
	LHES 4	Adult		LHES 13	4.0
	LHES 5	Adult		LHES 180	4.0 - 5.0
	LHES 6	Adult		LHES 186	5.5
	LHES 7	Adult		LHES 187	5.0
	LHES 8	Adult		OM 3265	2.5 - 3.0
	LHES 9	Adult		W 226	3.5
	LHES 10	Adult		W 229	2.5
	LHES 11	Adult	Pongo pygmaeus	LHES 1	Adult
	LHES 12	3.5 - 4.0		LHES 2	Adult
	UOP CV-100	0.75		LHES 3	Adult
	W2210	Adult		LHES 4	Adult
	10009	Adult		LHES 5	4.0
P. paniscus	LHES 1	Adult		LHES 6	11.0
	LHES 2	Adult		LHES 7	3.0
	LHES 3	Adult		LHES 8	6.5
	RG 11049	Adult		UOP CV-99	9.0

[1] KNM-ER 820 is designated as *Homo* aff. *H. erectus* (Wood, 1991), whereas OH 22 is denoted as (?)*H. erectus* by Tobias (1991). In this work we have denoted the latter specimen as cf. *H. erectus*.

[2] Observations made on casts of specimens are denoted by a (c). See the Methods section for a discussion of the use of casts and details of methods employed in determining their suitability for use.

[3] Age determinations derive from the following sources: Amud 7 (Rak et al., 1994); Arago II and XIII (de Lumley et al., 1982); Circeo III (Sergi, 1955); Ehringsdorf G (Koski and Garn, 1957; Legoux, 1961; Vlček, 1993); Ein Gev I (Arensburg and Bar-Yosef, 1973); Fish Hoek (Keith, 1931); Gibraltar 2 (Skinner, 1997; Stringer and Dean, 1997); Haua Fteah I (McBurney et al., 1953; Trevor and Wells, 1967); Haua Fteah II (Tobias, 1967); KNM-ER 820 (Bromage and Dean, 1985; Smith, 1986); KNM-WT 15000 (Smith, 1993); Krapina 53, 59, and 63 (Radovčić et al., 1988); Pech de l'Azé (Patte, 1957); Qafzeh IX (Vandermeersch, 1981); Qafzeh XI (Vandermeersch and Tillier, 1977; Tillier, 1984); Roc de Marsal 1 (Tillier, 1983b; Madre-Dupouy, 1992); Skhul 4 and 5 (McCown and Keith, 1939); Teshik Tash (Gremyatskij, 1949); Zhoukoudian B1, F1, G1, H1, and Skull 101 (Weidenreich, 1936, 1938-39). We assigned specimens AL 333-43b and SK 64 age determinations based on data in Bromage and Dean (1985) and Smith (1986). Note that age estimates in the literature may derive from different criteria or combinations of criteria for any single individual and that this complicates the age determinations reported herein (see Ferembach, 1970; Tillier, 1983a-b; Dean et al., 1986; Madre-Dupouy, 1991, 1992; Schwartz and Tattersall, 1995). Developmental ages for great apes were determined with reference to Dean and Wood (1981).

[4] Ehringsdorf G observations are from a cast of the new reconstruction of Ehringsdorf 7/8 (Vlček, 1993).

[5] Observations on Krapina 53 (mandible C) are supplemented by observations on Krapina 67 (KDP-9) as it is potentially antimeric to Krapina 53 (Radovčić et al., 1988).

[6] The taxonomic status of the Tabun C2 mandible is currently being questioned and the specimen may be referable to anatomically modern humans, as opposed to its inclusion within the Neanderthal group (see Quam and Smith, 1998; Rak, 1998b).

[7] Specimen numbering for Dar es Soltan 5 follows Ferembach (1976).

II. METHODS

1. Methodology for developmental age determinations

Developmental ages for the PHMA individuals are based on comparison of jaws and loose teeth to the dental eruption and calcification standards of Ubelaker (1984). All ages for this subsample were assigned by a single observer (GDR) and checked for accuracy by four independent investigators. For the UOP subsample, developmental ages represent a mean-age assessment derived from individual scores assigned to each tooth available per individual. Age determinations for the UOP subsample were assigned by a single observer (GDR). Individual tooth scores were obtained by comparison of images from either or both periapical and lateral head radiographs with the calcification and eruption sequence of Schour and Massler (1941). In both subsamples (PHMA, UOP) teeth were only scored on the basis of calcification, due to the known geographical variance in dental eruption pattern (El-Nofely and Isçan, 1989). Variation in age assignment related to the use of different aging methods is not significant given the age categories employed. The included age groups and their sample sizes are detailed in Table 2. Note that ranges specified in Table 2 result from our having collapsed the sample, which is aged in tenth year increments, into broader developmental age categories. The range specified does not include error values (i.e., ± x-years) for the age stages as the Schour and Massler (1941) study did not include them. Further details of the aging methods employed and an assessment of interobserver and intraobserver error in age assignments are provided by Richards (in prep.). Developmental ages for great apes were determined following Dean and Wood (1981) whereas those for *Australopithecus* and *Homo* derive from the literature or direct observation with reference to Bromage and Dean (1985) and Smith (1986) as detailed in Table 1.

Creed-Miles *et al.* (1996:148) evaluated medial ramal anatomy "...in *known age* modern humans..." (ital. in orig.) for comparisons with that of Neanderthals and AmHs. Logan and Kronfeld (1933), Grossman and Zuckerman (1955), Lewis and Garn (1960), Moorrees *et al.* (1963a, b), Nanda (1969), Demirjian *et al.* (1985), and Demirjian (1986) have observed, however, that developmental, or physiological, age is a measure which describes the status of an individual whereas chronological age conveys only a rough estimate of this status because of the range of development observed for any given age. Further, estimates of chronological age from the dentition will vary from ± 0.25 to ± 1-2.0 years depending on the age of the individual and the method used (Brauer and Bahador, 1942; Hägg and Matsson, 1985; Smith, 1991; Saunders *et al.*, 1993). Given that chronological ages are not available for fossil taxa and the potential to introduce substantial error in attempting to determine them, appropriately framed comparisons (see Koski and Garn, 1957) of modern and fossil taxa should only employ developmental age assessments.

2. Criteria used in assessing medial pterygoid tubercle occurrence rates

To evaluate the MPT character state we performed two interrelated studies. In the first study, we compiled a series of casts of subadult and adult Neanderthal individuals noted by Rak *et al.* (1994) as possessing MPTs (Amud 7, La Chapelle 1, La Ferrassie 1, Gibraltar 2, Kebara 2, Krapina 53 and 63, Pech de l'Azé, Roc de Marsal 1, Shanidar 1 and 2, Tabun C1, and Teshik Tash). We employed a composite definition of a MPT that is based on the original and amended definitions of a MPT (Rak *et al.*, 1994, 1996). The employed definition states that a MPT is a prominent tubercle which takes the form of a distinct lip in the upper-most portion of the attachment site of *m. pterygoideus medialis*. The MPT is said to differ from other muscle related tubercles as it is more prominent and reflects a superiorly directed gradual increase in tubercle size (Rak *et al.*, 1994). Using the observed range of expression of a MPT in the above individuals and employing this definition, we scored our recent *H. sapiens* series. In the latter series, we only included mandibles which retained both rami, and the feature was scored as present only in bilateral occurrences. The character was scored as absent: (1) when it fit the Rak *et al.* (1994, 1996) definition but was present on one ramus only; and (2) when it fell outside the observed range of variation, as determined by our assessment of the Rak *et al.* (1994) Neanderthal sample. In the case of fossil specimens we included all available individuals, most of which only retain a single ramus. This methodology potentially overestimates the frequency of MPTs in fossil hominids relative to the values for recent humans but is believed to follow the methodology of Rak *et al.* (1994).

In our second study, we examined the attachment site of the *m. pterygoideus medialis* in detail. This aspect of our work has as its foundation an assessment of the components which together result in bony morphology related to the *m. pterygoideus medialis*. One result of this methodological approach is the conclusion that the current definition of a MPT does not allow an accurate quantification of observed morphology. Resultantly, we did not calculate frequency data for taxa in the second analysis.

3. Procedures for collecting hard and soft tissue data

As previously stated, our initial examination was aimed solely at determining MPT occurrence rates in recent *H. sapiens* and Neanderthals following the studies of Rak *et al.* (1994, 1996). In our subsequent evaluation we expanded our sample to include all available subadult and adult representatives of the hominid and great ape taxa previously noted (Table 1). We also expanded our scope to include aspects of the medial mandibular ramus inferior to the *crista endocondyloidea* and posterior to the *fossa submandibularis* (*fovea submandibularis*). Osseous structures examined in detail include the: (1) *c. endocondyloidea*; (2) *s. colli*; (3) *l. mandibulae*; (4) *f. mandibulae-c. mandibulae*; (5) mylohyoid groove (*sulcus mylohyoideus mandibulae*); (6) *tuberculum pterygoideum superius* (*tps*); (7) *tubercula* and variously sized ridges and depressions/pits associated with the *m. pterygoideus medialis* attachment site; and (8) variously sized bony deposits in the region of the *m. pterygoideus medialis*, *ligamentum sphenomandibulare* (*sensu stricto* (*s.s. / s.l.*); see Terminological issues below), and deep cervical fascia insertion sites. Note that the above list includes structures which interact to create bridging of the mylohyoid groove and bridging and extension of the *l. mandibulae*. The latter is involved in the 'Horizontal-Oval' (H-O) character state of Kally (1955b).

Our study is not intended to be a detailed quantification of the morphology of each of the above structures. The focus is the morphology of the *m. pterygoideus medialis* insertion site. For this reason we do not define a series of 'types' to delineate variation in each of these structures nor do we provide metric assessment of size and shape characteristics. Such a detailed assessment is well beyond the scope of this study and we do not believe that such a work would currently be useful. Our study constitutes an *initial assessment* which will hopefully provide a basis for quantitative assessments. Given this approach, we provide a description of the general morphology and range of variation observed throughout ontogeny, where possible, for the listed structures. In all ontogenetic series examined, individuals were seriated within their respective age group and the range of variation noted. Not only were these subsets of the sample population referred to continually throughout our work, but either portions of or the complete aged series were continually re-examined to ensure the accuracy of specific observations. The level of detail in our description of any structure or region varies depending on the degree that it is related to understanding the primary character state under consideration, the MPT. Note that the level of emphasis on any structure is driven both by its perceived value to an overall understanding of the region and by its inclusion in earlier publications on the character state (see Discussion). In specific instances, particularly in our description of the fossil material, we do provide a more 'typological' assessment of certain structures. This was done in order to delineate specific morphological trajectories which may be of interest to subsequent ontogenetic and phylogenetic studies. In the specific instance of MPT variation in Neanderthals and AmHs we divide the observed ranges of variation into 'types' solely to underscore the fact that significant variation is present in these samples.

To augment our observations of the gross bony anatomy we dissected modern human cadavers. All dissections were carried out with the aid of a binocular microscope (10-40x) in order to identify, separate, evaluate, and describe fascial planes, ligaments, and musculotendinous attachments. To investigate the musculotendinous and tendon-bone interfaces of the *m. pterygoideus medialis* we initially attempted various blunt dissections to eliminate the muscle bundles but retain the tendinous attachments and insertions. This methodology was soon abandoned as it results in significant loss of tendon bundles connecting the larger tendons. Whereas digestion of the muscle by immersion in an acid solution could have been used, the experience of one of us (GDR) with this method shows it to provide unsatisfactory results. Given these facts, we determined that sectioning of the muscle while it was still attached to the bone would provide the best preliminary results. Individual muscles were cut into variously sized sections in either the coronal or transverse plane or they were cut either longitudinally or transversely in the plane of the main tendons. Observations on the internal structure of the *m. pterygoideus medialis* presented herein include those made by both blunt dissection and by sectioning. Overall this methodological approach is insufficient in providing a full understanding of the *m. pterygoideus medialis* anatomy. Our sample population is also confined to recent human adults.

Given the methodological approach detailed above and the lack of both subadult human and great ape soft tissue samples we sought amplification and clarification of relationships in the existing literature. Discussion of *m. pterygoideus medialis* anatomy in relation to mandibular tubercle morphology is complicated, however, by a lack of detailed comparative work. Whereas a series of recent papers reported on the *m. pterygoideus medialis* septa (Anton, 1993; Antón, 1994a, b, 1995, 1996), and these observations were employed in related studies (Antón, 1994a, 1995, 1996; Nagar and Arensburg, 2000), we have found the earlier works of Schumacher (1959, 1961, 1962, 1980, partial transl. in McDevitt, 1989), Schumacher *et al.* (1976), and Gaspard *et al.* (1973a, b) to be more detailed and useful. Using these earlier descriptions of musculotendinous anatomy and septal arrangements, we made a *preliminary* series of correlations with our human cadaver sample. Based on this correlative work, we provide a *tentative* scheme for *m. pterygoideus medialis* septum-to-tubercle relations which follows the septal numbering system of Schumacher (1959, 1961, 1962: Figures 1a-f, 2b). Further, we employ this numbering system throughout the human ontogenetic series. Note that correlations between septa and tubercles in this subadult series are based on comparative tubercle morphology throughout the ontogenetic series and reference to the adult series (tubercles and septa). Correlating musculotendinous with bony medial ramal anatomy for the great apes presents a greater problem. In this case we followed the work of Schumacher (1961, 1962) on *Pongo*. To our knowledge no data is currently available for subadult and adult *Pan* and *Gorilla* or subadult *Pongo*. We also made reference to the work of Gaspard *et al.* (1973a, b) on cercopithecoids. Whereas we have made a concerted effort to correlate bony morphology with musculotendinous anatomy, we do not believe that further clarification can be attained from the methods employed in our or the above mentioned studies. For this reason, we are developing protocols for sectioning of the *m. pterygoideus medialis* which will be used to produce three dimensional reconstructions of the muscle and musculotendinous-bone interface to further strengthen our correlations.

Observations on the *ll. sphenomandibulare* and *stylomandibulare*, deep cervical fascia, neurovascular bundles, buccal fat pad, and potential spaces associated with the mandibular ramus were made on our human cadaver sample. All dissections of this region were carried out under a dissecting microscope (10-40x). Dissections of bisected skulls proceeded from the midline laterally. Following removal of sufficient excess tissues, observations on the pterygoid muscles, the course and distribution of neurovascular bundles, and the origins and insertions of the *l. stylomandibulare* were made. During removal of the *m. pterygoideus medialis* (see above) we made a series of observations on its relationships to the *l. sphenomandibulare*, neurovascular bundles, deep cervical fascia, and buccal fat pad. Under high magnification (20-40x) we then investigated the structure, insertions, and relationships of the *l. sphenomandibulare* and deep cervical fascia to neurovascular and bony ramal elements.

4. Terminological issues and definitions

In our initial study we directly assess the validity of the MPT character state as defined by Rak *et al.* (1994, 1996) and, therefore, utilize the term MPT. In our second study it would be possible to use one of two terms, MPT or *tpi*, in reference to the superior-most tubercle of the *m. pterygoideus medialis*. As noted in the introduction, Creed-Miles *et al.* (1996) have suggested that the term *tpi* is a synonym for the MPT. We observed, however, that a *tpi* may involve septum 6, septa 6 and 4, or septa 6, 4, and 2^{III} of the *m. pterygoideus medialis* depending on the individual or taxon involved. Further, both our data and those of Creed-Miles *et al.* (1996) demonstrate that attachments for multiple structures occur in the area of the *tpi*. These structures vary in their effect on *tpi* morphology throughout growth. These facts render the term '*tpi*' essentially useless for detailed comparison of individuals or taxa. Because the term MPT refers to a character state which includes five morphological components in its definition (Rak *et al.*, 1994, 1996) it can only be employed in specific instances (i.e., our initial study; reference to studies employing the definition of Rak *et al.* 1994, 1996). Further, in some cases (cf. "Sinanthropus", G1; Amud 1; recent *H. sapiens*) the septal insertions reside in a depression which is bounded by a low rampart; in such cases use of the descriptors '*tpi*' or 'MPT' would have little meaning as this attachment variant is not a tubercle proper. Whereas we exclude the latter insertion 'types' from percentage occurrence of MPTs in recent *H. sapiens*, they cannot be excluded from consideration of the attachment site. Note, however, that the focus of our work is on the formation of tubercles. Further discussion of the morphological descriptor *tpi* and an assessment of statements attached to the MPT character state are provided in the Discussion. Therefore, in our second study we discuss the area impacted by the superior-most insertion sites of the *m. pterygoideus medialis* by reference to the specific septal attachments involved (see caution above: Figures 1a-f, 2b).

We employ the new term *tuberculum sulcus colli* (*tsc*) to denote a small tubercle that is located superior to the septum 6 attachment of the *m. pterygoideus medialis*, at the junction of the inferior border of the *s. colli* with the posterior ramal border (Figure 2a-b). The attachment site for septa in the superior portion of the muscle and the *tsc* are morphologically variable but the former (inclusive of depressions and tubercles) is invariably present whereas the *tsc* is absent in many individuals.

The *l. sphenomandibulare* (*s.s.*: = spheno-maxillary ligament of Hovelacque and Virenque, 1913; Patte, 1957) is a mesenchymal remnant of Meckel's cartilage and, as such, is embryologically distinct (Cameron, 1914-1915; Richany *et al.*, 1956; Bossy and Gaillard, 1963; Hamilton and Mossman, 1978). Richany *et al.* (1956) and Ishizeki *et al.* (1999) observed that, during growth, cells of Meckel's cartilage lose their identity and tend to become fibroblastic in nature, ultimately becoming surrounded by a fibrous tissue. In adults this fibrous tissue (ligament) is intimately related to a condensation(s) of loose connective tissue which supplements its extent (Hovelacque and Virenque, 1913; Bossy and Gaillard, 1963; Williams and Warwick, 1980), portions of which may be more appropriately called aponeuroses (DuBrul, 1980). Cave (1979) suggests that the latter thickenings develop in response to continuous or intermittent movement which necessitates augmentation and thickening of the relevant deep fascia. Due to high idiosyncratic variation in adults the form and attachment site(s) of this ligament-fascial sheet composite are both variously expressed on dissection and variously depicted in anatomy texts (Clemente, 1987; DuBrul, 1980; Williams and Warwick, 1980; Woodburn, 1978). Both Cameron (1914-1915) and Ouchi *et al.* (1998) suggest that at least a portion of this variation can be attributed to ontogenetic changes which result in age induced shape variations. Further, because of the *l. sphenomandibulare's* (*s.s.*) relation to fascial sheets surrounding the *mm. pterygoideus medialis* and *lateralis*, it has been referred to within the more inclusive term; 'interpterygoid fascia' (Barker and Davies, 1972), 'interpterygoid aponeurosis' (Hovelacque and Virenque, 1913; Gaspard *et al.*, 1973a; Billy and Vallois, 1977), or 'pterygomandibular fascia' (Gaughran, 1957; Wilson *et al.*, 1984). Given the above and with reference to Hovelacque and Virenque (1913), Gaughran (1957), Bossy and Gaillard (1963), and Alkofide *et al.* (1997) it is clear that the complexities of these tissues are in need of further clarification, especially in relation to bony attachment sites. In the remaining text, therefore, use of the term *l. sphenomandibulare* (*s.l.*) will refer to this combined ligamentous-connective tissue complex. Further, our gross observations on this tissue complex should be considered as a preliminary statement of anatomical relationships as we are only now in the early stages of histomorphological studies aimed at further clarification of these relationships.

5. Statistical procedures

Chi-square (X^2) and the Yates' correction for continuity (X_c^2) were calculated and employed in analysis of the frequency of occurrence of the MPT in our recent *H. sapiens* ontogenetic sample following Simpson *et al.* (1960) and Sokal and Rohlf (1987).

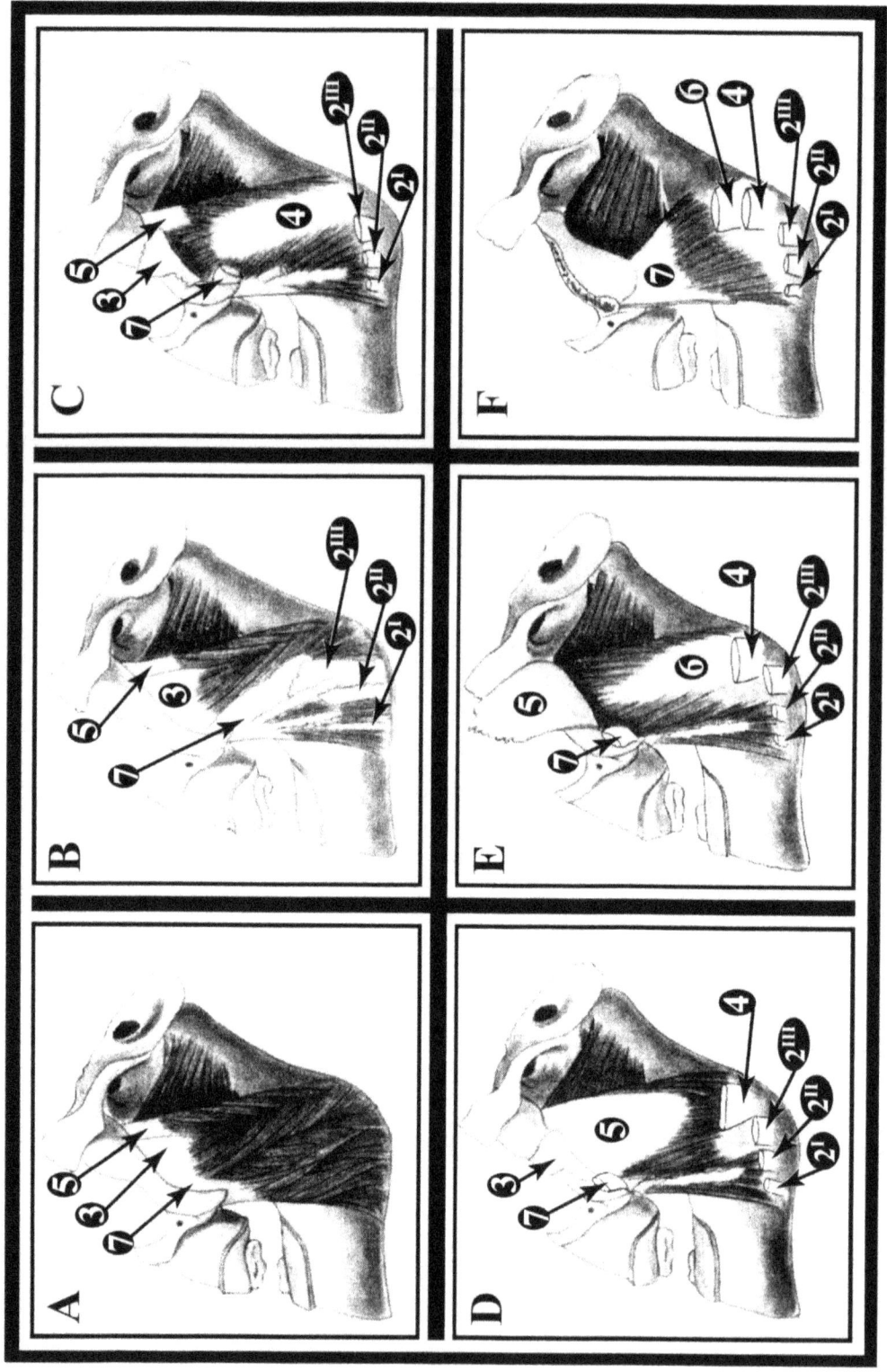

Figure 1a-f: Schumacher's (1959, 1961, 1962) numbering system for septa (tendons) of the *m. pterygoideus medialis* of a 6.0-year-old recent *H. sapiens*. Modified and redrawn from Schumacher (1962). Reprinted with permission from Urban and Vogel.

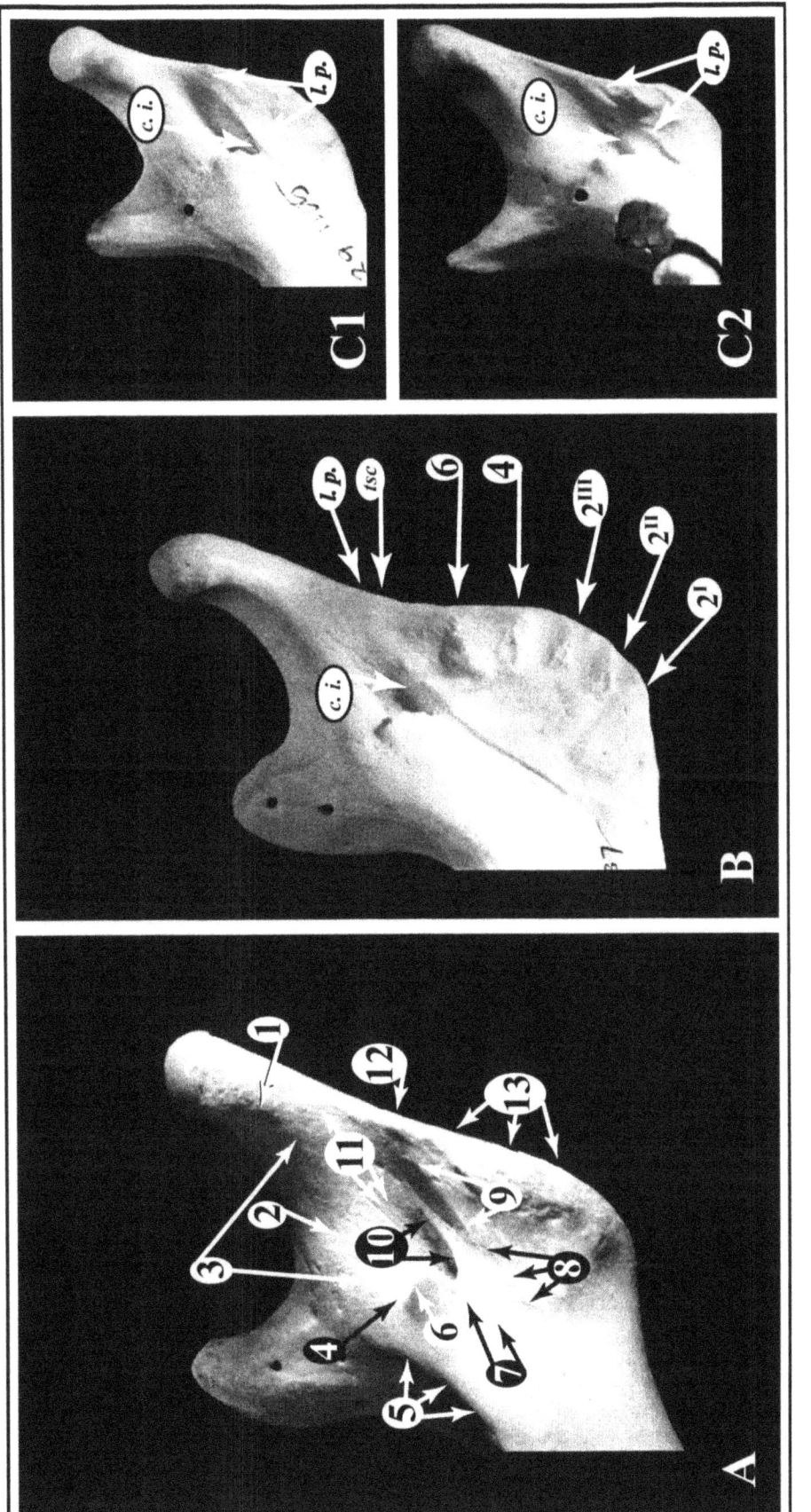

Figure 2a-c: Medial views of mandibular ramus of subadult and adult recent *H. sapiens*. In (a) morphological features of the medial ramus include the: (1) *tuberculum pterygoideum superiorus*; (2) groove for neurovascular bundle to deep temporal region (n-v. groove): (3) *crista endocondyloidea*: (4) lingular notch: (5) *crista pharyngea*; (6) *lingula mandibulae*; (7) and (8) anterior and posterior borders of the mylohyoid groove, respectively: (9) *linea pterygoidea (lp)*; (10) *crista intermedia (ci)*; (11) *sulcus colli*; (12) *tuberculum sulcus colli (tsc)*: and (13) general attachment region for the *l. stylomandibulare*. In (b) tubercles associated with septal insertions for the *m. pterygoideus medialis* are numbered following Schumacher (1959, 1961, 1962: see Figure 1a-f). The region interposed between the *l. pterygoidea* and the septum 6 insertion comprises an area of fleshy muscle origin-insertion and, in some cases, an 8th septal insertion. In (c) two variants of the relationship between the *c. intermedia* and *l. pterygoidea* are shown. Observe in (c1) how the anterosuperior aspect of the *l. pterygoidea* brings this crest into line with the *c. intermedia*. In our descriptions of this region such cases are described as only possessing a *l. pterygoidea*. In (c2) observe the more anteroinferior course of the *l. pterygoidea* and the position of the *c. intermedia* relative to both the *l. pterygoidea* and the *s. colli*.

RESULTS OF OBSERVATIONS AND DESCRIPTION OF MEDIAL RAMAL BONY AND SOFT TISSUE ANATOMY IN MODERN AND FOSSIL HOMINOIDS

I. ASSESSMENT OF THE MEDIAL PTERYGOID TUBERCLE CHARACTER STATE, AS DEFINED, IN RECENT *HOMO SAPIENS*

1. Introduction

In our initial assessment of the character state we address two questions: (1) do MPTs similar to those said to be present in Neanderthals occur in recent *H. sapiens*; and (2) if such MPTs are present, what is the frequency of occurrence and geographic distribution of the character in an ontogenetic sample of recent *H. sapiens*? Based on the Rak *et al.* (1994, 1996) definition and our assessment of the range of variation in their Neanderthal series we recorded the bilateral presence or absence of a MPT in recent *H. sapiens* ($N = 689$). This series comprises individuals ranging in age from newborn to adult. The number and percentage occurrence of the MPT in recent *H. sapiens* is detailed in Table 2 while the geographic distribution of the feature is detailed in Table 3.

2. Percentage occurrence of the character state by age group

Based on the above criteria, we found that MPTs are present in 22% of newborn, recent *H. sapiens*. The rate of occurrence rises sharply by the age of 0.5 years to 33%, reaching a high of 46% at 0.75 years. Whereas the percentage increase is high in these groups, Chi-square tests do not show either increase to be significant at $P \leq 0.05$. In succeeding age stages the rate of occurrence drops steeply at 1.0 year-of-age to 24% but rises again to 33% and 32% at 1.5 and 2.0 years of age, respectively. At the ages of 3.0 and 5.0 years the percentage occurrence falls to 22% and then 18%, respectively. While the decreases observed on a yearly basis are not significant the overall decreases from 0.75 to 4.0 or 5.0 years of age are significant at $P< 0.025$ ($X_c^2 = 5.44$ and 6.48, respectively). In general, the percentage occurrence continues to diminish in succeeding age stages to a complete absence of the MPT feature in our sample by the 10th postnatal year. In the 11th and 12th years the occurrence rises sharply to 18% and 20%, respectively, but falls below 9% again in the 15-18.0 year old age groups. None of the increases or decreases in percent occurrence after 5.0 years of age are significant at $P< 0.05$. In our adult group, which combines all ages > 20.6 years of age, the percentage occurrence is 31%.

3. Geographic distribution of the character state

Our ability to evaluate the geographic distribution of the occurrence of the MPT character state is limited by the lack of provenience data for 46% of the sample population and variation in the age ranges sampled in each region. The percentage occurrence ranges from 17% in India and our 'geographic origin unknown' group, to 24-25% in North and South America, and to 33% in our composite Europe-China group. All Chi-square determinations for these comparisons are non-significant with the exception of North America and 'geographic region unknown' at $P< 0.025$ ($X^2= 5.12$). Comparison of the occurrence rate by age stage for the two largest of these grouping, 'geographic origin unknown' ($N = 317$) and North America ($N = 290$), shows a pattern consistent with that seen in the composite *H. sapiens* sample. While these subsamples are not fully comparable in sample sizes and represented age stages, both ontogenetic subseries show a high occurrence in the early stages and very low percentages as the 10.0 year-old stage is approached. The North American subsample contains no individuals over the age of 15.0 years and, resultantly, it is not possible to test for comparability in later age stages.

Table 2: Number and percentage of presence or absence of an MPT[1] and sample sizes (*N*) by developmental age for recent *Homo sapiens* (*N* = 689)

Developmental age (in years)	Age range (in years)	N	MPT present	MPT absent
Birth	(newborn-0.2)	51	11 (22%)	40 (78%)
0.50	(0.3-0.6)	18	6 (33%)	12 (67%)
0.75	(0.7-0.9)	22	10 (46%)	12 (54%)
1.0	(1.0-1.2)	34	8 (24%)	26 (76%)
1.5	(1.3-1.6)	40	13 (33%)	27 (67%)
2.0	(1.7-2.2)	47	15 (32%)	32 (68%)
3.0	(2.3-3.6)	64	14 (22%)	50 (78%)
4.0	(3.7-4.6)	81	15 (19%)	66 (81%)
5.0	(4.7-5.6)	49	7 (14%)	42 (86%)
6.0	(5.7-6.6)	37	9 (24%)	28 (76%)
7.0	(6.7-7.6)	34	5 (15%)	29 (85%)
8.0	(7.7-8.6)	30	2 (7%)	28 (93%)
9.0	(8.7-9.6)	27	2 (7%)	25 (93%)
10.0	(9.7-10.6)	16	0 (0%)	16 (100%)
11.0	(10.7-11.6)	15	3 (20%)	12 (80%)
12.0	(11.7-13.6)	17	3 (18%)	14 (82%)
15.0	(13.7-17.6)	25	2 (8%)	23 (92%)
18.0	(17.7-20.6)	15	1 (7%)	14 (93%)
Adult	(> 20.6)	65	20 (31%)	45 (69%)

[1] Refer to the Methods section for scoring procedures and the Discussion section for an assessment of the value of these data in systematics.

Table 3: Number and percentage of presence or absence of an MPT[1] and sample sizes (*N*) by geographic region for recent *H. sapiens* (*N* = 689)

Geographic region	N	MPT present	MPT absent
Origin unknown	317	55 (17%)	262 (83%)
Mexico and South America	50	12 (24%)	38 (76%)
North America	290	72 (25%)	218 (75%)
India	23	4 (17%)	19 (83%)
Europe and China	9	3 (33%)	6 (67%)
Totals	**689**	**146 (21%)**	**543 (79%)**

[1] Refer to the Methods section for further details of the geographic origin of the included individuals. See also the Discussion section for an assessment of the value of these data in systematics.

II. DESCRIPTION OF BONY MEDIAL RAMUS ANATOMY IN AN ONTOGENETIC SERIES OF RECENT *HOMO SAPIENS* AND RELATED SOFT TISSUES OF ADULTS

1. Introduction

In our second study we expanded both the anatomical area and range of taxa under examination and compiled a broader series of observations. Here we present the results of our examination of the ontogeny of the medial mandibular ramus in recent *H. sapiens*, great apes, and fossil hominids. We supplement these data with observations on the hard and soft tissue anatomy from our adult human cadaver series. These data are presented so as to provide a basis from which to evaluate the impact of the ontogenetic trajectory(ies) of and morphological variation in the: (1) related ligamentous and fascial sheets, including the *ll. sphenomandibulare* and *stylomandibulare*; (2) associated neurovascular bundles; (3) *s. colli* and its delimiting borders; (4) *l. mandibulae-canalis mandibulae-f. mandibulae* complex; (5) formation of a flat to concave area between the *s. colli* and the superior-most bony attachment site of *m. pterygoideus medialis*; (6) relationship of the *s. colli* and associated soft tissue components with the superior-most bony attachment site(s) of *m. pterygoideus medialis*; and (7) muscle related bony topography (tubercles, depressions, etc.) associated with the *m. pterygoideus medialis*. Note that our observations on recent *H. sapiens* derive from two disjunct data sets. The ontogenetic data, inclusive of adults, is based solely on observations of dry bone specimens whereas the soft and related hard tissue data derives from cadaver specimens. Results provided should be considered as a preliminary statement on bony anatomy and soft tissue relationships as a complete analysis is beyond the scope of the current work.

2. Observations on ligaments and fascia of the medial ramus region

With tissue change due to fixation noted, in all individuals examined we found a more or less dense and morphologically complex connective tissue lining and attaching to the medial ramus. This sheet comprises: (1) the *l. sphenomandibulare* (*s.s.*); (2) a variable quantity of dense ligamentous bands; (3) a variably dense series of ligamentous sheets within which neurovascular structures reside; and, in some areas, (4) the periosteum. Entheses of the *l. sphenomandibulare* (*s.l.*) attach to either or both the fibroperiosteum of the medial ramus or bone. In both cases this more general tissue sheet is associated with bony tubercles or with short to long bony lines, although, the latter attachments to bone are associated with stronger markings. In many cases the ligamentous bands within this tissue sheet attach superiorly to either the *l. sphenomandibulare* (*s.s.*) or, more generally, the sphenoidal spine-pterygotympanic-squamotympanic fissure region as discussed in Hovelacque and Virenque (1913), Cameron (1914-1915), Richany *et al.* (1956), Bossy and Gaillard (1963), Burch (1966), Cave (1979), Alkofide *et al.* (1997), and Ouchi *et al.* (1998). Mandibular attachments of the *l. sphenomandibulare* (*s.s.*) and associated ligamentous bands-fascial sheets are complex (Hovelacque and Virenque, 1913; Berns and Sadove, 1962; Barker and Davies, 1972). Note that our observations are confined to regions relevant to the *m. pterygoideus medialis* insertion site but that bony attachments and tissue connections outside this specific region are detailed in Hovelacque and Virenque (1913). On microdissection of this tissue sheet we found the *l. sphenomandibulare* (*s.l.*) to comprise at least three separate fibrous layers joined together by loose areolar tissue. As a layered composite this fibrous sheet can be easily removed from the bone except at three main sites. We number and refer to these attachments from the lateral to medial-most layer as Sites 1, 2, and 3 of the *l. sphenomandibulare* (*s.l.*: Figure 3a-d). Note, however, that there are numerous, idiosyncratically expressed minor attachments of this sheet throughout the *fossa pterygoidea* (see below). The medial-most fibrous layer forms a continuous sheet which covers the entire *f. pterygoidea*. The main site of bony attachment of this layer is around the tubercle for septa 6 and 4 of the *m. pterygoideus medialis* (Hovelacque and Virenque, 1913; Barker and Davies, 1972; Billy and Vallois, 1977; Williams and Warwick, 1980) where it is pierced by tendon entheses associated with the muscle and so becomes part of the muscle's attachment. This represents our attachment Site 3 (Figure 3d). The intermediate layer also covers portions of the *f. pterygoidea* but differs from the latter layer in both its position and its bony attachment sites. The intermediate layer attaches to bone along the: (1) inferior border of the *s. colli* from the posterior ramal border to the posterosuperior border of the mylohyoid groove (comprises *linea pterygoidea* and *tsc*); (2) anterior and posterior borders of the mylohyoid groove; and (3) medial border of the *f. mandibulae* or, when present, the *l. mandibulae*. A small, raised tubercle is sometimes present at the posterior attachment site of the ligament for which we employ the term *tsc* (see Terminology section: Figure 2a-b). This constitutes our attachment Site 2 of the *l. sphenomandibulare* (*s.l.*: Figure 3c). Note that this layer also provides the lateral-most soft tissue cover for the medial-most extent of the mylohyoid groove. The lateral-most layer of the *l. sphenomandibulare* (*s.l.*) extends no further inferiorly than the base of the *s. colli*, but does line the *c. mandibulae* (Starkie and Stewart, 1931; Hamparian, 1973; Wadu *et al.*, 1997). This layer attaches to bone along the lateral-most surface of the medial border of the *f. mandibulae*, and when present the *l. mandibulae*, and extends inferiorly to the base of the *f. mandibulae*. Extending both anteriorly and posteriorly from the foramen this layer continues: (1) anteriorly as a fascial tube lining the *c. mandibulae*; and (2) posteriorly as a sheet which attaches within the *s. colli* for a variable distance along a crest which extends from the inferior border of the *f. mandibulae* (Figure 3b). We employ the term *crista intermedia* to refer to the latter crest (but see below) which is, in essence, an extension of the inferomedial wall of the *c. mandibulae* (Figure 2a). In recent *H. sapiens* the angle of this attachment site varies such that the course of the *c. intermedia* ranges from slightly

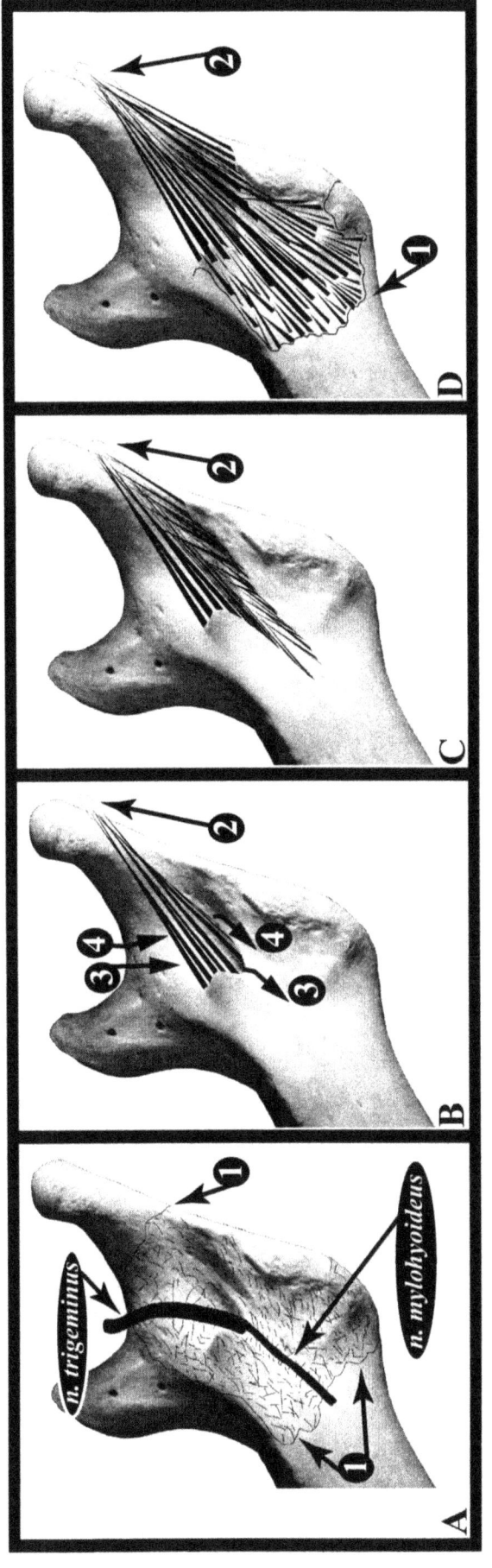

Figure 3a-d: Schematic representations of layers forming the *l. sphenomandibulare*-deep cervical fascia complex and their bony attachment sites. In (a) observe that a fibroperiosteal sheet lines the bone's surface. Cut edges of this sheet occur at (1). Figure (b) is a generalized depiction of the lateral-most ligamentous-fascial layer and its bony attachment sites (= Site 1). The cut superior end of the ligamentous sheet is noted at (2). Observe how the mylohyoid neurovascular bundle can course, minimally, either between the ligament's fibrous bands and over the *c. intermedia* (3) or it can take a more posterior course around this crest, thereby not piercing this insertion site of the ligament (4). In (c) and (d) are shown generalized depictions of the medial (Site 2) and intermediate (Site 3) ligamentous-fascial sheets and their bony attachments, respectively.

- 17 -

superolateral to the inferior border of the *s. colli* to coincidence with it (Figure 2c1-2). This series of lines, projections, foramina, and canals constitutes our attachment Site 1. Because this lateral-most layer takes a posterolateral course from the *f. mandibulae*, the mylohyoid neurovascular bundle is positioned slightly medial to this tissue layer (Figure 3a-b). This neurovascular bundle enters the mylohyoid groove through an opening in the ligament and is then covered medially by the intermediate and medial ligamental layers. The intermediate and lateral layers are continuous laterally with a connective tissue sheet (fibroperiosteum?) which covers the bone's surface in the *s. colli* and mylohyoid groove and lines the opening of the *f. mandibulae* and walls of the *c. mandibulae* (Figure 3a). Given this configuration the mylohyoid neurovascular bundle is encased between the fibroperiosteal layer, laterally, and the intermediate and medial layers of the *l. sphenomandibulare* (*s.l.*) complex, medially. It is important to note that fibers of the layers which comprise this ligamentous sheet reach their bony attachments at varying angles and that this creates a highly interwoven fabric. Further, given this angular variation and the fact that the layers are joined by loose connective tissue, small neurovascular bundles can run within the sheet, as opposed to piercing it. Currently we have only evaluated these layers below the level of the *c. endocondyloidea* and, resultantly, are unable to document their specific cranial attachment(s). Further, note that Weidenreich (1936) employs the single term *l. pterygoidea* to denote the superior-most bony attachment (= extent) of *m. pterygoideus medialis* and that this usage would include our ligament attachment Sites 1 and 2. We, however, restrict the term *l. pterygoidea* to that part of our attachment Site 2 posterior to the mylohyoid groove. The *l. pterygoidea*, then, delimits only the bony portion of the muscle's insertion area posterior to the mylohyoid groove and inferior to or coincident with the inferior border of the *s. colli* (Figure 2a). In some cases there is an anterosuperior expansion of the *m. pterygoideus medialis* such that the *l. pterygoidea* becomes coincident with the posterior border of the mylohyoid groove. Further details regarding the *c. intermedia* and *l. pterygoidea* are provided below.

Most of the *m. pterygoideus medialis* septa 6 and 4 attachment sites are associated with the posterior ramal border and have posterior surfaces which, in general, are angled anteromedially (Figure 4a-f). Given this positioning and configuration it appears likely that the *l. stylomandibulare* and superficial portion of the *m. masseter* muscle may also be involved in their production (Figure 2a). Note, however, that superficial insertion sites for the *m. pterygoideus medialis* (= septum 2^{I-II}) also extend into this area and, resultantly, are involved in shaping the posterior aspect of the more superior attachment sites (= septa 6 and 4 and, variably, septum 2^{III}: Figure 1a-f.). Further, whereas most textbooks of anatomy (cf. Clemente, 1987; DuBrul, 1980; Williams and Warwick, 1980; Woodburn, 1978) depict the *l. stylomandibulare* as running anteriorly from the tip of the *processus styloideus* of the *ossis temporalis* to the mandible, this is, in fact, not the case. Because this ligament is a thickening of the deep cervical (parotid) fascia its course

is controlled by the position of this fascia relative to the *p. styloideus ossis temporalis* and its associated muscle bundles. The *l. stylomandibulare*, as a thickening of this fascial sheet, follows the fascia's course to insert along the posterior ramal border at the level of the superior-most tendinous attachment of *m. pterygoideus medialis*. We observed significant idiosyncratic variation in this ligament's angular relationship to the posterior ramal border in dissections of adult humans. Portions of this variation may be related to the known variation in *p. styloideus ossis temporalis* length (Dwight, 1907; Zuckerman et al., 1962; Kaufman and Irish, 1970; Frommer, 1974; Correll et al., 1979). In some individuals with minimal growth of the process we found the ligament to extend posteromedially from the ramus whereas it extended anteromedially in some cases with more extensive growth. The latter variation may also result from differences in craniofacial hafting relative to cranial base flexion (*s.s.*) in the absence of significant *p. styloideus ossis temporalis* growth. The point of origin of the ligament differed by ≤ 5.0 cm along the sagittal plane. Given these data, the exact relationship of the *l. stylomandibulare* to the direction at which it 'restrains' the mandible is unclear. Further, we found that the ligament may attach to either the anterior surface of *m. stylopharyngeus* or to the bony process. In the former case the attachment was positioned anterior and inferior to the tip of the process whereas in the latter case the ligament was positioned anterior and superior to the tip. Observed variation in the ligament's origin further complicates an understanding of its relationship to tubercles for the *m. pterygoideus medialis*. Because our dissection sample did not include subadults, we are unable to describe the anatomical relationships in subadult recent *H. sapiens*.

3. Observations on neurovascular and related soft tissues of the medial ramus region

Major neurovascular structures associated with the superior aspect of the mandibular ramus include the: (1) maxillary artery and vein; (2) pterygoid venous plexus; (3) *nervus alveolaris inferior* and artery; (4) *n. lingualis*; (5) *n. mylohyoideus* and artery; (6) arteries to *m. pterygoideus medialis*; (7) parapharyngeal process of the parotid gland; and (8) pterygomandibular portion of the buccal fat pad (Hovelacque and Virenque, 1913; Gaughran, 1957; Murphy and Grundy, 1969; Latham and Scott, 1970; Hamparian, 1973). We confirmed the observations of Hovelacque and Virenque (1913) and Barker and Davies (1972) that each of these structures is associated, either individually or in combination, with the medial aspect of and openings in the *l. sphenomandibulare* (*s.l.*). Neurovascular structures enter a space between the: (1) *crista endocondyloidea*, superiorly; (2) *f. mandibulae*, anteriorly; (3) inferior aspect of the *s. colli* and medial borders of the mylohyoid groove, inferiorly; (4) *l. sphenomandibulare* (*s.l.*), medially; and (5) medial aspect of the ramus, laterally. The space created between the *l. sphenomandibulare* (*s.l.*) and the medial ramus is: (1) closed anteriorly; (2) intermittently open inferiorly; and (3) fully open superiorly and posteriorly due to the ligament being

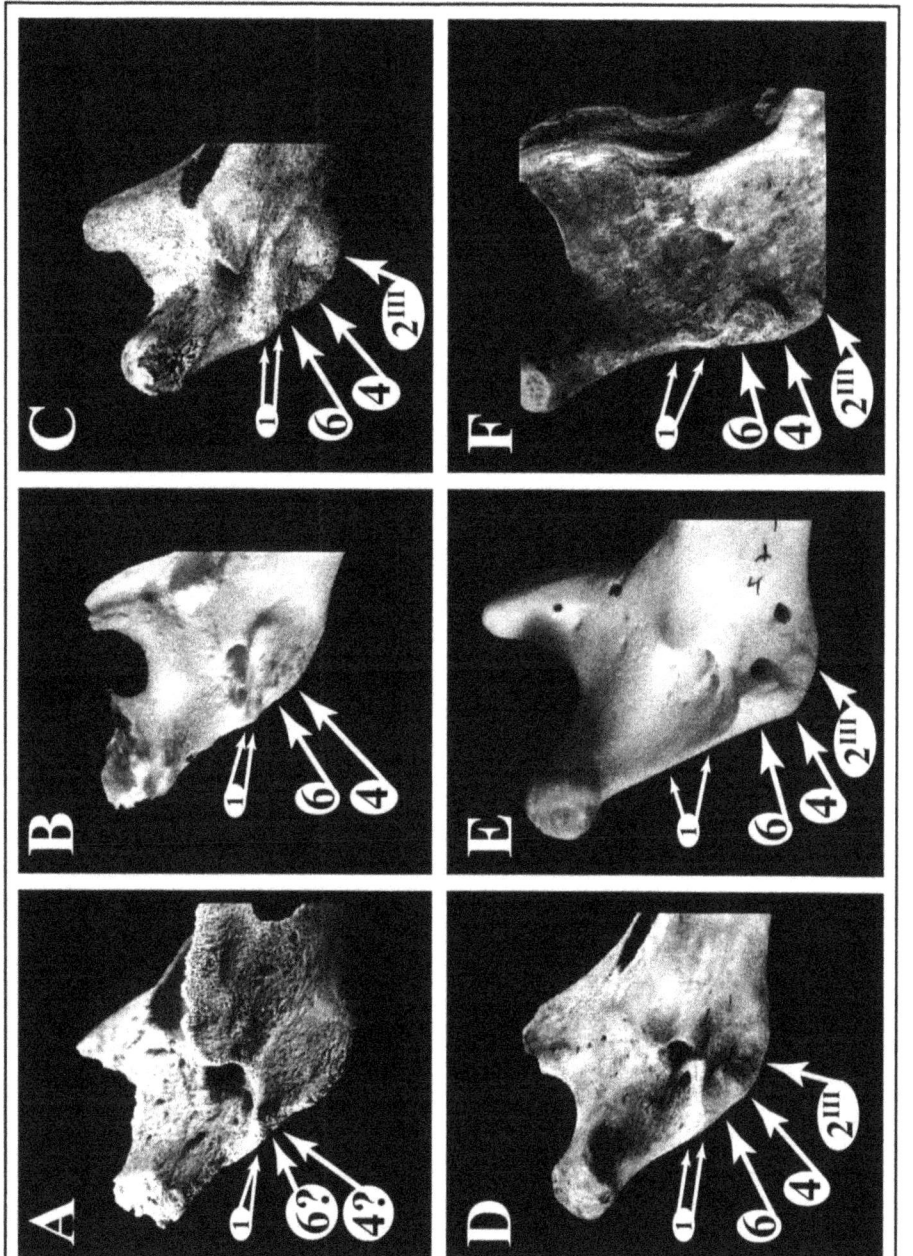

Figure 4a-f: Examples of recent *H. sapiens* subadults showing some of the variation in medial mandibular ramus features. Specimens are aged developmentally as follows: (a) newborn; (b) newborn to < 0.5 years; (c) 0.75 years; (d) 1.0 year; (e) 2.0 years; and (f) 8.0 years. Numbered arrows depict location of insertion sites for septa 6, 4, and 2^{III} of the *m. pterygoideus medialis*. Observe the relationship between the base of the *s. colli-l. pterygoidea* and the septa 6 and 4 insertion and the development of a flat to concave region between them (1). Also observe how the inferior *s. colli* border and the muscle insertion-tubercle are coincident in (a) but are seen to separate with increasing age in the series (b-f). Also note changes in the depth and degree of inferior *s. colli* shelving and the variation in development of the *l. mandibulae* in this series. Multiple openings for the major branches of the *n. trigeminus* are clearly visible in (a, c-e). Observe the triangular-to-rhomboidal shape of the septa 6 and 4 tubercles. Note in (e) the relationship of the *s. colli* to the septa 6 and 4 tubercle. This anatomy is consistent with that in individuals who possess a bifurcation of the major neurovascular bundle(s) which wrap around the posterior ramal border and result in the *l. mandibulae* attachments becoming coincident with the *m. pterygoideus medialis* insertion.

only attached at its anterosuperior, posterosuperior, and posteroinferior edges in these regions, respectively (Barker and Davies, 1972). These openings allow transmission of various neurovascular bundles. Note that our expanded definition of the *l. sphenomandibulare* allows for multiple openings in the inferior aspect of the ligament. This observation is consistent with that of Hovelacque and Virenque (1913), Bossy and Gaillard (1963), Barker and Davies (1972), and Wilson *et al.* (1984) but differs from Ossenbergs' (1974a, b).

We confirmed the observations of Hovelacque and Virenque (1913) and DuBrul (1980) that neurovascular structures of the superomedial ramal area are enclosed in variously dense connective tissue tubes. These tubes consist medially of the *l. sphenomandibulare* (*s.l.*) and laterally of the fibroperiosteal lining of the bone. Note that our understanding of the exact relationship of this lining to the ligament is currently unclear and that it may represent a portion of our lateral or intermediate layers. We found substantial variation in the number of tubes containing neurovascular tissue, the contents of any given tube, the position of these tubes on the ramus, and their degree of bony attachment. This variation results from differences in: (1) positioning of branch points of the nerves, arteries, and veins relative to the ramus; (2) positioning of these branch points relative to the *l. sphenomandibulare* (*s.l.*); and (3) the growth rate of these soft tissues relative to the developing bone. In general, most differences in the posterior region of the *s. colli* result from variation in the maxillary artery and vein, the pterygoid venous plexus, the *n. mylohyoideus* and artery, and the vascular supply to *m. pterygoideus medialis*. Further, the neurovascular bundle which enters the *s. colli* posteriorly is generally positioned above the superior-most attachment of the *l. sphenomandibulare* (*s.l.*; Site 2). In some cases, however, this bundle may approach the posterior ramal border as two separate bundles. In other cases this bifurcation occurs just anterior to the posterior border of the ramus. In the latter cases, the upper-most bundle takes the usual course while the lower-most bundle runs in a slightly inferiorly placed fascial tube. This second neurovascular bundle enters a potential space between attachment Sites 2 and 3 of the *l. sphenomandibulare* (*s.l.*). The resultant of this variant is that a substantial portion of the neurovascular bundle will be positioned in the space between the *s. colli* and the septum 6 attachment (cf. "Sinanthropus": Figure 4e). This configuration results in a more inferior positioning of the inferior border of the *s. colli* (= *l. pterygoidea*) and in some taxa may result in an otherwise non-observable *c. intermedia* (see below). A 'forced' inferior positioning of the ligament can also be caused by variation in the degree to which the parapharyngeal process of the parotid gland extends into this space.

4. Overview of hard and soft tissue relationships in the recent *Homo sapiens* series

In adult recent *H. sapiens* specimens the *s. colli* is delimited on three sides: (1) superiorly by the *c. endocondyloidea*; (2) anteriorly by the *f. mandibulae-l. mandibulae* complex; and (3) inferiorly by the change in topography from a concavity (cf. a sulcus) to a flat or concave ramal surface (Figure 2a). The superior sulcal border ends posteriorly at or just below the *tuberculum pterygoideum superius* (*tps*) and at or near the posterior ramal border (Figure 2a). The inferior *s. colli* border is marked by either one or two bony crests or lines. In the former case the inferior border runs as a continuous line from the posterior ramal border to the base of the *f. mandibulae*, being broken only by the mylohyoid groove (Figure 2c1). In the latter case there are two crests or lines, one which runs from the inferior aspect of the *f. mandibulae* into the sulcus as a sharp crest and one which runs inferomedial to the latter, being continuous from the posterior ramal border to the mylohyoid groove (Figure 2c2). Although Weidenreich (1936) notes high idiosyncratic variation in the expression of the inferior *s. colli* border, he only employs the single term *linea pterygoidea* to denote this border. Further, Weidenreich (1936) employs a taxon specific (i.e. "Sinanthropus") term, the *crista intermedia*, to denote a short crest he observed in the anterior aspect of the *s. colli* (cf. mandible G1). Based on our comparative data we consider the *c. intermedia* to be a partially formed extension of the medial wall of the *c. mandibulae* and to be homologous to the more superior and laterally-directed crest we observed forming a portion of the inferior border of the *s. colli* in recent *H. sapiens* (= in part, attachment Site 1 of the *l. sphenomandibulare* [*s.l.*]). Note that the configuration of the *c. intermedia* in "Sinanthropus" mandibles is consistent with a *crista* variant caused by a normal neurovascular pattern variation. The term *c. intermedia* is, therefore, used throughout to refer to a sharp crest which originates from the inferomedial aspect of the *f. mandibulae* and which then extends posteriorly a variable distance into the *s. colli* or which forms a portion of the inferior sulcal border (Figure 2a-c). In some recent *H. sapiens* and in all "Sinanthropus" this crest is truncated by a superoinferiorly oriented neurovascular or vascular groove. In cases where the *c. intermedia* and *l. pterygoidea* are coincident we only employ the latter term (Figure 2c1). The latter combination of structures generally produces a low, rounded line on the bone whereas an isolated *l. pterygoidea* generally produces a low, sharp line.

In subadult recent *H. sapiens* the *s. colli* is not a true sulcus (Figure 4a-e). Whereas the delimiting boundaries are the same as in adults, the 'sulcus' is actually a rather broad and deep depression. This feature is normally deepest anteriorly but in some term infants the posterior region is deeper. The depressed region comprising the *s. colli* consumes the entire distance from the *f. mandibulae* to the posterior ramal border (Figure 4a-e Vs Figure 4f). Note that in term infants the *f. mandibulae* is only a slight pit within this larger depression with multiple '*c. mandibulae*' running anteriorly from this pit (Chávez-Lomelí *et al.*, 1996; Richards *et al.*, in prep.: Figure 4a-e). At this time the ramal aspect of the *c. mandibulae* is only in its earliest stages of development (Chávez-Lomelí *et al.*, 1996; Wadu *et al.*, 1997).

Morphology of the subadult *s. colli* appears to be related in part to the increased area needed to accommodate minimally the: (1) multiple branches of the *n. alveolaris inferior* and associated vessels (Carter and Keen, 1971); (2) pterygomandibular extension of the buccal fat pad (Murphy and Grundy, 1969; Sperber, 1981); and (3) maxillary vein and pterygoid venous plexus. It is probable that the basic morphology of this region is established in fetal life and reflects also the direct association of the developing membranous portion of the mandible with degenerating first branchial arch cartilage. In many fetal to newborn infants this depression forming the *s. colli* is extreme and results in or is associated with an equally extreme shelving of the inferior sulcal border (Figure 4a-d). Because of the depth of the depression the *s. colli* borders are generally strongly expressed and especially so in the case of the inferior border. This extreme projection of bone results in a more medial positioning of the attachment site of *m. pterygoideus medialis* (Figure 4a-d). In these cases this arrangement places the medial extent of the superior septal attachments in very close proximity to the inferolateral border of the lateral pterygoid plate. With growth this depression is remodeled such that it becomes more sulcus-like, having in the early phases a fossa-like anterior component and a less deep, sulcus-like posterior component (Figure 4a-f). In the adult condition the relationships are variable but generally the anterior component is less deep whereas the posterior component may be nearly flat (Figure 5a-e). In adults, the anterior component is associated with the: (1) *n. alveolaris inferior* and artery; (2) *n. mylohyoideus* and artery; and (3) pterygomandibular extension of the buccal fat pad. Idiosyncratically expressed ontogenetic factors, then, are likely to be responsible for much of the extensive variation observed by Weidenreich (1936) in recent *H. sapiens s. colli* morphology.

In recent *H. sapiens* the morphology of the *l. mandibulae* region is characterized by: (1) positioning of the superior opening of the *f. mandibulae* at or near the medial-most projection of the *c. endocondyloidea*; (2) a lingular tip that projects medially from the *c. endocondyloidea*; (3) a superoinferiorly convex and mediolaterally concave region between the *c. endocondyloidea* and the lingular tip (= lingular notch); and (4) a variably extended bony plate which arises from that portion of the medial-most cortical plate which forms the medial wall of the *f. mandibulae-c. mandibulae* (Figures 2a, 4a-f, and 5a-e). Note that in its most attenuated state that minimal bone is formed at the posteroinferior corner of the *l. mandibulae*. This results in a wide opening to the anterosuperior aspect of the infundibulum of the mylohyoid groove (Figure 5d). Note that a posteriorly positioned *l. pterygoidea* produces a similar effect but one which occurs at the posterosuperior opening to the groove. The presence of this type of lingular morphology indicates that bone forming the *l. mandibulae* is a separate skeletal unit from that forming the medial wall in the mandibular foramen-canal region. In recent *H. sapiens* adults the medial wall of the *f. mandibulae-c. mandibulae* is variably expressed superoinferiorly, ranging from coincident with the *s. colli*'s inferior border to ca. 2.0 cm below that border. Further, note that the *c. intermedia* is the posterior extension of this aspect of the *f. mandibulae-c. mandibulae*. In infants the *l. mandibulae* is generally expressed as a small triangular extension of the medial-most cortical plate forming the wall of the *f. mandibulae-c. mandibulae*. This plate extends posteriorly over the *s. colli*. With growth the angle between the superior and posterior borders of the *l. mandibulae* generally becomes more obtuse, although, in some individuals they may retain a more acute angular relation (Figure 4a-f). Note that posterior extension of the entire lingular plate will have less effect on this angle than growth of the inferior aspect of the lingular plate alone. The degree to which the notch between the lingular plate and the *c. endocondyloidea* is developed is related to the amount of posterior extension of the superior *l. mandibulae* and the degree to which the *l. mandibulae* extends medially.

In fetal to newborn recent *H. sapiens* there is, generally, little to no space between the inferior border of the *s. colli* and the superior bony attachment site of the muscle (Figure 4a-b). This morphology is consistent with Schumacher's (1959, 1962) observation that septum 6 of the *m. pterygoideus medialis* was not apparent in his fetal to newborn sample (Figure 6a-d). From the bony anatomy we consider the developing septum 6 superior insertion site to be essentially coincident with the *l. sphenomandibulare* (*s.l.*) in most individuals of this developmental age (Figure 4a-b: but see discussion). Separation of the ligament and septum 6 occurs during growth such that the muscles insertion site becomes positioned inferior to the *s. colli* and, resultantly, the *tsc* (Figure 4b-d, f). Initially the bony insertions for septa of *m. pterygoideus medialis* run inferomedially from the *s. colli* border (Figure 4a-b). In individuals possessing strongly marked superior attachments of the muscle in conjunction with strong medial projection of the inferior sulcal border, separation of these structures initially results in a superoinferiorly short and inferomedially slanting ledge between the two structures (Figure 4c-d). In adults this region is morphologically variable but is generally a concave to flat, anteriorly pointing wedge-shaped area which varies in its superoinferior height (Figure 5a-e). This region may contain a substantial portion of the neurovascular bundle, particularly veins. Once clear separation of the *s. colli* and septal insertion site(s) occurs, in most cases, the bone will be slightly to substantially concave as it reaches the superior-most delimiting border of the tendinous attachment of the *m. pterygoideus medialis* (Figures 4b-e and 5b-e). Note that this concavity may result from either or both lateral movement (resorption) of the medial ramal border relative to the attachment site or medial extension of the site (apposition). The relationship between these two growth processes and the form of the attachment is currently unclear. In individuals with a bifurcated neurovascular bundle this concavity does not appear to result, however, from the muscle mass arching over the bundle as a superior concavity occurs in the presence of bifurcated and non-bifurcated neurovascular bundles. We cannot, however, fully exclude the *l. sphenomandibulare's* (*s.l.*) attachment Site 3 from a role in creating this concave bony configuration. Note, however, that the distance between the *s. colli* and the attachment site

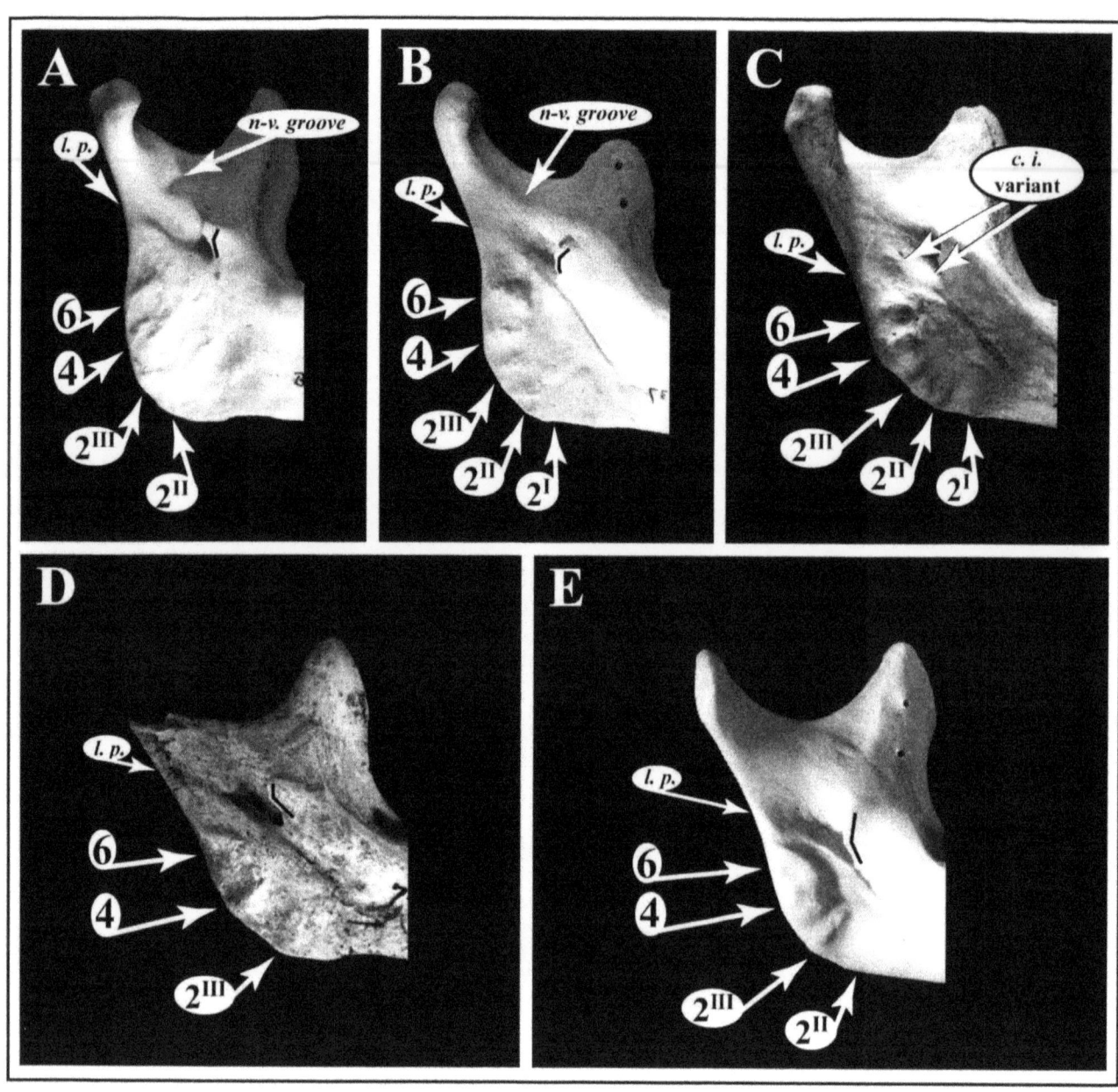

Figure 5a-e: Examples of recent *H. sapiens* adults showing some of the variation in medial ramal features. Numbered arrows depict the location of insertion sites for septa 6, 4, and 2^{I-III} of the *m. pterygoideus medialis*. Although tubercles associated with septa 6, 4, and 2^{III} represent a morphological continuum they are here classified as Type 1 (a-b) and Type 2 (c-e) for descriptive purposes. Observe how the insertion sites for these septa present as individual tubercles (b) or as 'coalesced' tubercles with 'infilling' of the intertubercle region(s) as in (d-e). Black bars have been added on the *l. mandibulae* to help delineate angular variations in the superior and inferior portions of its posterior aspect. In (d) note the attenuated form of the posteroinferior portion of the posterior lingular border. Note in (a-e) the degree of variation in the size of the space between the *l. pterygoidea* and the superior aspect of the septa 6 and 4 tubercle. Also observe the angular variation in the septa 6, 4, and 2^{III} insertions and their relationship to the mylohyoid groove and *l. mandibulae* regions. Abbreviations in this and subsequent figures are as listed in Figure 2.

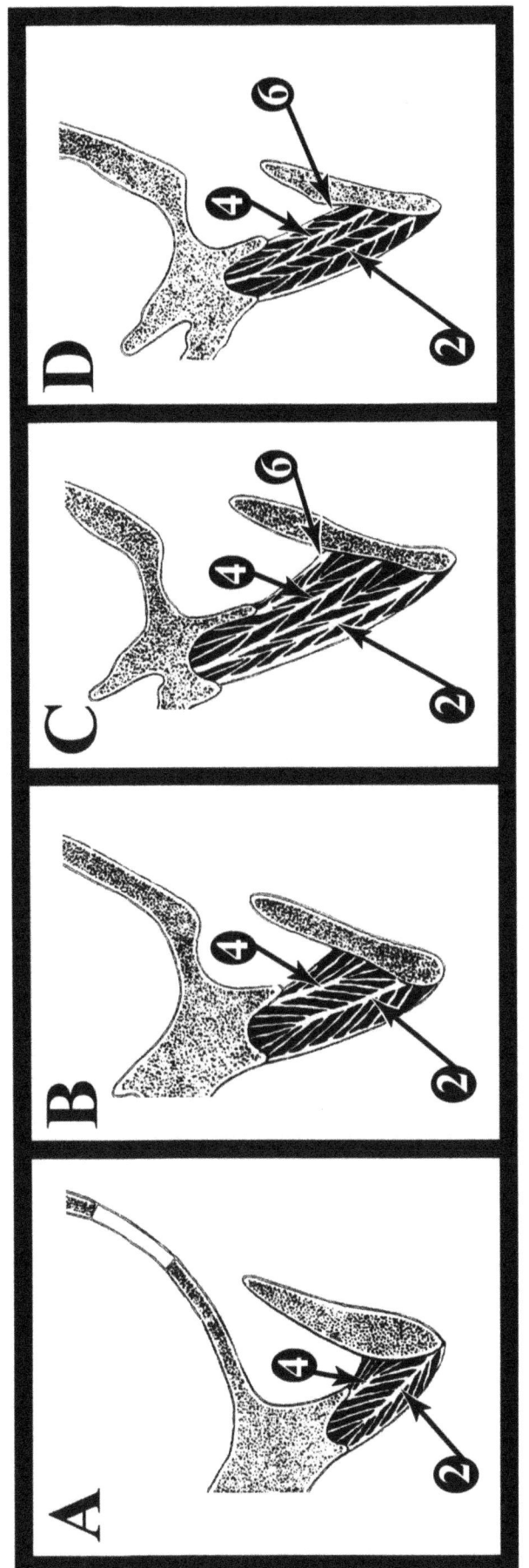

Figure 6a-d: Schumacher's (1962) ontogenetic sequence showing development and placement of major *m. pterygoideus medialis* septa in the: (a) newborn; (b) complete deciduous dentition; (c) complete permanent dentition; and (d) edentulous stages. Whereas Schumacher only found a septum 6 to occur in later age stages we consider it to be present in early age stages (refer to text Discussion for further details). Modified and redrawn from Schumacher (1962). Reprinted with permission from Urban and Vogel.

is generally occupied by fleshy muscle fibers in adults (Figure 2b) but occasionally may also include a small septum 8 insertion which is associated with a minor tubercle. Of note in some of the latter cases is that the fleshy attachment has a distinctly different angulation (septum 7 fibers?) than the remaining posterior head and that this may account for these supplementary tubercles. The situation in our dry bone sample of subadults is less clear, as fleshy muscle and small tendon entheses in this region mainly insert periosteally, thereby leaving no clear bony traces of the muscle's superior-most extent evident on gross observation.

The morphology of septal attachments in the superior aspect of the *m. pterygoideus medialis* is variable in both subadults and adults (Figures 4 and 5). Note that our focus here is on development of tubercles in the superior aspect of the attachment site but that other individuals present with septal associated depressions. In fetal to newborn mandibles the superior bony attachment of the muscle generally presents as a roughened elevation under the posteroinferior edge of the *s. colli* (Figure 4a-b). The superior extent of attachment is at the medial-most extent of the inferior border of the *s. colli*. In most newborns it is possible to discern a small tubercle in the superoposterior aspect of the muscle's attachment site which is generally continuous with the inferior sulcal border (Figure 4a-b). This tubercle generally presents with a clear septum 4 attachment ridge but it may also show development of a septum 6 ridge. In the first months after birth these bony septal attachments separate from the sulcal border and, resultantly, septa 6 and 4 ridges are the norm (Figure 4c-f). During the latter process the sulcal overhang becomes less prominent, tubercle size increases, or a combination of these factors occurs. As separation of the two structures continues the superior edge of the tubercle is initially an inferomedially slanted ledge. With growth the tubercle presents with a concave superior surface, in nearly all tubercles examined. As a clearly separate tubercle develops the observed range of variation is similar to that seen in adults (Figures 4 and 5). In many cases the early postnatal condition is still present in individuals aged 3.0-4.0 years of age whereas in others a strong multi-septum associated tubercle already exists prior to or by 1.0 year of age. In all cases the tubercle is anteroposteriorly short with substantial variation in its medial extent (Figure 4c-f). Strong medial projection of tubercles appears to be accomplished in the superoinferior extent of the attachment by bone deposition between septa 6 and 4 (Figure 4c-f). In these cases the superior and inferior tubercle borders are slightly marked by anteroposteriorly oriented elevations associated with the latter septa (Figure 4c-f). With continued growth the tubercle becomes well separated from the *s. colli* but there appears to be little change in tubercle extent, at least through the early juvenile stages (Figure 4a-f). Note that the degree of separation of septa 6 and 4 at the posterior border of the ramus is approximately 5.0 mm by ca. 1.5 years of age and increases to about 10.0 mm in adults. In both subadults and adults, septa 6 and 4 either converge at their anterior extent or parallel each other. The former situation results in triangular shaped attachments whereas the latter results in rhomboidal ones (Figures 4c-f and 5a-e). In cases where the bony ridges associated with septa 6 and 4 do not converge, we found on dissection that the septa do tend to converge anteriorly. In the latter cases septum 4 tends to arch anterosuperiorly around septum 6, as also observed by Schumacher (1962), but the bony attachment does not fully reflect this configuration.

The bony attachment of *m. pterygoideus medialis* in adults presents as a continuation of the observed subadult pattern. The anteroposteriorly directed ridges for attachment of septa are elongated during mandibular growth, muscle hypertrophy, or both. Whereas there are generally only one or two ridges visible in the superior aspect of the attachment site in infants more ridges appear in the inferior aspect as the individual matures. In most individuals the degree of prominence of bony insertions for the superior septa of *m. pterygoideus medialis* decreases from septum 6 to 2^{III} (Figures 4c-f and 5). In the more superior aspects of the attachment, Weidenreich (1936) observed the *l. pterygoidea* to be represented by an obliquely coursing and relatively straight line and Patte (1957) noted that it is more inferiorly placed in infants relative to adults. Weidenreich (1936) also observed a high degree of variability in the line. We have observed the *l. pterygoidea* to range from an inferiorly inclined oblique line to a line which is horizontal and positioned parallel to or coincident with the *s. colli* in both infants and adults (Figure 2c1-2). The latter variant appears to be related to mylohyoid groove and *l. mandibulae* bridging, as discussed further below.

The general pattern of tubercles formed in the *m. pterygoideus medialis* insertion site can be described for adults. Whereas there is a morphological continuum in tubercle form, we are dividing the continuum into two types to facilitate discussion of fossil taxa. The first tubercle type (Type 1) occurs when the septum 6 ridge dominates that of septum 4 (Figure 5b). These tubercles: (1) are anteroposteriorly elongated; (2) arch superiorly over a concavity; (3) have a superior aspect which gradually thins to terminate superomedially in a sharp, fine edge; and (4) are slightly rounded and roughened on their medial aspect. The degree to which the superomedial 'free' edge of the tubercle is extended is highly variable. In some cases these tubercles are associated with pits which occur in the superior concavity. Such tubercles are associated with the superior-most of the main septa of *m. pterygoideus medialis* and, as such, are continuous with the space below the inferior border of the *s. colli*. This space is filled with fleshy fibers related to the origin of septum 7 and insertions of other minor tendons. This type of tubercle may extend to the posterior ramal border or it may be somewhat isolated anterior to that border. Note that in Type 1 tubercles there is an association of septum 6 with septum 4 but the latter attachment is very weak relative to that of septum 6 (Figure 5a-b).

The Type 2 condition results from a more equal association of septa 6 and 4 and, in some cases, septum 2^{III} may be variously merged with septum 4. In this condition a morphologically diverse series of tubercles results (Figure 5c-e). This tubercle type: (1) is anteroposteriorly elongated;

(2) is superiorly concave; (3) generally has a blunt superior border (i.e. lacks superior lipping); (4) either slopes gradually into the ramus at the inferior extent or ends more abruptly at an inferiorly placed concavity; (5) is always associated with the posterior border of the ramus; and (6) varies in the degree of bony deposition between the septal attachment sites. In these cases tubercle morphology appears to reflect the number of sites which have coalesced or failed to differentiate and migrate. In cases where septa 6 and 4 are not strongly developed the tubercle presents with a septum 6 ridge which slopes inferiorly into the ridge-base for septum 4; this is the minimal expression (Figure 5c). As noted, the general outline of the tubercle will be triangular to rhomboidal due to variation in the angular arrangement of septa. From this basic configuration bone deposition at the septal ridges combined with deposition between the septa appears to be the process which produces a variety of subtriangular to rhomboidal, variably projecting raised plateaus with concave-to-blunt superior and anterior borders (Figure 5a-e). The inferior border is also concave unless the septa 6 and 4 ridges are associated with septum 2^{III}, in which case it generally fades gradually into the ramus (Figure 5e). These tubercles are usually not associated directly with pits in the superior concavity. Further, the area between septa 6 and 4 can be filled with fleshy muscle fibers, with a combination of fleshy muscle and tendinous fibers, or solely by tendon. The degree of bony infilling between these septa varies but its maximum expression occurs when the interseptal space is filled to the height of the septal ridges (Figure 5c Vs 5d-e). As noted, processes giving rise to this bony infilling are clearly multifactorial, as opposed to simple bone deposition due to *m. pterygoideus medialis* induced tension on the fibroperiosteum, as noted by Hoyte and Enlow (1966) and as discussed further below.

The two tubercle 'types' can also be distinguished by the manner in which tendons of the muscle insert into the periosteum and bone and by the positioning of associated fleshy muscle fibers. Note, in both tubercle types, that septa 6 and 4 and, possibility, septum 2^{III} are associated with a fibrocartilaginous entheses and that details of these attachments will be discussed further below. Basically, Type 1 tubercles are associated with tendon entheses which insert directly into the bone. These entheses insert into the tubercle and superior concavity at varying angles, resulting in a highly interwoven fabric, as noted for complex tendons by Elliott (1965). Based on the observed distribution of tendon fibers it is clear that this tubercle is related to a broad portion of the *mediolateral* extent of septum 6 of the *m. pterygoideus medialis*. The superoinferior extent of fibers reaching this area is more restricted, however, with the curved tubercle reflecting the extent and direction of contributing tendinous fibers. When present, pits associated with these tubercles contain very short fleshy muscle fibers which attach superiorly to the tendon web and to periosteum (fibrocartilage?) inferiorly. Because the *m. pterygoideus medialis* is a multipennate muscle with strong linkage of the intramuscular septa the level of fascicular involvement will be greater than that indicated solely by the individual septal attachments, as noted by Antón (1995, 1996) and explicated by Schumacher (1962).

Type 2 tubercles are associated with septa comprising densely packed ovate bundles of tendinous tissue (fascicles) which vary in cross-sectional area. Many of these ovate tendons have lateral surfaces which are flattened (i.e. oval medially to flat laterally). The general arrangement of fascicles comprising septa 6 and 4 is to have large ovate (ovate-flat) bundles attaching at the posterior border and for increasingly smaller bundles to then extend anteriorly from these to the anterior extent of the tendon insertion region. The size of the fascicles, then, decreases both inferiorly and anteriorly from the posterosuperior-most attachment of septum 6. In some cases, the posterior-most fascicles coalesce as they approach the ramus such that they form a solid mass at the bone surface. In the general arrangement, fascicles attach to variably sized superiorly inclined tubercles. In the latter case, the degree of tendon coalescence appears related to the degree of bony infilling between the septa and to the medial extent of the tubercle. Whether these variants result from genetic, epigenetic (*sensu* Atchley, 1993), or nonheritable idiosyncratic variation is unclear. Further, these tubercles have slightly roughened or undercut surfaces for tendinous or fleshy attachments around their periphery which vary in degree relative to tubercle height (= medial extent). In tubercles of this type, entheses may only insert into the periosteum or they may be strongly embedded into the concave area of bone, but they generally present with varying degrees of this attachment continuum. Further, many of the lateral-most musculotendinous bundles attaching to the anterolateral tubercle face have a different orientation then that of the main muscle mass. These tendons vary from weakly expressed flat tendons to strongly expressed round ones. A curious variation appears in these tendons as many have a doubled 'insertion'. Fibers extending from the muscle's origin insert by way of tendinous fibers in the region between the anterior mylohyoid groove border and the *crista pharyngea*. However, from this 'insertion' the tendon fibers change direction and 'insert again' at the anterolateral base of the septum 6, 4, and 2^{I-III} tubercles. Many of the directional changes in these bundles create angular changes in the range of ± 90°. These musculotendinous bundles appear to be associated with mylohyoid groove and, potentially *l. mandibulae* bridging. The *m. pterygoideus medialis* contains two portions, sometimes referred to as heads (Scott and Dixon, 1972; Van Eijden *et al.*, 1995), and a substantial number of these lateral-most musculotendinous bundles can be traced to the superficial head of *m. pterygoideus medialis*. Note that further work is required to determine whether these tendons with 'doubled insertions' do not actually consist of a musculotendinous bundle which inserts into the anterior insertion/origin of an as yet unrecognized tendon attached between the septal related tubercles of the *m. pterygoideus medialis* and the region anterior to the mylohyoid groove. We have observed what appear to be isolated tendons in this region but our methods do not currently allow us to further clarify the nature of these structures.

III. DESCRIPTION OF BONY MEDIAL RAMUS ANATOMY AND RELATED SOFT TISSUES IN ONTOGENETIC SAMPLES OF GREAT APES

1. Introduction

To evaluate the ontogeny of medial ramal structures in great apes we examined small samples of *Gorilla gorilla*, *Pan paniscus*, *P. troglodytes*, and *Pongo pygmaeus*. Observations are provided on the morphology of the *c. endocondyloidea*, *f. mandibulae*, *c. mandibulae-l. mandibulae*, *m. pterygoideus medialis* insertion, and posterior ramal border. Because we did not dissect great ape specimens ourselves, correlations between observed bony morphology and soft tissue anatomy are made with reference to literature descriptions.

2. Overview of hard and soft tissue relationships in ontogenetic samples of great apes

In great apes the *c. endocondyloidea* may be straight or slightly concave anteriorly. This structure is a relatively weak to strongly defined crest above the *f. mandibulae-s. colli* in the sequence *Pongo*, *Gorilla*, *P. troglodytes*, and *P. paniscus*, respectively. In *Pongo* this crest is generally short while it tends to be stronger and to run a longer course in *Gorilla* and *P. troglodytes*, respectively (Figure 7a-d). In adult recent *H. sapiens* the *c. endocondyloidea* tends to be a short, weakly expressed crest that is concave and truncated by a vertically oriented shallow groove (Figure 5a-b).

Dissimilarity also exists in the bony attachment sites for the *l. sphenomandibulare* (*s.l.*) between great apes and recent *H. sapiens*. In most cases the *c. intermedia* is relatively long and well delineated in *P. troglodytes*, but in no case did we observe this crest to reach past mid-ramus (Figure 7a-d). Alternatively, *Gorilla* and *Pongo* generally have shorter crests. In one *Gorilla* subadult the *s. colli* was absent and the *f. mandibulae* presented with a smoothly rounded opening without cresting. Differences observed in *P. troglodytes* appear to result, in part, from a more posteriorly located bifurcation of the mylohyoid neurovascular bundle relative to the *f. mandibulae* (Figure 7c). Great apes, in general, present with a *c. intermedia* that is distinct from the *l. pterygoidea* although, these structures were observed to be coincident in some *Gorilla* and *Pongo*, as in some recent *H. sapiens*. In no case, however, did we observe the *c. intermedia* to enter the *s. colli* (Figure 7a-d). Based on the bony anatomy we consider the *l. sphenomandibulare* (*s.l.*) attachment sites to be generally similar to those of recent *H. sapiens*. Differences in attachments sites in great apes do exist, however, with Site 1 being more prominent in *P. troglodytes*, but less so in *Gorilla* and *Pongo*, and Site 2 and 3 apparently being co-incident (Figure 7a-d).

The relationship of the *c. endocondyloidea* to the *f. mandibulae* in great apes tends to isolate the foramen below the medially projecting crest and results in a short but more sharply defined superior border to the *s. colli* (Figure 7a-d). In recent *H. sapiens* the superior border is not marked by a sharp crest (Figure 5a-e). In all great apes examined (*N* = 48) the superior opening of the *f. mandibulae* was found to be positioned inferior to the *c. endocondyloidea* whether or not the *crista* was lightly or strongly projecting. Further, in all these cases a notch was absent at the superior aspect of the *f. mandibulae* and the superomedial wall of the *c. mandibulae* did not extend or arch medially (Figure 7a-d). These observations indicate that great apes possess a simple medial wall to the *c. mandibulae*, a more complex secondary division of this wall, or *l. mandibulae*, is absent. Given our observations we concur with Weidenreich (1936) and Swindler and Wood (1973) that great apes do not possess a *l. mandibulae*.

As in recent *H. sapiens* the *s. colli* of great apes can be divided into anterior and posterior components. The basic configuration of the anterior component of the *s. colli* in adult great apes is a short and narrow, sharply defined sulcus whereas the posterior component is, generally, a lightly-marked narrow to broad sulcus (Figure 7a-d). In some *Gorilla* the posterior sulcal component can, however, be strongly marked. The posterior component terminates at the posterior ramal border at a level similar to that of recent *H. sapiens*. Further, the sulcal components are generally separated medially by a slightly to well marked raised or not depressed area (Figure 7b). In subadult *Pongo* the anterior sulcal component was sometimes observed to be very vertically oriented but in no case did we find a marked posterior component. In adult *Pongo* the sulcus tends to become more open anteriorly whereas the posterior component is narrow, shallow, and arcs posterosuperiorly. Relative to *Pongo*, subadult *Gorilla* and *P. troglodytes* have a more posteriorly opening *f. mandibulae*. Adult *P. troglodytes* are generally similar to *Pongo* in sulcal morphology although the sulcus tends to be more broad. Placement of the *f. mandibulae* and, resultantly, the *s. colli* is significantly more anterior relative to the *c. pharyngea* in *P. troglodytes* than in either *Gorilla* or *Pongo*.

Of the great apes, *s. colli* morphology of *P. troglodytes* subadults (*N* = 7) is most similar to that of recent *H. sapiens*. It tends to be deep and have a medially projecting lower border, although, this border is generally not as strongly projecting as in recent *H. sapiens*. Because our sample lacks individuals of late fetal to newborn age we cannot confirm, however, that the lower sulcal border in *P. troglodytes* infants is continuous from the *f. mandibulae* to the posterior ramal border, as in human infants. Further, in the age range observed, the sulcus of *P. troglodytes* subadults shows some significant differences relative to humans. In *P. troglodytes*, the anterior component is a deep sulcus while the posterior component is a broad depression (Figure 7a-d). As noted, the two sulcal components are separated by a slightly raised area whereas they are separated by a shallow groove in humans. Further, with growth the anterior component of the *s. colli* in *P. troglodytes* becomes a well delineated sulcus while the posterior component is maintained as a shallow depression. We observed the former configuration to exist in individuals having fully erupted M1/1 but in all specimens the latter condition existed by the adult stage. As noted in infant *P. troglodytes*, the posterior sulcal component is broad and deep and this accentuates the attachment Site 2 (and 3?) of the *l. sphenomandibulare* (*s.l.*). Further, this configuration is very similar to that found in recent *H. sapiens* infants, but note that in neither case is the ligamentous attachment strongly demarcated by bony elevations.

We have not found a *tsc* in subadult or adult great apes. Given the general absence of significant bony attachment sites for the *l. sphenomandibulare* (*s.l.*) along the middle to posterior aspect of the *s. colli*, this finding is not unexpected (Figure 7a-d). In infants and adults the Site 2 attachment of the *l. sphenomandibulare* (*s.l.*) and the superior-most extent of the muscle (= *l. pterygoidea*) are nearly coincident with the tubercle(s) for superior septa in the age range observed (> 2.5 years: Figure 7b-d). A potentially similar ligament-muscle arrangement appears to be present in some fetal to ca. 0.5 year-old humans. With growth, morphological changes observed between the inferior border of the *s. colli* (Site 2; *l. pterygoidea* and *tsc*) and the superior septal attachment site of *m. pterygoideus medialis* in recent *H. sapiens* were not observed in great apes. The latter result most probably reflects significant differences in positioning of the functional components related to medial ramal anatomy as discussed below.

The relationship between the *s. colli* and the superior aspect of the attachment site for the *m. pterygoideus medialis* differs between great apes. Noting intraspecific variation, *P. troglodytes* generally possesses a more horizontal orientation of the attachment site relative to the more vertical one in *Gorilla*, *Pongo*, and many *P. paniscus*. The latter attachment orientation is most similar to hominids. In infant *P. troglodytes* the superior-most bony attachment is near to or coincident with the inferior border of the *s. colli* and tends to be similar to that described above for human infants (Figure 7a-d). Some *P. troglodytes* infants ($N = 4$, 59%) have either strong medial shelving of the *s. colli's* inferior border or retain a portion of this shelving with the resultant that the septal attachment site strongly projects medially at its superior-most extent. Medial shelving of the region is not retained in older individuals and may result from remodeling of the *s. colli's* posterior component (Figure 7a-d). In adult great apes the *m. pterygoideus medialis* attachment is a broad, flat field which is generally demarcated superiorly by a developed tubercle(s). This tubercle(s) differs significantly from that observed in *Australopithecus* and *Homo*, however, not only in its relationship to the *s. colli* but also in morphology. Given the bony evidence, we consider the observed tubercle(s) to be produced by septum 6 and, in some cases, by involvement of secondary septa occurring between septa 6 and 4. The potential for minor contributions from septum 4 cannot, however, be excluded in all cases. The general pattern of tubercle formation in great apes is for anteroposteriorly short ovate, to sub-triangular raised areas to occur in the superior-most aspect of the attachment site (Figure 7a-d). Tubercles were always observed to involve the posterior ramal border, as noted for *Pongo* by Bluntschli (1929). In many cases these superiorly placed tubercles strongly project medially but are generally associated with other equally large tubercles within the muscle's attachment area. We have not observed a tubercle in the superior attachment area of great apes which obtains the superoinferior or anteroposterior expansion seen in adult *Homo*. However, tubercles similar to those observed in both recent and fossil *Homo* subadults do occur. Relative to other great apes, only *P. troglodytes* appears to consistently have large tubercles in the superior aspect of the *m. pterygoideus medialis* attachment site. It is unusual in adults, however, for the latter tubercles to appear as isolates, as strong tubercles can be found along the full course of the posterior ramus.

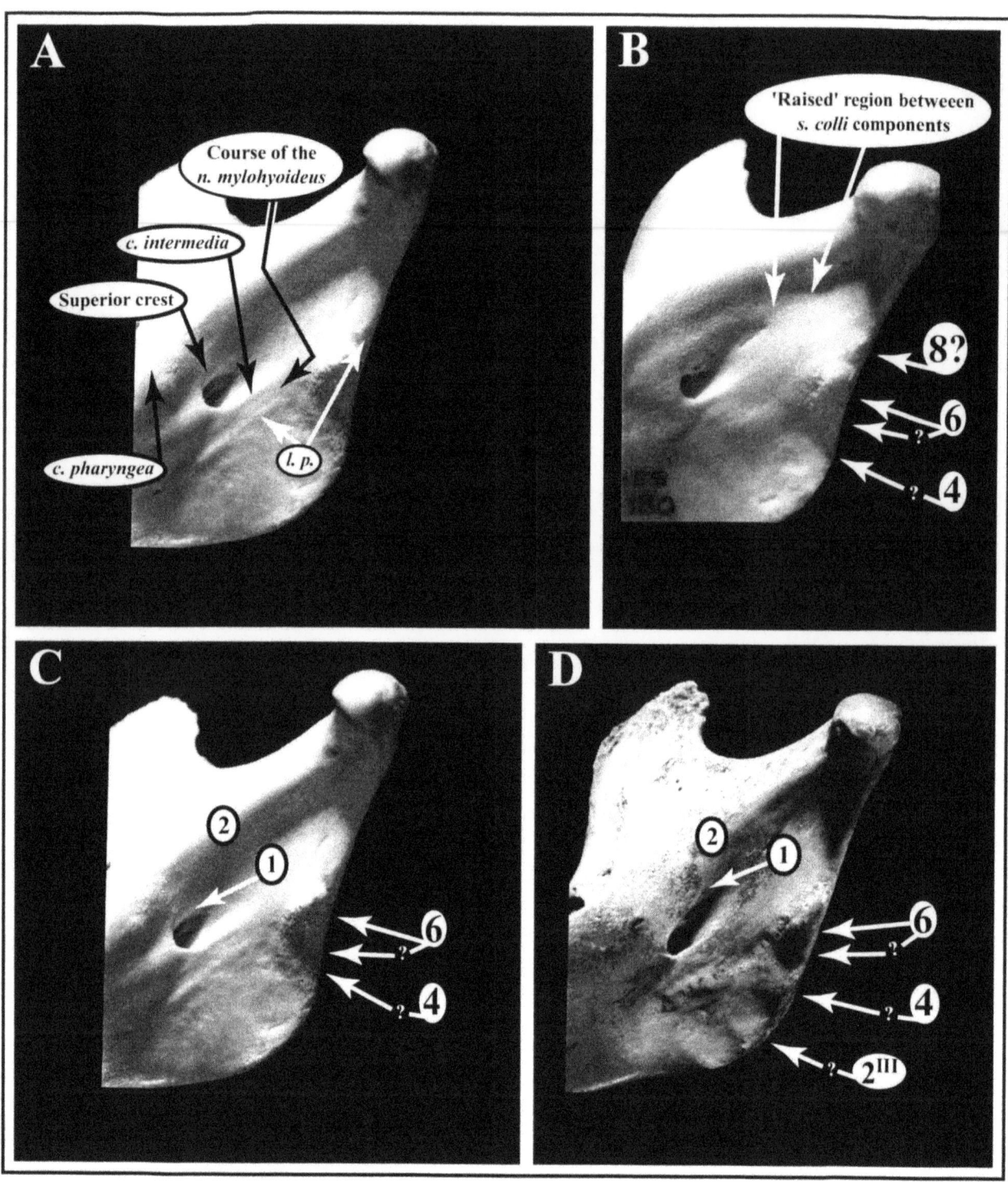

Figure 7a-d: Examples of *P. troglodytes* subadults showing some of the variation in medial ramal features. Numbered arrows here depict the probable location of insertion sites for septa 6, 4, and 2^{I-III} of the *m. pterygoideus medialis*. Figure 7a shows the location of features discussed in the text. Observe the: (1) configuration of the *c. endocondyloidea*; (2) position of the *f. mandibulae-c. intermedia* complex and its relationship to the *l. pterygoidea*; (3) position of the mylohyoid groove; (4) *c. pharyngea* to *c. mandibulae* orientation; (5) 'raised' region in the middle of the *s. colli*; (6) lack of a strongly marked *l. pterygoidea* insertion in the middle to posterior portion of the ramus; and (7) horizontal (superoinferiorly short) orientation of the *m. pterygoideus medialis* insertion. Also note that the *l. pterygoidea* and septum 6 (and 8?) are coincident, i.e. lack an intervening space. Further, note the relationship of the *c. intermedia* to the *l. pterygoidea* and the lack of a *l. mandibulae*. In this taxon, and apes in general, we do not see a clear splitting of the medial cortical plate to form the *l. mandibulae* as seen in hominids. Observe in (d-e) how the *f. mandibulae* has a superior (1) and inferior crest extending from it and the foramen's position below the projecting *c. endocondyloidea* (2).

IV. DESCRIPTION OF BONY MEDIAL RAMUS ANATOMY IN ONTOGENETIC SAMPLES OF PLIO-PLEISTOCENE HOMINIDS

1. Introduction

To evaluate the structural associations and range of variation in medial ramal structures, inclusive of the superior attachment of *m. pterygoideus medialis*, and their value to taxonomic assessments and phylogenetic reconstructions we expanded our sample of subadult and adult fossil hominids ($N = 74$). Taxonomic groups in this series include: (1) *A. afarensis*, $N = 10$; (2) *A. africanus*, $N = 4$; (3) *A. robustus*, $N = 4$; (4) *A. boisei*, $N = 2$; (5) *H. habilis* (s.l.), $N = 1$; (6) *H. erectus* (s.l.), $N = 13$; (7) ArHs, $N = 6$; (8) Neanderthal, $N = 20$; (9) AmHs, $N = 13$; and (10) *H. sapiens* ssp. indet., $N = 1$. Our ability to evaluate morphological details of the medial ramus in this sample is highly affected by taphonomic factors. Only 22 (29.7%) individuals retain portions of the right and left rami and only 13 (17.6%) of these retain sufficient detail to evaluate the bilateral occurrence of the *tsc* and muscle related tubercles.

2. Description of the bony medial ramus in fossil hominids

2.1. *Australopithecus afarensis*

In *A. afarensis* the medial ramus is poorly preserved but the *c. endocondyloidea*, *s. colli*, and *m. pterygoideus medialis* attachment areas in this taxon are clearly derived relative to great apes. The *c. endocondyloidea* is strongly expressed posteriorly but by mid-ramus it becomes broad and flat (AL 288-1, 333w-16, 333w-1e, 333-100, Mak VP-1/83, 1/12), except in AL 333-43b and 333w-52 and Mak VP-1/2 (Figure 8a-e). The subadult specimen AL 333-43b has a deep, anteroposteriorly restricted depression in the *c. endocondyloidea* at mid-ramus (Figure 8a) whereas AL 333w-52 has a strongly developed *c. endocondyloidea* which exhibits only a slight anterior concavity. The Mak VP-1/2 specimen lacks any prominence of the posterior-aspect of the *c. endocondyloidea*, probably resulting from a slightly posteroinferiorly rotated condylar neck-condylar head relative to all other *A. afarensis* (Figure 8b-d). Details of the *s. colli* region differ in some individuals in the Hadar sample relative to those in the Maka sample. Preserved anatomy of AL 288-1 and AL 333-43b shows the *s. colli* to have a short, near vertical anterior component which opens into a broad, anteriorly-open depression. Further, the posterior component in AL 288-1 and AL 333-43b comprises both this broad depression and a short, horizontal portion inferior to the condyle (Figure 8a-b). Preserved portions of the posterior component appear similar in AL 333w-1e and 333w-16. In AL 333w-52 the anterior component appears similar to other Hadar individuals as does the posterior secondary flexure whereas the posterior *s. colli* component differs in being deep and narrow. In AL 288-1 the *f. mandibulae* and *s. colli* are isolated from the *f. pterygoidea* (Johanson et al., 1982). The inferior border of the *s. colli* in this specimen comprises two distinct, but generally coincident, ridges the *c. intermedia* and *l. pterygoidea*. This composite inferior *s. colli* border is essentially continuous from the *c. pharyngea* to near the posterior ramal border. Further, the inferior border of the *s. colli* in AL 288-1 forms a relatively high ridge which results in a *s. colli* with a short and horizontal posterior component and a longer and inferiorly sloping anterior component. The latter morphology creates a superiorly-open 'trough' for the contained neurovascular bundle (Figure 8b). Note that Johanson et al. (1982) suggest that the *c. intermedia* bounds the *s. colli* and continues anteriorly as a sharp crest to join the *c. pharyngea*. They also note that a *l. pterygoidea* is not present in AL 288-1. We differ from these authors by considering the specimen to exhibit a strong superoanteriorly directed extension of the *l. pterygoidea*. This configuration is considered by us to obscure the *c. intermedia* by incorporating it into the muscle-associated *l. pterygoidea*, as demonstrated herein for recent *H. sapiens* and other taxa as noted below. The subadult AL 333-43b presents with a configuration similar to AL 288-1, as does AL 333w-52, with the exception that the inferior *s. colli* border is not as developed in the infant (Figure 8a). The opening of the *f. mandibulae* and lingular region are not preserved in AL 288-1 and AL 333-43b (Figure 8a-b).

The Maka specimens preserve a slightly different pattern relative to those from Hadar in several regards. The inferior border of the *s. colli* is weak (Mak VP-1/2 and 1/12) to lightly marked (Mak VP-1/83: Figure 8c-d). The *f. mandibulae* and *c. intermedia* are preserved only in Mak VP-1/83 (Figure 8c). In the latter specimen the *f. mandibulae* opens posteriorly and the superior aspect of the foramen is positioned on the lower-third of the *c. endocondyloidea*. Further, the Mak VP-1/83 specimen presents with a small *l. mandibulae* and possesses a minimally developed lingular notch. The medial wall of the *f. mandibulae-c. mandibulae* is well formed and reaches to the level of the *s. colli*. In this individual the anterior sulcal component is linear, deep, and not as vertically oriented as in AL 288-1 and 333-43b (Figure 8a-c). The posterior component is a broad, shallow depression that retains its depth until near the posterior ramus, where it shallows dramatically and exhibits a slight angular difference as found in AL 288-1, 333-43b, 333w-1e, and 333-16 (Figure 8a-c). Significantly, in this Maka specimen the sulcal components are separated by a slightly raised area similar to that observed in great apes (Figure 8c). Preserved anatomy in Mak VP-1/2 and 1/12 indicates an extremely shallow *s. colli*. The sulcus comprises a near vertical anterior component which opens into a long, horizontally oriented, and superiorly placed posterior component (Figure 8d). There is a clear difference in the overall depth of the *s. colli* between these two groups with the Hadar sample generally being more deep. Significantly the *c. intermedia* and *l. pterygoidea* in Mak VP-1/83 are well separated with the latter structure being continuous with the posterosuperior border of the mylohyoid groove. The *c.*

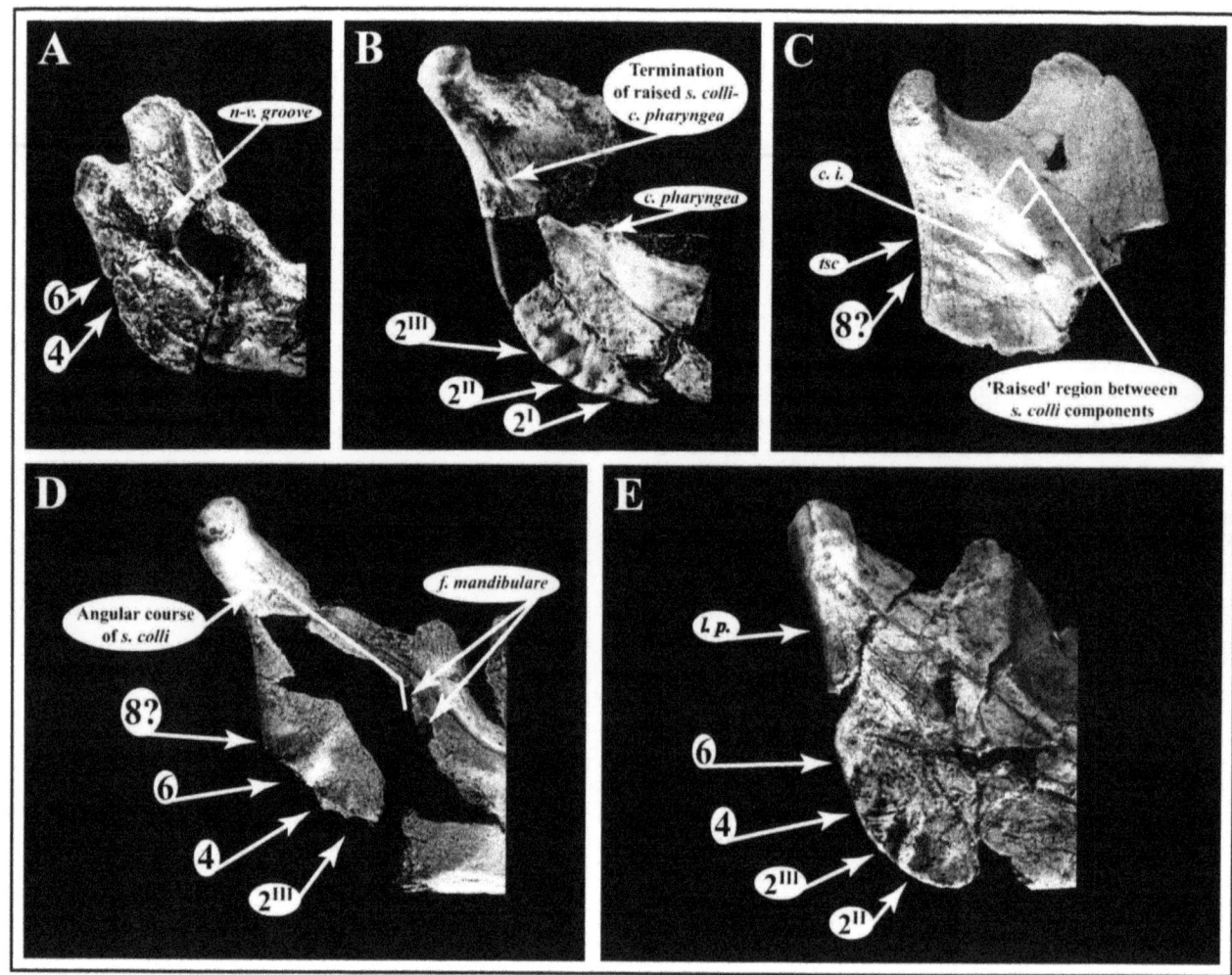

Figure 8a-e: Medial mandibular ramus anatomy in *A. afarensis* (a-d) and *A. africanus* (e). Specimens figured are from left to right: AL 333-43b, reversed; AL 288-1; Mak VP-1/83; Mak VP-1/2, reversed; and Sts 36. In this and subsequent figures numbered arrows depict the location of insertion sites for septa 6, 4, and 2^{I-III} of the *m. pterygoideus medialis*. In (a) note the depth of both the *s. colli* and the neurovascular groove in the *c. endocondyloidea* in the subadult AL 333-43b. In (b) observe how the *l. pterygoidea* is continuous from the *c. pharyngea* to near the posterior ramal border. Note in (c) the position of the *f. mandibulae* relative to the *c. endocondyloidea* and how the *c. intermedia* is both separate from the *l. pterygoidea* and resides within the *s. colli*. In (c-d) note what appears to be the presence of an 8th septal insertion site. Compare the configuration of the above structures in *A. afarensis* (b-d) to those in *A. africanus* (e).

intermedia lies in the *s. colli* and is separate from and above the *l. pterygoidea* (Figure 8c). The mylohyoid groove arises from the anterior-most aspect of the *f. mandibulae* and, although bridged in AL 288-1, it is open in AL 128-23 and Mak VP-1/2, 1/12, and 1/83 (Figure 8a-d).

A *tsc* is only present in Mak VP-1/83. Whereas AL 288-1 and, to a lesser degree, AL 333-43b have a strong Site 2 attachment which could indicate the presence of a *tsc*, the inferior *s. colli* border ends before reaching the posterior ramal border (Figure 8b). The *m. pterygoideus medialis* attachment site is well marked in AL 288-1 and 333-108 but very faint to slightly marked in the series Mak VP-1/83, 1/12, and 1/2 (Figure 8a-d) A very weak indication of the septa 6 and 4 attachments are present in AL 333-43b whereas the area is not preserved in AL 288-1 (contra Rak *et al.*, 1994) or Mak VP-1/83, and the tubercle site is damaged in AL 333-108. Portions of septa 6 and 4 tubercles are preserved in Mak VP-1/2 (strong) and Mak VP-1/12 (slightly less marked). The latter specimens have tubercles with concave superior borders (the former exhibits minor lipping) which are well separated from the *s. colli* (Figure 8d). Further, all Maka specimens have a small, triangular-shaped tubercle (= septum 8?) located in the space between septum 6 and the *s. colli* (Figure 8d). The latter secondary tubercles range from faintly to strongly marked in the series: Mak VP-1/83, 1/2, 1/12 (Figure 8c-d). Excepting AL 288-1 and 333-108 the region inferior to the septa 6 and 4 tubercle site is not preserved and, resultantly, it is not possible to determine the degree of development of more inferiorly placed tubercles (= septum 2^{I-III}). It is significant to note that the Maka specimens, generally, have a strong septa 6 and 4 tubercle (White *et al.*, 2000) but a relatively weak *m. pterygoideus medialis* attachment overall. The latter is especially notable as they possess a secondary septal attachment site in the region above septum 6.

2.2. *Australopithecus africanus*

In *A. africanus* the *c. endocondyloidea* is curved and not strong in Sts 52b but more marked in Sts 36. In Sts 36 and 52b, Stw 498, and MLD 40 the *s. colli* has a strongly depressed anterior component which is superoinferiorly tall and which broadens and shallows posteriorly (Figures 8e and 9a). The relationship of the anterior and posterior *s. colli* components is similar in AL 288-1 and Sts 52b whereas Sts 36 differs. In the latter specimen the anterior component is tall and deep whereas the posterior component is extremely shallow (Figure 8e). These similarities and differences between AL 288-1 and Sts 36 and 52b may be due mainly to a weakly expressed *c. endocondyloidea* in Sts 52b. In MLD 40 and Stw 498 the anterior component is similar to Sterkfontein individuals but it is more vertically angled; the posterior component is not preserved (Figure 9a). In MLD 40, Sts 52b, and Stw 498 there is clear evidence of a *l. mandibulae*, as indicated by the presence of a medially extended tip and slightly developed lingular notch (Figure 9a). Both MLD 40 and Stw 498 present with less developed *l. mandibulae* than that found in Sts 52b. The lingular region in Sts 36 lacks both of these features (Figure 8e). In all these specimens the medial wall of the *f. mandibulae-c. mandibulae* is well formed and reaches to the level of the *s. colli*. The inferior border of the *s. colli* in *A. africanus* comprises the *c. intermedia* and *l. pterygoidea* and is continuous from the *f. mandibulae* to near the posterior ramal border (Figures 8e and 9a). This sulcal border presents as a low ridge which is only slightly developed relative to the Hadar specimens, being most similar to those observed in the Maka individuals (Figure 8c-d and Figures 8e and 9a). The inferior *s. colli* border differs from *A. afarensis*, in general, as it is slightly concave near the mylohyoid groove but less concave from that groove to the posterior ramal border. The mylohyoid groove runs over a low ridge forming the *s. colli*'s inferior border, as opposed to truncating it. The configuration of the *s. colli* differs from that found in *A. afarensis* but is more similar to that found in later hominids. Neither a *tsc* nor a significantly developed tubercle(s) for the *m. pterygoideus medialis* can be discerned in the superior aspect of the muscles insertion site in these specimens (Figures 8e and 9a).

2.3. *Australopithecus robustus*

The *c. endocondyloidea* in the *A. robustus* individuals SK 12 and 23 and SKW 5 is curved and broken by a vertical groove, but not strongly expressed. The *f. mandibulae* in SK 12 and 23 is superoinferiorly narrow but slightly more open in SKW 5. The *f. mandibulae* in SK 12 and 23 is positioned within a swelling of the base of the *torus triangularis*. This positioning results in or provides for the *l. mandibulae* expression to range from essentially absent (SK 12) to weakly expressed (SK 23). In SK 64 and SKW 5 a rudimentary *l. mandibulae* is present but its development most probably reflects an immature status in these subadult individuals. In all cases the medial wall of the *f. mandibulae-c. mandibulae* is well developed. The *s. colli* is superoinferiorly narrow and more linearly continuous from the *f. mandibulae* to the posterior ramal border. In the former feature this group is more similar to *A. afarensis* but differs significantly in other details from both *A. afarensis* and *A. africanus*. As in some *A. afarensis* and all *A. africanus* the *c. intermedia* and *l. pterygoidea* are continuous, excepting in SKW 5. The latter crest-line forms a low ridge as in *A. africanus* but it does not possess the concavities of the latter taxon. Neither a *tsc* nor a developed tubercle in the superior attachment area are apparent in *A. robustus* specimens SK 12 or 23. In SKW 5, a *tsc* is absent but a strong septa 6 and 4 associated, sub-triangular tubercle is present. Further, the tubercle's main medial expanse is well separated from the *s. colli*. This tubercle is consistent with those occurring in *Homo*. As in the Maka specimens (Mak VP-1/2, 1/12, and 1/83), a small secondary tubercle is located just superior to the septum 6 insertion. A slight separation of the *c. intermedia* and *l. pterygoidea* occurs in this specimen but this may be related to a young developmental age.

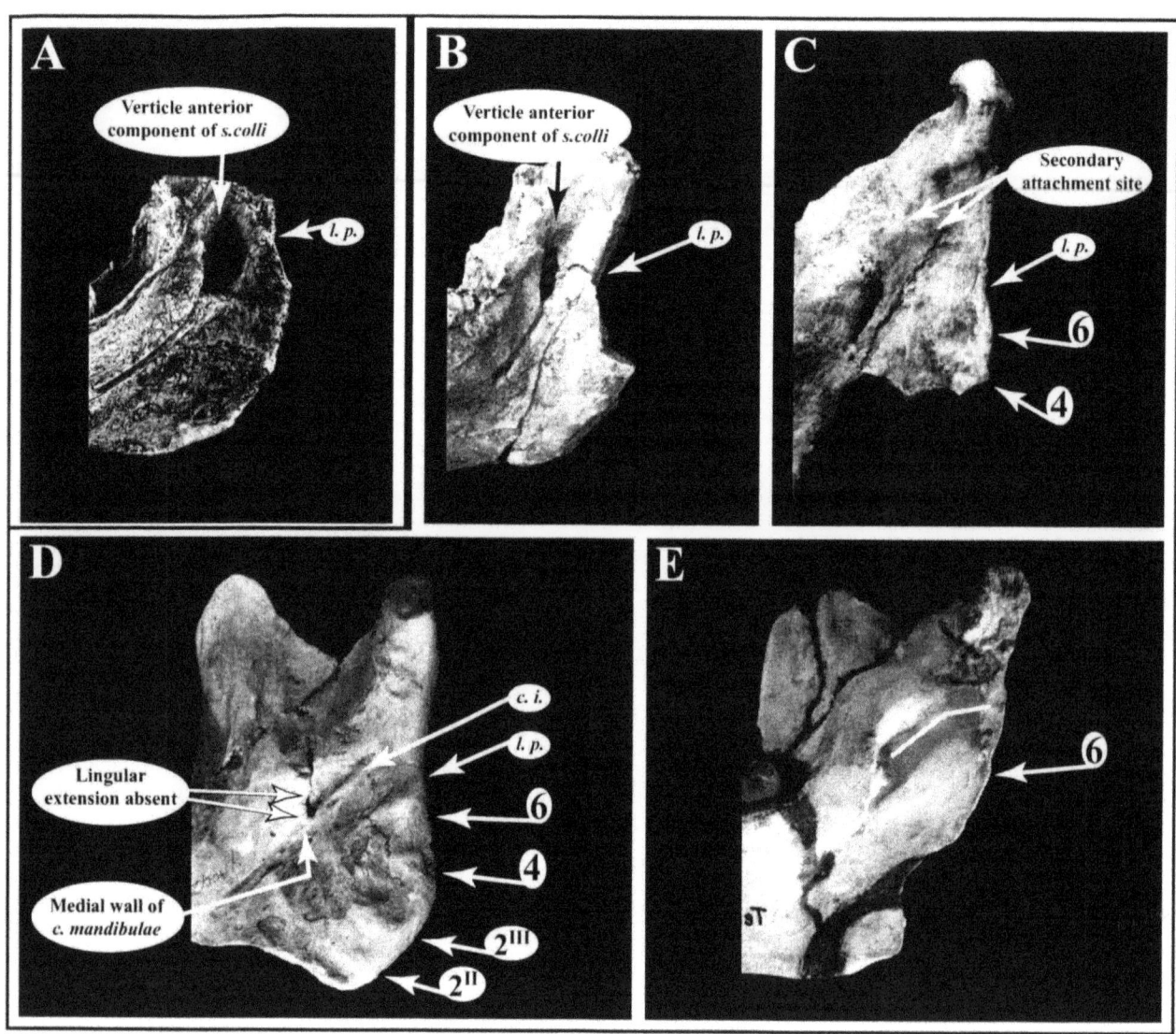

Figure 9a-e: Medial mandibular ramus anatomy in: (a) *A. africanus*: Stw 498, reversed; (b) *H. habilis* (*s.l.*): OH 13; and (c-e) *H. erectus* (*s.l.*): KNM-BK 67; Zhoukoudian G1; and Ternifine 2, reversed. Note in *A. africanus* (a) and *H. habilis* (b) the vertical orientation of the anterior *s. colli* component-*f. mandibulae* complex and how the orientation changes to less vertical in *H. erectus* (c-e). The medial extension of the *l. mandibulae* and a deepening of the lingular notch are minimally expressed in (a-c) and (e) but more strongly expressed in (d). In Figure 9c note what appears to be a secondary *l. sphenomandibulare* (*s.l.*) attachment. Also observe the lack of posterior extension of the *l. mandibulae* in (c-d) and how the medial wall of the *c. mandibulae* is, therefore, left uncovered by this lingular extension. In (c) note the development of a raised septa 6 and 4 tubercle and compare this to the areally vast insertion site for septa 6, 4, and 2^{III} in Figure 9d which is only slightly raised and composed of ridges and depressions.

2.4. Australopithecus boisei

In *A. boisei* the *c. endocondyloidea* is strongly expressed in the Peninj mandible whereas it is broad and flat in KNM-ER 729. The *f. mandibulae* is round and positioned under a projecting *c. endocondyloidea* in Peninj but it is more superoinferiorly ovate and not covered by the *crista* in KNM-ER 729. A true *l. mandibulae* is not present in these individuals. Whereas these specimens differ substantially in the degree of *c. endocondyloidea* development we do not consider this to affect lingular expression. The *s. colli* in Peninj is similar to that of *A. robustus*. The *s. colli* of KNM-ER 729 differs from the pattern observed in other 'robust' *Australopithecus*, but is similar to Mak VP-1/2 and 1/12, in having a very shallow anterior component which lacks any prominence of the superior (*c. endocondyloidea*) and inferior border (*c. intermedia* and *l. pterygoidea*). In *A. boisei* specimens KNM-ER 729 and Peninj, weakly developed *tsc*'s are apparent. As observed in other *Australopithecus*, excepting *A. africanus*, a small secondary tubercle is present in the space above the septal 6 attachment site. The Peninj mandible preserves superiorly placed tubercles bilaterally and presents with only slight development of the left tubercle and an amorphous development of the right.

2.5. Homo habilis (sensu lato)

In *H. habilis* (*s.l.*: OH 13) the *c. endocondyloidea* is curved, weakly expressed, and traversed by a vertically oriented groove (Figure 9b). Although the posterior ramus is damaged, the majority of the *s. colli* is preserved. The anterior sulcal component is vertically oriented, deep, and anteroposteriorly narrow (Figure 9b). This morphology differs from *A. africanus* as in that taxon the anterior sulcal component broadens posteriorly whereas OH 13 maintains a relatively narrow sulcus (Figure 9a-b). The preserved posterior region indicates that this component was probably very shallow (Figure 9b). Specimen preservation is such that it precludes confirmation of a *c. intermedia*, although, given the narrow and vertical nature of the anterior sulcal component, this feature was most likely present. The *f. mandibulae-s. colli* is superoinferiorly elongate and when combined with its extreme anterior positioning results, in part, in the lack of a developed *l. mandibulae*. Development of a lingular notch is not extensive. The medial wall of the *f. mandibulae-c. mandibulae* is positioned below the inferior border of the *s. colli* due to either or both the extreme verticality of the *f. mandibulae-s. colli* or a superior extension of the *l. pterygoidea* (Figure 9b).

2.6. Homo erectus (sensu lato)

Our *H. erectus* (*s.l.*) sample comprises: (1) KNM-BK 67; (2) KNM-ER 820 and 992; (3) KNM-WT 15000; (4) OH 22; (5) SK 15; (6) Ternifine 2 and 3; (7) Thomas Quarry 1; and (8) Zhoukoudian B1, F1, G1, and H1. Subadult anatomy is preserved in KNM-WT 15000 and Zhoukoudian B1 and F1. The youngest individual, KNM-ER 820, only preserves details of the lingular and anterior *s. colli* region.

In KNM-ER 820, medially directed development of the *l. mandibulare* and the depth of its associated notch are minimal. The *l. mandibulare* also does not project posteriorly at its superior or inferior extent. Of interest is that a slight groove for the *n. trigeminus* is present on the *c. endocondyloidea* just posterosuperior to the lingular tip. This morphology is similar to that in KNM-BK 67 but differs from the more open concavity of the *crista* present in *H. habilis* (OH 13) and other *H. erectus* specimens examined. A *c. intermedia* is not preserved but was probably present, given the orientation of the *f. mandibulae* and *l. pterygoidea*. The anterior *s. colli* component is vertically oriented. The general configuration of the preserved morphology is consistent with both *H. habilis* (*s.l.*) and *H. erectus* (*s.l.*).

The subadult Zhoukoudian specimens are similar in developmental age (8.0-9.0 years) and morphology. In these individuals, the *c. endocondyloidea* resembles that described for recent *H. sapiens*; it has a strong medial concavity. The *s. colli* in mandible F1, however, resembles the condition noted in much younger human infants. The sulcus is relatively broad and deep, especially anteriorly, and its lower border is well marked and medially flaring. Mandible B1, alternatively, retains the broad and deep anterior component but lacks the strong flaring of the inferior sulcal border. A *tsc* is not present in either B1 or F1. In both mandibles a *l. pterygoidea* is present but only mandible B1 exhibits some prominence of the *m. pterygoideus medialis* superior attachment site. An incipient *c. intermedia* is present in both B1 and F1. In the slightly older subadult KNM-WT 15000 the *c. endocondyloidea* is more developed and does not exhibit a medial concavity. The inferior sulcal border runs from the posterior ramal border to become continuous with the posterior border of the mylohyoid groove. This configuration of the *c. endocondyloidea* and inferior sulcal border creates a narrow and well delineated *s. colli*. The sulcus has a slightly depressed anterior component which extends past mid-ramus and a lightly marked posterior component. This configuration differs from others in this and earlier groups by combining a narrow sulcus with a linear and strongly anteroinferiorly inclined *s. colli*. The *c. intermedia* and *l. pterygoidea* are nearly coincident, but the former is still present bilaterally. Whereas the morphology of this area may be related, at least in part, to the individual's developmental age it is unlikely to account for all observed differences given our assessment of the development of this region. In the superior attachment area for the *m. pterygoideus medialis* a triangular-shaped, depressed area exhibits slightly marked ridges for septa 6 and 4. A *tsc* is not present in KNM-WT 15000.

The *c. endocondyloidea* morphology in KNM-BK 67 and Zhoukoudian G1 and H1 is similar to that of other Pleistocene *Homo* groups and consistent with that defined here for recent *H. sapiens* (Figure 9c-d). The *s. colli* region morphology in KNM-BK 67 is unique in some aspects (Figure 9c). In this specimen, as in OH 22 and the *H. habilis* specimen OH 13, the anterior *s. colli* component is nearly vertical. It appears that a *c. intermedia* is present in KNM-BK 67 but fossil preservation and cast quality preclude confirmation. The Baringo specimen differs from OH 13 and 22, however, in not having a developed border to the posterior aspect of the *s. colli*'s anterior component. It also possesses a linear series of developed rugosities in the superoposterior portion of the *s. colli*. This feature delimits the base of the neurovascular bundle which enters the *s. colli* from the posterior ramal region (Figure 9c). If one considers the *s. colli* to be directly associated with the main neurovascular bundle, then the posterior sucal component is nearly horizontal and intersects the anterior component at an angle of ~ 90°. It is clear that this series of rugosities results from a secondary insertion of the *l. sphenomandibulare* (*s.l.*) which is located well superior to its normal insertion site(s). A developed inferior border to the *s. colli* is absent in KNM-BK 67 and there is no indication of a developed *l. pterygoidea*. The *s. colli* (*s.s.*) consists of a neurovascular groove, superiorly, and a broad depression which both opens into the *f. pterygoidea* and surrounds the septa 6 and 4 insertion site. It is probable that a significant portion of the neurovascular bundle and parapharyngeal process of the parotid gland were contained in this depression. Of note is that preserved portions of OH 22 not only lack the broad depression found in KNM-BK 67 but indicate an extremely flat *c. endocondyloidea* and shallow anterior sulcal component. Given the verticality of the anterior component in both these specimens, it is probably this shallowness which established the basis for mylohyoid groove-*l. mandibulae* bridging in OH 22.

In Zhoukoudian specimens G1 and H1 the anterior sulcal component is seen to be split into two unequal portions, a small upper and a large lower sulcus, by the *c. intermedia* (Figures 9d and 10a). The trajectory of the upper sulcus is subvertical (H1 > G1) as it angles only slightly to moderately posteriorly whereas the lower sulcus is oriented posterosuperiorly. The sulcal pattern in G1 and H1 indicates that the neurovascular bundle split into two subequal bundles as it crossed the posterior ramal border (Figure 10a). The inferior *s. colli* border in G1 and H1 is displaced inferiorly due to this neurovascular pattern. Given this *s. colli* configuration a clearly defined space between the sulcus and the septum 6 attachment does not exist in either the subadults or these adult individuals (Figures 9c and 10a). A separate *tsc* is not present (Figure 10a). Specimens G1 and H1 present with septa 6 and 4 attachment sites which are not 'tubercles' but slight depressions bounded by low, raised walls (Figures 9c and 10a: cf. KNM-WT 15000). This attachment variant is also found in AmHs, Neanderthals, and recent *H. sapiens* and is discussed further below.

Although the medial rami of SK 15 and KNM-ER 992 are incomplete, their *m. pterygoideus medialis* attachment regions are preserved and can be described in relation to adult *H. erectus* (*s.l.*) specimens other than Zhoukoudian G1 and H1. In SK 15, development of a septa 6 and 4 tubercle is moderate, whereas it is moderate-to-strong in KNM-BK 67. In the latter individual a rhomboidal tubercle exists which is fractured at its base and, resultantly, it is not possible to know if septum 2^{III} is involved or the degree of tubercle prominence relative to other *m. pterygoideus medialis* tubercles (Figure 9c). In SK 15, although showing significant crushing of the ramus (Robinson, 1953), a subtriangular septa 6 and 4 associated tubercle is preserved. A composite of the rami of KNM-ER 992 shows a low *tsc* and a septa 6 and 4 tubercle, which is well separated from the *s. colli*, to be present. Preserved portions of the septa 6 and 4 tubercle on the right side indicates a tubercle with only a moderate anteroposterior extent. The inferior tubercles (septum 2^{I-II}) are not as strongly marked on the right rami as the septa 6 and 4 tubercle, although they are more strongly marked on the left.

The Ternifine 2 and Thomas Quarry 1 individuals differ from other adults in this taxonomic group. The *c. endocondyloidea* of both specimens is similar in being weakly expressed (Figure 9e). In Ternifine 2 the *s. colli* has a long and deep, vertically oriented anterior component and a very short, shallow, and horizontally oriented posterior component. The difference in orientation of the sulcal components is minimally marked (Figure 9e). The *f. mandibulae*-*s. colli* region is damaged in Ternifine 3 but observable morphology is consistent with that of Ternifine 2 as also observed by Arambourg (1963). The Ternifine 2 mandible presents with a *s. colli* and *m. pterygoideus medialis* attachment site which is most similar to that of SK 15 (Figure 9e). The *s. colli* in Thomas Quarry 1 is similar to the Ternifine 2 mandible except that the posterior component is longer and more horizontal. A short, slightly raised *c. intermedia* is present in Thomas Quarry 1 whereas the crest is incorporated into the *l. pterygoidea* in Ternifine 2 (Figure 9e). The superior extent of the *m. pterygoideus medialis* is damaged in Ternifine 2 but it is clear that the septa 6 and 4 insertion was not well developed (Figure 9e). The Thomas Quarry 1 mandible is similar to Ternifine 2 and KNM-ER 992 in possessing a weakly developed *m. pterygoideus medialis* insertion. The septa 6 and 4 insertion in this specimen is minimally marked by the posterior-most fibers of the septa. This specimen does show separation of the septum 6 insertion from the *s. colli*, although it is not wide. A small *tsc* is present in Thomas Quarry 1 but the region is not preserved in either Ternifine 2 or 3.

Morphology of the *l. mandibulae* is similar in the subadult specimens KNM-ER 820 and KNM-WT 15000 and in the adult specimens KNM-BK 67 and 992 and OH 22. The *l. mandibulae* is minimally developed in its medial extent and shows an increased but still shallow lingular notch relative to earlier taxa (Figure 9c). In the Zhoukoudian subadult (B1, F1) and adult (G1, H1) mandibles the *l. mandibulae* strongly projects medially and there is a strong lingular notch (Figure 9d). Ternifine 2 and 3 and Thomas Quarry 1 present with *l. mandibulae* morphology generally consistent with that of the Zhoukoudian G1 individual (Figure 9d-e).

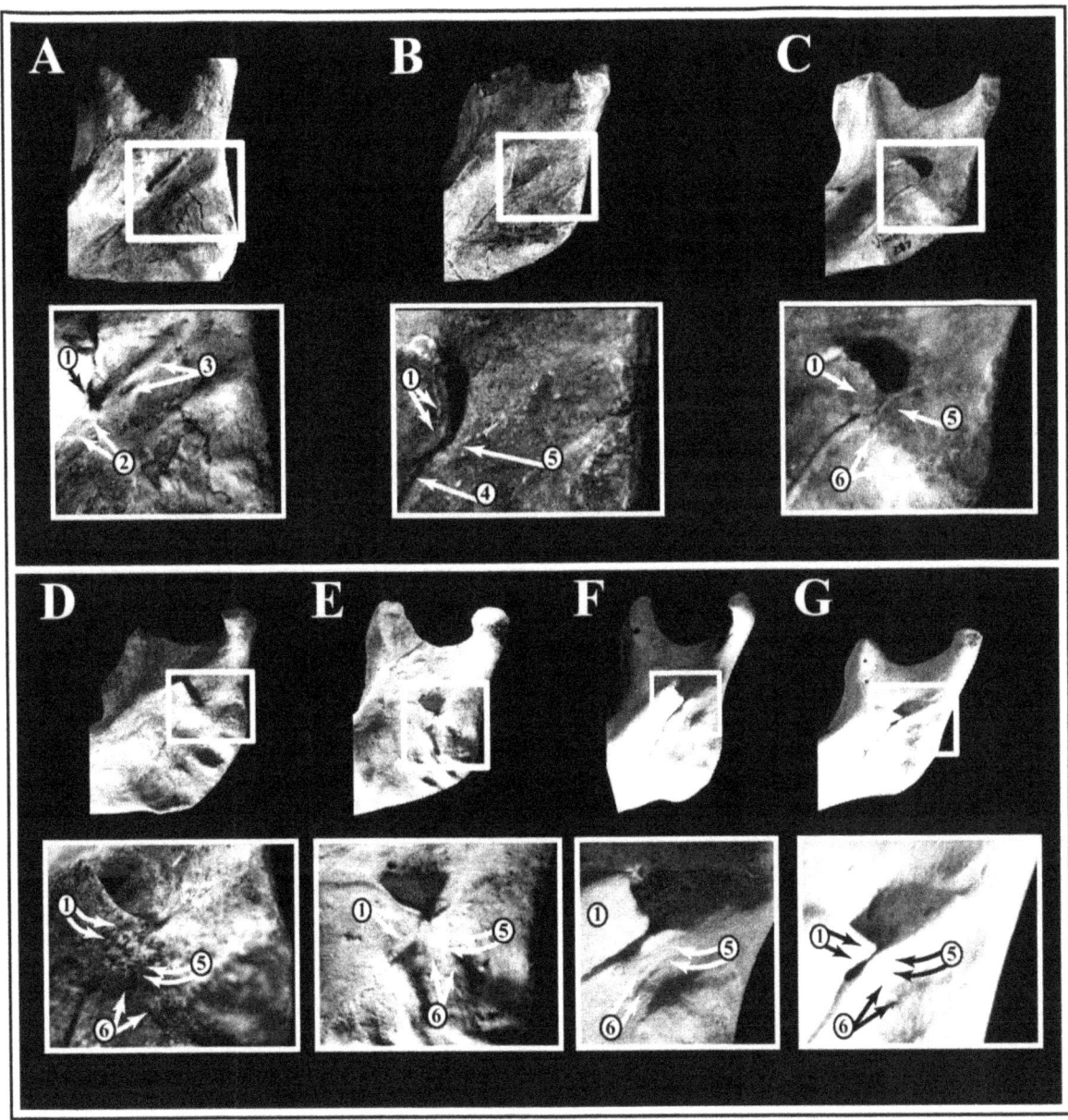

Figure 10a-g: Close-up views of the *f. mandibulae-l. mandibulae* complex in hominids. From left to right specimens figured are: (a) Zhoukoudian G1; (b) Arago XIII; (c) Vindija 207; (d) Zafarraya; (e) Zhoukoudian 101; (f) recent *H. sapiens* adult; and (g) recent *H. sapiens* subadult (7.0-8.0 years of age). In (a) observe how the medial wall of the *c. mandibulae* (2) is uncovered due to a lack of posterior extension of the *l. mandibulae* (1). Also note the presence of a strongly expressed *c. intermedia* (3) in this individual and its relationship to the inferiorly positioned *l. pterygoidea*. In (b) note how the *l. mandibulae* (1) is now posteriorly extended so that it covers the medial wall of the *c. mandibulae* and part of the mylohyoid groove (4), thereby approximating the anterosuperiorly extended *l. pterygoidea* (5). Observe in (c-g) the relationship between the *l. mandibulae* (1) and the *l. pterygoidea* (5). In this relationship we have only found cases where the *l. mandibulae* is overlapped by (d) or abuts to the *l. pterygoidea* (c). This is presumably due to the muscle being forced 'over' the medial aspect of the ligament. Also note in (c-g) how extensions from the septa 6 and 4 tubercle (6) are oriented such as to meet or cross over the *l. mandibulae*. Observe how the condition in Neanderthal mandibles (c-d) is similar to the condition seen in AmHs (e) and recent *H. sapiens* adults and subadults (f-g), respectively. The conditions depicted in (c-g) involve the same structures but differ in the degree to which factors involved in producing the morphology are expressed. Whether this phenotypic difference is related to the level of genetic penetrance, differences in function, or a combination of these factors is not known. We believe that recognition of variation in expression of these features will provide greater understanding of relationships than that possible by considering the multi-component H-O character in a simple, dichotomous fashion.

2.7. Archaic *Homo sapiens*

Our ArHs sample consists of: (1) Arago II and XIII; (2) Ehringsdorf F and G; (3) Mauer; and (4) Montmaurin 1. The Ehringsdorf G specimen is the sole subadult in this series (Figure 11a). This specimen presents with a *c. endocondyloidea* and *s. colli* which are very similar to that described for Thomas Quarry 1. The *l. mandibulae* is not well developed medially nor is the lingular notch. A *c. intermedia* is probably coincident with the *l. pterygoidea* but descriptions and cast quality preclude confirmation. There is a distinct *tsc* and a large, medially projecting septa 6 and 4 tubercle (Figure 11a).

Adults in this group present with *c. endocondyloidea* morphology generally consistent with that described for recent *H. sapiens* (Figures 10b and 11a-d). Configuration of the anterior component of the *s. colli* in Arago II and XIII, Mauer, and Montmaurin 1 is similar to that observed in the Ternifine 1-3 and Thomas Quarry 1 individuals, although it is slightly less vertically oriented (Figures 9e and 11b-d). The anterior *s. colli* component in Ehringsdorf F differs slightly from other ArHs specimens by being superoinferiorly concave and more deeply excavated. Excepting Mauer and Montmaurin 1, the posterior component of the *s. colli* in this group differs from that found in *H. erectus* (*s.l.*) as it is more distinct (Figures 9c-e and 11b-d). In *s. colli* morphology Mauer differs only slightly from the basic configuration found in Arago II and XIII and Montmaurin 1 due to superior extension of the anterosuperior aspect of the *l. pterygoidea* (Figure 11b-d). Given the *l. pterygoidea*'s extension the anteroinferior border of the *s. colli* is strongly marked and walled-off from the *m. pterygoideus medialis* attachment region anteriorly. This condition results in a more narrow and well defined sulcus which is partially bridged below the *f. mandibulae* on the right ramus (Figure 11b). A short *c. intermedia* is present in Montmaurin 1 and possibly also in Arago II (Figure 11d). In Arago XIII and Mauer the anterior extension of the *l. pterygoidea* into the posterior mylohyoid groove region apparently redirects forces imposed on the *l. sphenomandibulare* (*s.l.*) to the former structure as a bony *c. intermedia* is absent (Figures 10b and 11b-c). This results in the superoposterior border of the *c. mandibulae* being very short and becoming continuous with the *l. pterygoidea* at the posterosuperior edge of the mylohyoid groove in these specimens (Figures 10b and 11b-c). This difference creates a more discrete boundary between the *s. colli* and the *f. mandibulae*. The *l. mandibulae* morphology of Arago II, Mauer, and Montmaurin 1 is generally similar; these specimens present with a medially projecting lingular tip and have a developed lingular notch (Figure 11b, d). Alternatively, Ehringsdorf F and G and Arago XIII are more similar to *H. erectus* (*s.l.*) by only showing minor development of lingular features (Figure 11c). Earlier, Smith (1978) concluded that it was not possible to determine if *l. mandibulae* bridging was present in the Ehringsdorf F mandible. Given the observed lingular region morphology, we concur with Jidoi et al. (2000) who concluded that bridging is not present in this specimen.

With the exception of Mauer and Montmaurin 1, all specimens in the ArHs group present with small *tsc*'s. Excepting the latter specimen, the attachment site for *m. pterygoideus medialis* extends relatively high on the ramus and may be related to producing the superoinferiorly short *s. colli* (Figure 11b-c). In Montmaurin 1 a *tsc* cannot be confirmed and the muscle does not extend as far superiorly (Figure 11d). The *l. pterygoidea* forms the inferior border of the *s. colli* and is well marked in all specimens (Figure 11b-d). The relationship of the inferior *s. colli* border to the septal 6 attachment is such that a relatively moderate to broad area exists between the sulcus and the attachment (Figure 11b-d). The latter intervening space was clearly filled with idiosyncratically expressed fleshy attachments and minor tendons. Septa 6 and 4 tubercles range from slight to strongly marked in the series: Arago II, Arago XIII, Ehringsdorf G, Mauer, and Montmaurin 1. Tubercle formation in the latter specimen is at the maximum end of the size range for normal individuals, fossil or recent (Figure 11b-d). Further, in the latter specimen the right tubercle shows involvement of septum 2^{III} whereas the left does not. Tubercle development in Mauer is complicated by taphonomic factors (erosion?) involving the right tubercle. However, both sides clearly show septa 6 and 4 tubercles with some development of the septum 2^{III} attachment (Figure 11b: Schoetensack, 1908; but contra Billy and Vallois, 1977). Although the septal attachments are less clear in Mauer, the right tubercle appears less well developed than the left tubercle. Arago XIII has a septa 6 and 4 associated tubercle which is not significantly different from the remainder of the *m. pterygoideus medialis* related tubercles (Figures 10b and 11c). All remaining specimens have septa 6 and 4 tubercles which are more developed than those in the remainder of the attachment site.

2.8. Neanderthals

2.8.1. Subadult Neanderthals

Our subadult Neanderthal sample comprises Gibraltar 2, Krapina 53, Pech de l'Azé, Roc de Marsal 1, and Teshik Tash (Figure 12a-c). Development of the *c. endocondyloidea* ranges from curved and weakly expressed to bar-like and relatively strongly expressed in the series: Gibraltar 2, Pech de l'Azé and Krapina 53, Teshik Tash, and Roc de Marsal 1. Development of a vertical groove in the *c. endocondyloidea* is weak in Teshik Tash and Roc de Marsal 1 (Figure 12a, c). Excepting Krapina 53, all subadult specimens in this group present with the modern *f. mandibulae-l. mandibulae* pattern; there is strong medial projection of the lingular tip and the presence of a lingular notch (Figure 12a-c). The Krapina specimen lacks the latter features. Morphology of the *s. colli* ranges from a broad depression encompassing the distance from the *f. mandibulae* to the posterior ramal border in Gibraltar 2 and Krapina 53 to a more defined sulcus in Pech de l'Azé, Roc de Marsal 1, and Teshik Tash (Figure 12a-c). Development of the inferior *s. colli* border ranges from slightly developed in Krapina 53 and Teshik Tash to strong in Pech de l'Azé and Roc de Marsal 1. Excepting Gibraltar 2, the *l. pterygoidea* forms the inferior sulcal border in all

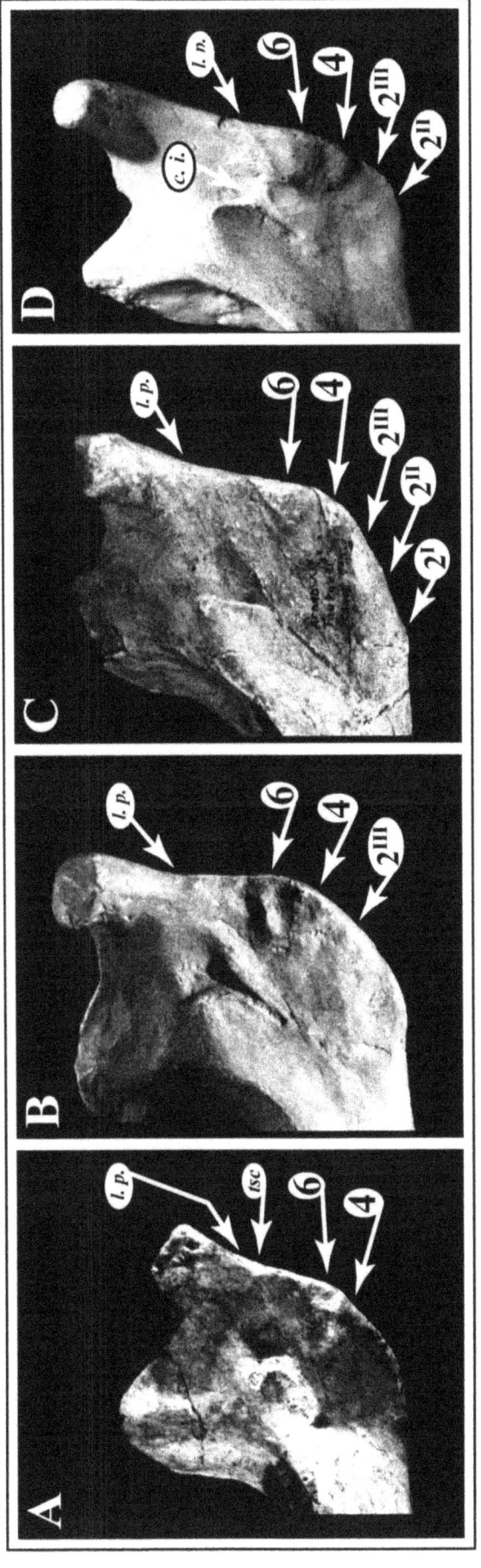

Figure 11a-d: Medial mandibular ramus anatomy in archaic *H. sapiens*. Specimens figured are from left to right: (a) Ehringsdorf G, reversed; (b) Mauer, reversed; (c) Arago XIII; and (d) Montmaurin 1. In (b-c) note the posterosuperior height of the *m. pterygoideus medialis* insertion and the large distance between the *l. pterygoidea* and the septum 6 insertion. Observe in (c) how the *l. pterygoidea* is anterosuperiorly extended relative to the condition in (c-d). Note that in (d) the *c. intermedia* does not extend into the *s. colli* as occurs in "Sinanthropus" specimens (cf. Zhoukoudian G1). Whereas this feature is variable, this configuration is similar to that found in some Neanderthal specimens wherein the *c. intermedia* is short, abruptly courses medially, and quickly fades into *f. mandibulae*. In the ArHs subadult (a) note the well developed septa 6 and 4 insertions, how the anterior tubercle extends into the posterior mylohyoid groove region, and the lack of a developed *l. mandibulae*. Based on our ontogenetic series of recent *H. sapiens* subadults and given the developmental age of this individual (11.0–12.0 years of age) the configuration of these structures would be inconsistent with the development of lingular bridging, although its later formation cannot be completely ruled out.

these individuals (Figure 12a, c). Gibraltar 2 differs from others in this group by having a short *c. intermedia* and a very lightly marked *l. pterygoidea* which together form the inferior sulcal border (Figure 12b). There is a tendency in this group to wall off the anteroinferior aspect of the *s. colli*, thereby making the sulcus appear prominent. The only opening in the inferior sulcal border is that for the mylohyoid neurovascular bundle proper (Figure 12a-c). This process is apparent in all specimens excepting Gibraltar 2 (Figure 12b). Orientation of the mylohyoid groove differs in Pech de l'Azé as it is distinctly more horizontal relative to the more vertical orientation observed in this group (Figure 12a).

All subadult individuals show development of a *tsc* and have septa 6 and 4 tubercles (Figure 12a-c). Note that the septal arrangement in Krapina 53 differs from others in this group. The area interposed between the inferior border of the *s. colli* and the superior tubercle is generally smooth in these subadults (Figure 12a-c). Such regions in recent *H. sapiens* indicate the presence of periosteally attached fleshy muscle fibers. In Pech de l'Azé development of the septa 6 and 4 attachments is weak whereas inferior septa ($2^{\text{I-III}}$) are more prominent. The septa 6 and 4 tubercle in Gibraltar 2 is essentially identical to that in Ehringsdorf G (Figures 11a and 12b). In Teshik Tash and Roc de Marsal 1 the septa 6 and 4 tubercle is both large and medially projecting but the two specimens differ morphologically. In Roc de Marsal 1 the ramus is fractured inferiorly but the preserved portion possesses a septa 6, 4, and 2^{III} tubercle (Figure 12a). This individual is unique in our fossil subadult sample as the septum 6 insertion has the appearance of a Type 1 tubercle. Teshik Tash presents with bilaterally developed tubercles but the left differs from the right by involvement of the septum 2^{III} insertion (Figure 12c).

2.8.2. Adult Neanderthals

In our adult Neanderthal sample the *c. endocondyloidea* is well developed, straight, and bar-like in Amud 1, Circeo III, Kebara 2, La Quina H5, Tabun C2, Vindija 207, and Zafarraya. Alternatively, the *c. endocondyloidea* is curved and less well developed in La Chapelle, La Ferrassie 1, Régourdou 1, Saint Césaire, Tabun C1, and Krapina 59 and 63 (Figure 13a-e). A vertical neurovascular groove is present on the *c. endocondyloidea* in La Chapelle, Régourdou 1, Tabun C1 and C2, Krapina 59 and 63, and Vindija 207 (Figure 13a-e).

The *s. colli* is anteroposteriorly short in Circeo III, Kebara 2, Krapina 59 and 63, La Ferrassie 1, Tabun C1 and C2, and Zafarraya whereas it is relatively long in Amud 1, La Chapelle, La Quina H5, Régourdou 1, Saint Césaire, and Vindija 207 (Figures 10c-d and 13a-f). This sulcus is only slightly depressed in the 'anterior' component in all specimens except Tabun C2 and Vindija 207. Note that in these specimens the majority of the anterior component is covered and what constitutes the observable 'anterior' component is actually in the mid-sulcal region (Figure 10c-d). Excepting the latter specimens, overall *s. colli* depth is very shallow irrespective of sulcal length (Figures 10c-d and 13a-f). The inferior border of the *s. colli* in all these specimens is essentially continuous with the inferior aspect of the medial border of the *f. mandibulae* (Figures 10c-d and 13a-f). Excepting Circeo III, La Quina H5, Régourdou 1, Saint Césaire, Shanidar 1, Tabun C1, and La Chapelle the *l. pterygoidea* is a continuous bony line that is not broken by the mylohyoid neurovascular bundle (Figure 13a-f). Note that some confusion exists regarding the morphology of the *l. pterygoidea* in Tabun C2 with McCown and Keith (1939) considering it to be continuous with the *l. mandibulae* whereas Tillier *et al.* (1989) and Tillier (1991) consider its connection to the *l. mandibulae* to be absent or attenuated, at most. In those specimens possessing an unbroken inferior border, the neurovascular structures enter the *f. pterygoidea* via a short to long canal comprising the mylohyoid groove and a sheet of bone which covers the groove's medial aspect (Figure 13c, d, and f). Note that: (1) Saint Césaire presents with a slight variant of the usual neurovascular pattern; and (2) that the pattern of the *l. mandibulae* and mylohyoid groove bridging in this group is variable (see discussion). All adult specimens present with the modern *f. mandibulae-l. mandibulae* pattern excepting Amud 1 which has a *l. mandibulae* positioned below the *c. endocondyloidea* and which lacks a lingular notch (bilaterally?: Figure 13a). With the exception of Régourdou 1 and Saint Césaire, all specimens in this group have a *tsc*.

As in other taxa, tubercles related to the superior aspect of the *m. pterygoideus medialis* are present but variably expressed in this group (Figure 13a-f). Whereas tubercle morphology forms a continuum from weak to strongly expressed, we recognize five categories for descriptive purposes. Group one consists of Amud 1 (Figure 13a). This specimen presents with a weakly expressed septa 6 and 4 tubercle which is barely distinguishable from other tubercles in the *m. pterygoideus medialis* attachment area. This tubercle type is similar to that observed in KNM-WT 15000 and "Sinanthropus" (Figures 9d and 13a). Of note in this context is that a slight concavity exist just above the septum 6 ridge in Amud 1 and this imparts a false impression of tubercle development (Figure 13a). In this case it is important to examine the full extent of the tubercle (see discussion). Group two consists of Circeo III and Régourdou 1, the rami of which are both damaged at or just below the septa 6 and 4 insertion (Figure 13b). Régourdou 1 shows a very weakly expressed septum 6 related elevation whereas Circeo III presents with a slightly raised septa 6 and 4 tubercle. Group three consists of Kebara 2, Krapina 63, and Tabun C1 (Figure 13c). These specimens present with: (1) subtriangular tubercles which are related to septa 6 and 4, with septum 6 being dominant; (2) little to no integration of septa 6 and 4 such that the interseptal area is concave; and (3) septum 6 tubercles which are slightly to strongly concave superiorly such that the tubercles appear 'hook-shaped'. Kebara 2 is somewhat unique in this group as it presents with a Type 1 tubercle which has a number of pits in the superior concavity (Figure 13c). The latter morphology also occurs in Roc de Marsal 1 (Figure 12a) and in some recent *H. sapiens*. In this group, only Krapina 63 shows some involvement of septum 2^{III} in tubercle formation. Group four consists of Krapina 59, La Chapelle, La Ferrassie 1, Shanidar 1, Saint

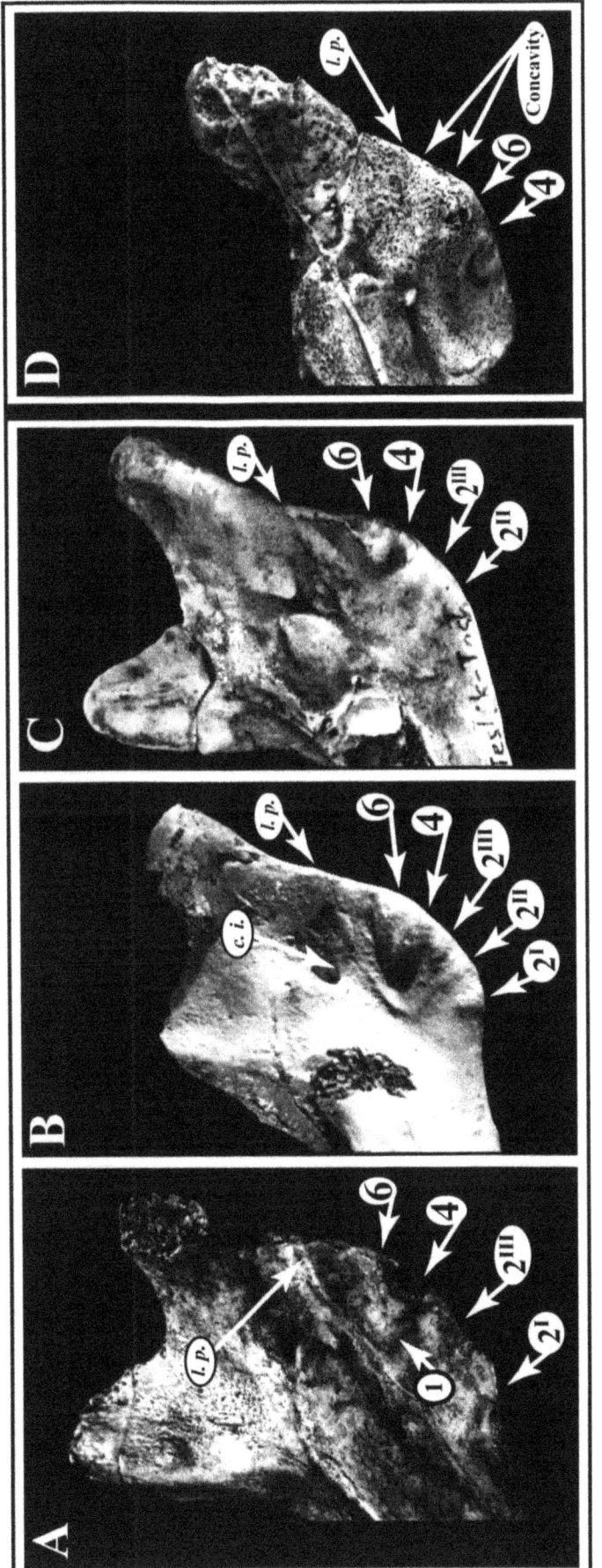

Figure 12a-d: Medial mandibular ramus anatomy in Neanderthal (a-c) and *H. sapiens* (d) subadults. Specimens figured are from left to right: (a) Roc de Marsal 1; (b) Gibraltar 2; (c) Teshik Tash; and (d) Amud 7. Observe in both (b) and (c) the presence of a distinct *c. intermedia*. Note in (a) the presence of small, round pits above the septum 6 insertion and an extension of the septal attachments at (1). Such pitting is also seen in Kebara 2 and recent *H. sapiens*. Note the difference in *l. mandibulae* development and positioning of the *l. pterygoidea* in (a) and (b). Also note the general size of the septa 6 and 4 tubercle relative to the size of the ramus and its position relative to the *s. colli* in subadults. Based on our cross-sectional data, tubercle size appears to remain stable over broad spans of developmental time and as the tubercle migrates during growth. In (d) note the deep and extended *s. colli*; the slight concavity between the *s. colli* and the septa 6 and 4 tubercle; and the slight medial extension and development of the *l. mandibulae* and lingular notch, respectively.

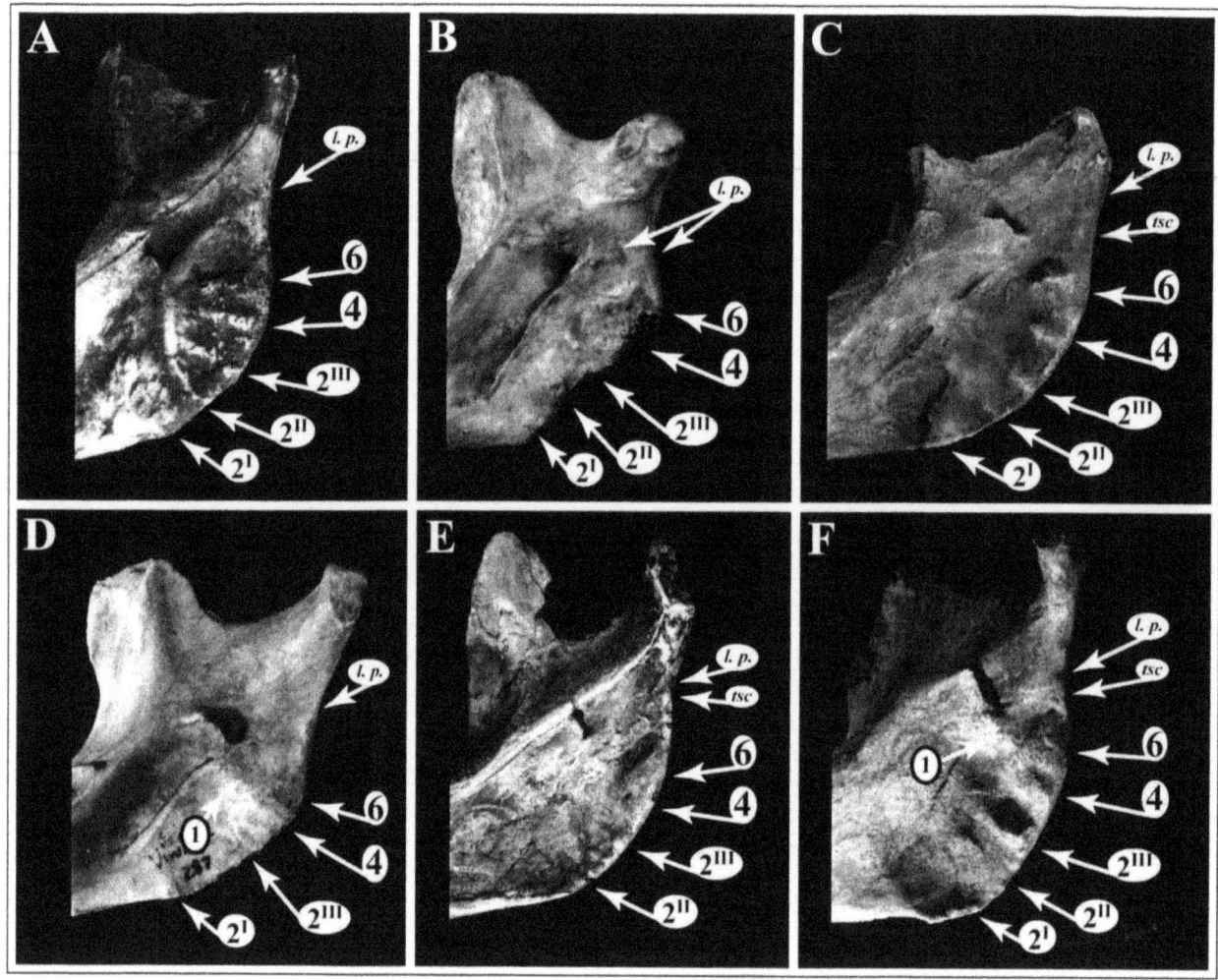

Figure 13a-f: Examples of Neanderthal adults showing some of the variation in medial ramal features. Specimens shown are from left to right: (a) Amud 1, reversed; (b) Régourdou 1; (c) Kebara 2; (d) Vindija 207; (e) La Quina H5, reversed; and (f) Zafarraya. Observe the range of variation in degree of development and coalescence of *m. pterygoideus medialis* related septal insertions. Note the lack of a pattern of: (1) superiorly directed hypertrophy of the septal insertions; and (2) concavities on the superior aspect of the septa 6 and 4 tubercle. In (a) note the presence of a depression superior to the septum 6 insertion and in (c) the presence of pits (cf. Roc de Marsal 1) above the septum 6 insertion. Individuals in (d and f) clearly show the extension of the septal attachments into the lingular region. In (a-f) note the variation in *l. mandibulae* morphology and extent and the length of the *s. colli*. Observe in (a) the lack of medial extension of the *l. mandibulae* and its positioning below the *c. endocondyloidea*.

Césaire, and Vindija 207 (Figure 13d). The tubercles of these individuals are related to septa 6 and 4, are subtriangular, and lack strong concavities along the superior and inferior tubercle margins. The tubercles differ from those of Group three: (1) by being slightly more developed and medially projecting; and (2) by having a filled interseptal space which creates a slightly concave-to-convex medial surface (except La Ferrassie 1). In La Ferrassie 1 the septa 6 and 4 attachment ridges do not show an infilling of the interseptal space, a condition found in many recent *H. sapiens*. Of interest is that the latter specimen presents bilaterally with well developed pits above but co-incident with the septum 6 ridge. This configuration is indicative of the intimate relationship between muscle attachment site depressions and tubercles (see van der Klaauw, 1963). Shanidar 1 presents with a left side tubercle similar to that of Group three whereas the right side is more similar to those of this group. Saint Césaire and Vindija 207 present with amorphously expressed, sub-triangular tubercles, most similar to the Krapina 53 subadult and many recent *H. sapiens* (Figure 13d). Note that in: (1) La Chapelle the tubercles are asymmetric bilaterally and that there is some integration of septa 2^{III} with septa 6 and 4; (2) La Ferrassie 1 the tubercles are symmetric but with only minor involvement of septum 2^{III}; and (3) Krapina 59 only the region above the septum 2^{III} tubercle is preserved. Group five consists of La Quina H5, Tabun C2, and Zafarraya (Figure 13e-f). Tubercles in this group differ from those of Group four by having well defined superior and anterior concavities; some also have inferior concavities (i.e. lack integration of septum 2^{III}). Medial extension of the septa 6 and 4 tubercle in this group varies from moderate to strong in the sequence: Tabun C2, La Quina H5, and Zafarraya (Figure 13e-f). Tubercle formation in the latter specimen is at the maximum end of the size range, being nearly identical to Montmaurin 1 as also noted by Billy and Vallois (1977: Figures 11d and 13e-f). Both KNM-BK 67 and SK 15 present with tubercles of similar shape to these and in relative size are positioned between Tabun C2 and La Quina H5 (Figures 9c and 13e). All Group five specimens present with an increased development of the septum 2^{III} tubercle (Figure 13e-f). The septa 6 and 4 tubercle in Zafarraya is isolated from the septum 2^{III} tubercle (Figure 13f) whereas bilateral differences exist in the degree of fusion of septum 2^{III} with septa 6 and 4 in Tabun C2 and La Quina H5. The latter specimen shows fusion of septa 6, 4, and 2^{III} on the right side (Figure 13e) but on the left side septum 2^{III} is separate. Bilaterally, medial projection of the tubercles is slightly greater in La Quina H5 than in Tabun C2. Further, Tabun C2 has significant development of *m. pterygoideus medialis* tubercles in the inferior aspects of the muscle attachment site. All tubercles of Groups 2 through 6, with the possible exception of Krapina 53, Saint Césaire, and Vindija 207, most likely reflect involvement of the *l. stylomandibulare*.

2.8.3. Morphology of the superior aspect of the medial pterygoid tubercle

In the definition of a MPT, Rak *et al.* (1994) note that the superior border of the *m. pterygoideus medialis* insertion formed a distinct lip in their Neanderthal sample (= La Chapelle, La Ferrassie 1, Kebara 2, Krapina 53 and 63, Shanidar 1 and 2, and Tabun C1). Our expanded sample shows that other individuals attributed to this group do not present with this feature (Amud 1, Circeo III, Gibraltar 2, Krapina 59, La Quina H5, Pech de l'Azé, Régourdou 1, Saint Césaire, Tabun C2, Teshik Tash, Vindija 207, and Zafarraya: Figures 12b-c and 13a-b, d-f). Further, our examination of La Chapelle, La Ferrassie 1, Krapina 53, and Shanidar 1 shows that they lack significant lipping of this border whereas Shanidar 2 and Tabun C1 only show lipping unilaterally. Strong lipping of the superior aspect of the tubercle only occurs in Kebara 2, Krapina 63, and Roc de Marsal 1 with the latter two specimens only preserving single rami (Figures 12a and 13c). Further, note that a high percentage of septa 6 and 4 or septa 6, 4, and 2^{III} tubercles in all taxa present with some degree of concavity along their superior surface (Figures 9c-d, 11a-d, 12a-c, and 13b-c, e-f).

2.8.4. Morphology of the medial aspect of the medial pterygoid tubercle

In defining the MPT character state Rak *et al.* (1994:320) also state that "...Neandertals display muscle markings that gradually increase in intensity as they ascend the ramus" and that they differed from "...modern humans, where in even the most robust individuals the medial pterygoid insertion markings are more homogeneously distributed throughout the area of muscle insertion on the internal face of the gonial angle...". We evaluated the *m. pterygoideus medialis* tubercles in the *f. pterygoidea* of our Neanderthal series ($N = 20$). The ramus is damaged in both the Krapina 53 subadult and in Roc de Marsal 1. In Krapina 53 there is no clear development of muscle related tubercles inferior to the septum 2^{III} attachment. Gibraltar 2 and Roc de Marsal 1 possess greater development of the 2^{I} tubercle than that for 2^{II} whereas Pech de l'Azé presents with greater development of superficial septa 2^{I-III} than that of septa 6 and 4 (Figure 12a-b). Note that the ramus is damaged in Roc de Marsal 1 but that preserved portions indicate tubercle development for superficial septa was similar to that of Gibraltar 2. In Teshik Tash there is slight unilateral development of the septum 2^{III} tubercle whereas inferior septa are not well developed (Figure 12c). The ramus inferior to the septa 6 and 4 attachment is not preserved in Circeo III, Régourdou 1, and Saint Césaire (Figure 13b). Inferiorly placed tubercles (= septum 2^{I-II}) are either not significantly different from the septa 6 and 4 attachment (Amud 1) or are not developed to any real extent in Krapina 59 and 63, Shanidar 1, Tabun C1, and Vindija 207 (Figure 13a, d). In La Chapelle, La Ferrassie 1, La Quina H5, and Zafarraya there is variable development of the septum 2^{III} tubercle but the remainder of the attachment area is not well marked by tubercles (Figure 13e-f). Only in Kebara 2 and Tabun C2 is there evidence of a gradual increase in tubercle size from the anteroinferior aspect of the *m. pterygoideus medialis* attachment to the superior aspect of the septum 6 insertion (Figure 13a-f). It is possible that Rak *et al.* (1994) consider the gradual increase to be limited to the superior most tubercle in the attachment site. If such is the case then the following apply: (1) virtually all specimens examined show a superiorly directed increase in insertion site markings from septa 2^{III} to 6 - this applies to both tubercles and depressions (Figures 4c-f, 5a-e, 9d, 11a-d, 12a-c, 13a-f, and 14a-c); (2) many individuals noted by Rak et al. (1994, 1996) as displaying this morphology (cf. Gibraltar 2, Krapina 53, La Chapelle, Teshik Tash; Figure 12b-c) do not show a gradual increase in tubercle size but rather show a localized increase in the septa 6 and 4 insertion, the normal condition; and (3) many septa 6 and 4 tubercles do not present with a gradual inferior to superior transition in tubercle size but have abrupt transitions at the septum 4 or 2^{III} base (Figures 12a-c, and 13e-f).

2.9. Anatomically modern *Homo sapiens*

Our AmHs sample consists of: (1) Border Cave 2 and 4; (2) Dar es Soltan 5; (3) Ein Gev I; (4) Fish Hoek; (5) Haua Fteah I and II; (6) Omo-Kibish 1; (7) Qafzeh IX and XI; (8) Skhul 4 and 5; and (9) Zhoukoudian 101. Qafzeh XI represents the only subadult in this group. The *c. endocondyloidea* is weakly expressed and curved. The right *s. colli* is strongly angled inferiorly from the posterior ramus but becomes horizontal at mid-ramus whereas the left side is more continuously angled anteroinferiorly. The sulcus is deeply depressed anteriorly but weakly expressed posteriorly. The *l. pterygoidea* is weakly expressed. The specimen is damaged in the *s. colli* region but a *c. intermedia* was most certainly present. A septa 6 and 4 tubercle is weak to moderately developed on the right but less apparent on the left ramus. Qafzeh XI present with a modern *f. mandibulae-l. mandibulae* pattern.

In our adult AmHs sample the *c. endocondyloidea* is only well developed, straight, and slightly bar-like in Skhul 5 whereas in the remaining sample it is curved and less well developed (Figure 14a-c). A vertical groove is present on the *c. endocondyloidea* in all specimens except Border Cave 4 and Skhul 5 (Figure 14a-c). In Dar es Soltan 5, Qafzeh XI, and Skhul 5 the *l. mandibulae* pattern is similar to that in Amud 1 wherein the *l. mandibulae* lies inferior to the crest's medial-most extent or under the *c. endocondyloidea* and it does not project medially nor does it possess a lingular notch (Figures 13a and 14b). This was probably also the case in Qafzeh IX and Skhul 4. Lingular region morphology in Dar es Soltan 5 gives a false impression that a true lingula is present. A small tubercle exists slightly above the posterosuperior edge of the medial border of the *c. mandibulae* which imparts a lingula-like morphology. All other individuals in this group have a *l. mandibulae* pattern consistent with that in most recent *H. sapiens*. The anterior component of the *s. colli* is deep in almost all specimens whereas the posterior component is shallow (Figure 14a-c). Only Dar es Soltan 5 differs slightly as the *s. colli* remains deep into the initial portion of the posterior component where it then shallows dramatically. Excepting Ein Gev I, Dar es Soltan 5, Omo-Kibish 1, and, possibly Qafzeh IX, the *s. colli* is relatively anteroposteriorly short and horizontally disposed. Expression of the latter features reaches a maximum in Zhoukoudian 101 (Figures 10e and 14a-c). Of note in the latter specimen is the posterior extension of the *l. mandibulae* and superoanterior extension of the *l. pterygoidea* which result in incipient bridging of the lingular region (Figures 10e and 14c). Asymmetry of *s. colli* expression in the latter specimen and Qafzeh IX is apparent as the left sides are similar while the rights differ from the contralateral side and between these individuals. Omo-Kibish 1 presents with a short *s. colli* which is vertically oriented and which runs a straight course from the *f. mandibulae* to the posterior ramal border. Haua Fteah II presents with a short *c. intermedia* similar to some ArHs whereas Ein Gev I is most similar to modern humans. Excepting the latter specimens and Omo-Kibish 1 (not preserved), this group is similar to Neanderthals in incorporating the *c. intermedia* into the *l. mandibulae-l. pterygoidea* (Figure 14a-c). Note that in specimens which lack a developed *l. mandibulae*, such as Dar es Soltan 5, the *c. intermedia* (an extension of the *c. mandibulae*) is still present. The *l. pterygoidea* is weakly expressed in Border Cave 4, Ein Gev I, Qafzeh IX, and Skhul 5 whereas Border Cave 2, Dar es Soltan 5, Fish Hoek, Haua Fteah I and II, and Zhoukoudian 101 are more strongly marked (Figure 14a-c). In general, this group differs from most ArHs but is similar to Neanderthals in possessing a superiorly extended anterosuperior aspect of the *l. pterygoidea*. The latter extension results in a more horizontal appearance to the *s. colli* (Figure 14a-c). An exception to the latter is Dar es Soltan 5 which has a long, slightly vertically oriented *s. colli* and anteroinferiorly oriented *l. pterygoidea*.

Poor specimen preservation precludes a full assessment of the area of the *tsc*, but Border Cave 4, Haua Fteah I and II, Omo-Kibish 1, and Zhoukoudian 101 all lack the feature. Expression of tubercles in the superior attachment area for the *m. pterygoideus medialis* ranges from very weak to moderately strong in the following sequence: Skhul 5, Haua Fteah I, Haua Fteah II, Qafzeh IX, Border Cave 4, Ein Gev I, Omo-Kibish 1, Skhul 4, Dar es Soltan 5, and Fish Hoek (Figure 14a-c). The attachment site in Zhoukoudian 101 differs in that the septum 6 insertion is a depression whereas the septa 4 and 2^{III} sites combine to form a moderately developed tubercle on the right and a slightly developed one on the left side (Figure 14c). With the above exception all tubercles are related to septa 6 and 4. Dar es Soltan 5, Ein Gev I, Fish Hoek, and Skhul 4 present with septa 6 and 4 insertions which differ significantly from the remaining septal attachments. In Omo-Kibish 1 the septal attachments are relatively strong but they are equally developed. Dar es Soltan 5 is of interest as it presents with a strongly marked insertion area. Insertion tubercles for septa 2^{I-III} are large whereas those for septa 6 and 4 are areally expansive, bounded anteriorly by a well developed ridge with tubercles, but not medially extended. Clearly the septa 6 and 4 insertions were very well developed but not associated with strong tubercle development.

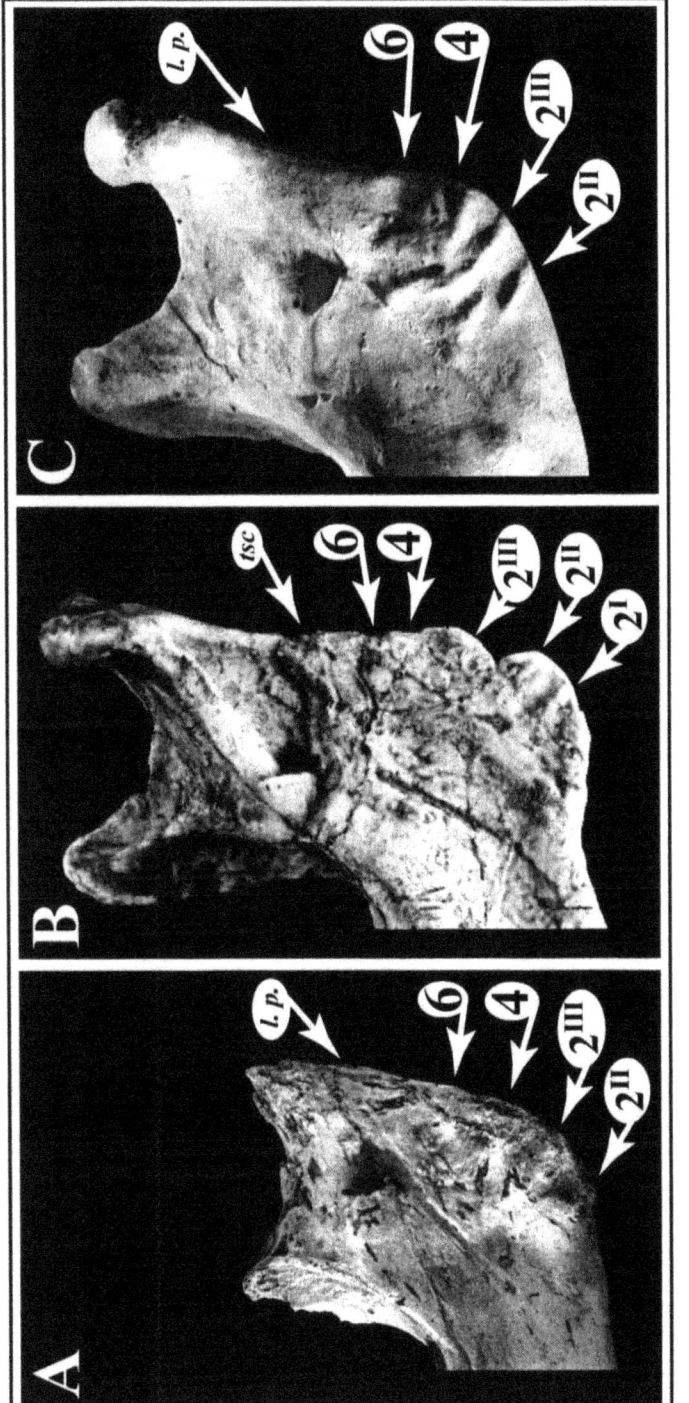

Figure 14a-c: Examples of anatomically modern *H. sapiens* adults showing some of the variation in medial ramal features. Specimens figured are from left to right: (a) Border Cave 4; (b) Skhul 5, reversed; and (c) Zhoukoudian 101. In both (a) and (b) note the lack of strong development of the septa 6 and 4 insertions. In Zhoukoudian 101 the septum 4 and 2^{III} insertions are associated with developed tubercles whereas the septum 6 insertion is not. A similar configuration is found in the Vindija 207 Neanderthal. Note the similarities in configuration of the *l. mandibulae* and positioning of the *l. pterygoidea* in these individuals relative to that of Neanderthals. Also note the position of the *l. mandibulae* relative to the *c. endocondyloidea* in (b) and compare this to that of Amud 1 (Figure 13a). The placement of the *c. intermedia* is such that it is linearly coincident with the *l. pterygoidea*, as found in some ArHs, most Neanderthals, and many recent *H. sapiens*.

2.10. *Homo sapiens* ssp. indet.

Our taxonomic category *H. sapiens* ssp. indet. consists of the Amud 7 infant. The *c. endocondyloidea* is damaged but appears to have been weakly expressed and curved (Figure 12d). Morphology of the *l. mandibulae* is similar to that found in similarly aged recent *H. sapiens* infants and, based on somewhat older subadults, to that of *H. erectus* (*s.l.*) and Neanderthals (Figures 4a-f and 12a-c). The *s. colli* is a deep depression that runs from the *f. mandibulae* to the posterior ramal border (Figure 12d). The posterior component is somewhat wider than the anterior component, as discussed for some recent human infants. A *c. intermedia* is not present, as is the case for many similarly aged recent *H. sapiens* infants. The *l. pterygoidea* is relatively strong near its confluence with the mylohyoid groove but near mid-ramus the line turns superiorly and becomes less well marked. This weak line reaches the posterior border but does not terminate in a true *tsc* (Figure 12d). What appears as a *tsc* is actually the result of a topographic change at the *s. colli*-septum 6 junction and is matched in recent *H. sapiens* infants. The apparent *tsc* is slightly accentuated by the loss of cortical bone at this junction (Figure 12d). The area between the inferior border of the *s. colli* and the tubercle is an inferomedially slanting ledge which is slightly concave (Figure 12d). The superior attachment site presents with a strong but relatively restricted septum 6 associated tubercle which receives a minor contribution from septum 4. The attachment presents as an isolated Type 2 tubercle (Figure 12d). Further, the configuration of the tubercle's posterior aspect indicates involvement of septum 2^{III} and possibly the *l. stylomandibulare*.

2.11. Bilateral occurrence of medial ramal features and limitations of the fossil record

The bilateral configuration of tubercles related to the superior attachment of the *m. pterygoideus medialis* can only be evaluated in 14 of the fossil individuals. This sample comprises: (1) ArHs [$N = 2$]; (2) Neanderthals [$N = 9$]; and (3) AmHs [$N = 3$]. With the exception of La Chapelle, La Ferrassie 1, Fish Hoek, Kebara 2, and Zafarraya, the right and left septum 6 and 4 insertions differ to a significant extent. The right side tubercle is larger in La Quina H5, Montmaurin 1, Qafzeh XI, Shanidar 1, Tabun C1 and C2, and Zhoukoudian 101 whereas the left is larger in Mauer and Teshik Tash. Note, however, that the right tubercle in Mauer is substantially smaller than the left and that at least a portion of this appears to be the result of taphonomic factors. As noted above many tubercles which are restricted to association with septa 6 and 4 on one ramus were found to incorporate the septum 2^{III} attachment on the contralateral side. The coalescence of septal insertions will give the appearance of a superiorly directed gradual increase in tubercle size and result in a loss of more evenly spaced insertion sites.

DISCUSSION OF THE ONTOGENY OF MEDIAL RAMAL BONY AND SOFT TISSUE ANATOMY IN MODERN AND FOSSIL HOMINOIDS

I. THE MEDIAL PTERYGOID TUBERCLE IN RECENT *HOMO SAPIENS* AND AN INTRODUCTION TO THE NECESSITY FOR A BROADER ASSESSMENT

1. Assessment of the recent *Homo sapiens* data

To examine the validity of the MPT character state as a Neanderthal autapomorphy we evaluate it both as defined and as a part of a broader anatomical-morphological complex. Given the character state definition and variation in the specimen series considered to display the character (Rak *et al.*, 1994, 1996) we found that a MPT (= *tpi*, in part) occurs in our recent *H. sapiens* ontogenetic series at a frequency of from 0.0% to 46.0%. Review of the percentage occurrence by developmental age clearly shows the MPT character state to vary ontogenetically, with newborns to 4.0-year-olds displaying consistently high occurrence rates (19.0-46.0%) and 5.0-18.0-year-olds displaying generally lower and more variable rates (0.0-24.0%: Table 2). Whereas her work is not directly comparable, a similar result was obtained by Coqueugniot (1999) in her analysis of a mixed European - Middle Eastern ontogenetic sample. The character state in our adult sample has an occurrence rate of 31.0%. This result differs significantly from that obtained by Coqueugniot (1999) who recorded only a 2.0% occurrence rate in adults. Whereas this result may reflect geographic differences, we believe it to result from methodological differences. Our data are generally consistent with values obtained by Creed-Miles *et al.* (1996) for subadults chronologically aged at <3.0 years of age and their statements regarding later age stages and with adult values obtained by Quam and Smith (1998). Note, however, that the description of a *tpi* in subadults provided by Creed-Miles *et al.* (1996) introduces doubt as to whether they actually differentiate between inferior *s. colli* relief and the *tpi*, as noted by Rak *et al.* (1996). We found the occurrence rate of a MPT, as defined by Rak *et al.* (1994, 1996), to vary geographically from 17.0% to 33.0% (Table 3) and to have a mean of approximately 25.0% in recent *H. sapiens*. The latter value is consistent with the value of 24.4% determined by Quam and Smith (1998). Note that our ontogenetic series for each geographic region are not fully comparable as they do not contain equal numbers of individuals in each age group. This fact may result in significant shifts in the percentage occurrence of the feature for any geographic region. Given the general consistency of our values with those obtained by other investigators, we consider our results sufficient for demonstrating the occurrence of the character state in relatively high percentages in all modern human populations.

In the process of establishing the range of tubercle variation in the Rak *et al.* (1994, 1996) Neanderthal sample, we observed a broad range of morphology. We also noted that the definition of a MPT did not clearly describe observable morphology. Given these observations we consider it imprudent to pursue analyses aimed at enhancing our understanding of frequency differences related to geography beyond those presented. Based on these observations we consider that our recent human data is of value only for demonstrating that the defined character state is not autapomorphic for Neanderthals.

2. Rationale for the need of a broader assessment of medial ramal anatomy

In defining the MPT character state Rak *et al.* (1994, 1996) and Hovers *et al.* (1995) included a: (1) positional-relational component; (2) shape component; (3) size component; (4) statement to account for the size component; (5) statement regarding tubercle homology; and (6) taxonomic-phylogenetic statement. Aspects of some of these components and statements have been reassessed by Antón (1995, 1996), Richards and Plourde (1995), Creed-Miles *et al.* (1996), Rak *et al.* (1996), and Coqueugniot (1999). The positional-relational component came into question when: (1) Creed-Miles *et al.* (1996) synonymized the term 'medial pterygoid tubercle' of Rak *et al.* (1994) with Bluntschli's (1929) term '*tuberculum pterygoideum inferius (tpi)*' and Weidenreich's (1936) definition of a *tpi*; and (2) Rak *et al.* (1996) subsequently identified a second tubercle superior to the largest of those involved in the MPT character state as the *tpi*. Note that the synonymy by Creed-Miles *et al.* (1996) referred only to adults. We consider that Weidenreich's definition of a *tpi*, and its restatement by Patte (1957), leaves little doubt as to the correctness of Creed-Miles *et al.*'s (1996) *positional* synonymy of the *tpi* with the superior aspect of the muscular region involved in the MPT character state. Note that some of the above confusion relating to this region results from Weidenreich's (1936) misidentification of the *tpi* in figures of both "Sinanthropus" and great ape specimens. In our analysis we do not, however, employ the term *tpi* as its definition (Bluntschli, 1929; Lenhossék, 1920; Weidenreich, 1936; Patte, 1957) is insufficient to allow detailed comparison of hominoids (see Methods). Since the MPT character state carries with it the above noted components and statements it cannot be equated with a single tubercle; the terms '*tpi*' and 'MPT' are not synonymous (contra Creed-Miles *et al.*, 1996). Note that we employ both terms in the following text where necessary and that, in general, they refer to aspects of the septa 6, septa 6 and 4, and septa 6, 4, and 2^{III} insertion sites of the *m. pterygoideus medialis*.

Features of bone arise and are modified throughout ontogeny as *parts* of functioning anatomical systems. Given this fact and the above, verification of the proposed character state requires, then, a broader ontogenetic investigation of morphological relationships between bony, neurovascular, ligamentous, and musculotendinous features of the medial mandibular ramus in recent *H. sapiens*, great apes, and fossil hominid taxa. The need to apply this level of detail to gain an understanding of the complexity of mandibular shape characteristics was earlier noted by Dullemeijer (1974). Application of this methodological approach provides not only resolution of problems related to the homology of *m. pterygoideus medialis* insertion tubercles but also provides a framework within which we address broader questions related to mandibular ontogeny, relationships of skeletal units to their functional matrices, and the application of ontogenetic data to questions of evolutionary history.

II. OVERVIEW OF THE ONTOGENY OF RECENT *HOMO SAPIENS* MEDIAL RAMUS MORPHOLOGY

1. Overview of the development of medial ramal morphology

Given the mosaic nature of ontogenetic processes which produce soft and hard tissues of the craniofacial region it should be expected that significant differences will exist between immature and mature individuals (Schaeffer, 1935). In recent *H. sapiens* fetuses and infants we document that the *s. colli* is actually a broad depression which encompasses the entire distance from the *f. mandibulae* to the posterior ramal border (Figure 4a-e). This depression is both superoinferiorly and anteroposteriorly concave and results, in part, from: (1) positioning of Meckel's cartilage relative to the developing membranous portion of the fetal mandible; and (2) a size discrepancy in later (i.e. post-fetal) developmental ages between the bony mandible and neurovascular bundles within and medial to the sulcus. Further, this relatively large soft tissue mass positions the *l. sphenomandibulare* (*s.l.*) more medially, relative to the mandibular ramus, in these groups as compared to adults. This combination results in a deep, superoinferiorly concave *s. colli* with strong medial projection of its inferior border as noted by Creed-Miles *et al.* (1996: Figure 4a-e). Attached to a superoinferiorly restricted region of this medially projecting inferior *s. colli* border are the: (1) *l. sphenomandibulare* (*s.l.*); (2) fascia covering the superior extent of the *m. pterygoideus medialis*; (3) fibers of the *m. pterygoideus medialis* from septa 6, 4, and 2^{III}; and (4) *l. stylomandibulare*. Because of both the idiosyncratically expressed size discrepancy between soft and hard tissue in the *s. colli* region and the growth rate differences between neural and facial structures, the space available for *m. pterygoideus medialis* attachment is limited. It appears that medial extension of the inferior *s. colli* border provides for or results in a larger attachment area and helps position the bone in close proximity to the lateral pterygoid plate. Such a positioning would reduce the distance between the muscle's origin and insertion that would need to be bridged by the developing musculotendinous primordia. It is also possible that there is a rapid laterally directed movement of portions of the ramus during early growth which is not matched by the attachment site that creates, in part, the observed projection.

Support for our suggestions regarding the reasons for strong medial extension of portions of the *m. pterygoideus medialis* insertion site comes from embryological studies of muscle development. These studies have demonstrated that muscle and tendon primordia arise independently of the bone (Edgeworth, 1935; Scott, 1951, 1954, 1957; Rayne and Crawford, 1971; Shellswell and Wolpert, 1977; Spyropoulos, 1977; Williams and Warwick, 1980; Sperber, 1981) and that attachment to bone is a relatively late developmental event (Long, 1947; Gasser, 1967; Rayne and Crawford, 1971; Sperber, 1981). Further, muscle reattachment studies have shown that osteogenic tissue will extend out toward an isolated muscle mass with the subsequent redevelopment of the muscle-bone interface (Chierici and Miller, 1984). Given the relative size of the pterygoid plate-to-medial ramus space in fetal to newborn humans (Sperber, 1981; Scott, 1954) a portion of the *s. colli* shelving and lateral expanse of the lateral pterygoid plate (Schumacher, 1962) is, then, probably related to these developmental processes. The epigenetic nature of this process gives rise to a high degree of idiosyncratic variation in expression of these bony features in recent *H. sapiens* (Weidenreich, 1936; Patte, 1957; Creed-Miles *et al.*, 1996).

The *s. colli* comprises anterior and posterior components. Shortly after birth the broad depression forming the *s. colli* becomes more sulcus-like and a reorganization of the relationship between the two sulcal components occurs (Figure 4a-f). The anterior component becomes relatively deeper, and the posterior component becomes relatively shallower (Figures 4a-f and 5a-e). A review of the anatomy of this region must preface discussion of the possible significance of this change.

The superior border of both sulcal components is formed by the *c. endocondyloidea*. This crest is weakly expressed, strongly anteroposteriorly concave and broken in its middle-to-posterior region by a shallow vertical groove (Figure 5a-b). The concavity allows for or results from the necessity to accommodate, minimally, the pterygoid venous plexus and pterygomandibular extension of the buccal fat pad (Murphy and Grundy, 1969). The morphological complexity of the pterygoid plexus and the critical role played by its relationship to the *mm. pterygoideus medialis* and *lateralis* is discussed in Deplus *et al.* (1996) whereas the role of the buccal fat pad is discussed in Latham and Scott (1970). The vertical groove in the *c. endocondyloidea* results from or provides for the dense, cord-like neurovascular bundle to the deep temporal region. Both of these bony features are related to the posterior component of the *s. colli*, although the pterygoid plexus is also related to the superior aspect of the bony anterior component. Given the course of the *n. alveolaris inferior* we do not, however, consider the weak medial extension and highly curved nature of this crest to be related to providing space for the nerve.

The remaining portion of the posterior component of the *s. colli* is related, minimally, to the inferior alveolar and maxillary arteries, portions of the pterygoid venous plexus, and extensions of the pterygomandibular portion of the buccal fat pad. The inferior border of the posterior component is formed by a variably expressed bony line, the *l. pterygoidea*, related to our attachment Site 2 of the *l. sphenomandibulare* (*s.l.*) and the superior-most insertion of *m. pterygoideus medialis* (Figures 4a-f and 5a-e). The posteroinferior-most extent of the posterior component may also be marked by a *tsc* (Figure 2a-b). The posterior component border courses anteriorly and may become continuous with the posterior edge of the mylohyoid groove.

Note, however, that the *l. pterygoidea* may not continue anteriorly on a linear course to the groove but may course anteroinferiorly from the posterior ramal border. This variation in the *l. pterygoidea* results in a highly variable distance between the anterior and posterior borders of the superior aspect of the mylohyoid groove (Figure 2c1-2).

The anterior component is related to the inferior alveolar and mylohyoid neurovascular bundles. These neurovascular bundles are surrounded by portions of the pterygomandibular extension of the buccal fat pad and the fat covered bundles are then individually enclosed in fascial tubes (Starkie and Stewart, 1931; Murphy and Grundy, 1969; Latham and Scott, 1970; Hamparian, 1973; Wadu *et al.*, 1997) that make up part of the lateral layer of the *l. sphenomandibulare* (*s.l.*). Latham and Scott (1970) note that the composite of encapsulated fat in this fibrous framework forms a tissue complex capable of resisting compressive forces.

Given these factors, the ontogenetic change in *s. colli* component morphology is potentially related to reduction and localization of the buccal fat pad as its role in early craniofacial growth (Latham and Scott, 1970; Rabkin, 1952; Sperber, 1981) is reduced. It is clear, however, that inclusion of that portion of the buccal fat pad that wraps the nerve results in or is provided for by the formation of the deep anterior sulcal component. Larnach and Macintosh (1971) quantified the depth of the *s. colli* in adult recent *H. sapiens* as a single structure, finding it to range from slightly (22%), to moderately (54%), to deeply depressed (24%).

The bony anteromedial and inferomedial borders of the anterior sulcal component include the *l. mandibulae*, mylohyoid groove, and *c. mandibulae-c. intermedia* (Figure 2a-c). All these structures provide for the mandibular attachment(s) of the *l. sphenomandibulare* (*s.s.* / *s.l.*: Figure 3a-d). As noted above, the inferior borders of the anterior and posterior components may become continuous, in which case the *c. intermedia* is generally partially or fully covered by the *l. pterygoidea* (Figure 2c1-2). This can result from either a widening of the anterior sulcal component which forces the *l. pterygoidea* inferiorly (cf. *A. africanus*, Sts 52b) or by an anterosuperior expansion of the *m. pterygoideus medialis* attachment site (cf. Neanderthals, AmHs, recent *H. sapiens*). In the first case the *c. intermedia* is generally exposed whereas in the second case the *crista* is generally incorporated into the *linea*.

To our knowledge only Larnach and Macintosh (1971) have attempted to determine *c. intermedia* occurrence rate in *H. sapiens*, finding only a unilateral trace in one of 169 mandibles. These authors' use of Weidenreich's (1936) definition of the *c. intermedia* probably accounts for the general absence of this normal variant, with *m. pterygoideus medialis* expansion accounting for most of the remainder. Understanding the frequency of occurrence of this character state, as delineated by Weidenreich (1936), requires that positioning of the *l. pterygoidea* relative to the *c. intermedia* be considered as these structures are responding to different functional components and expression of the former character will modify the expression of the latter.

In our ontogenetic series of recent *H. sapiens* we observed the *m. pterygoideus medialis* to have two main bony attachment points near the inferior border of the *s. colli* in fetal to newborn individuals. The upper-most of these attachment sites, the *l. pterygoidea*, defines the superior-most bony extent of the *m. pterygoideus medialis*. The bony indication of this attachment is highly variable and ranges from virtually absent to a thin, but distinct, bony line or crest (Figure 4a-f). The latter may be accentuated by superior flaring of the attachment as it extends the inferior *s. colli* border and by an apparent deepening of the concavity of the *f. pterygoidea*. The second main attachment area is initially coincident with or only slightly below the *l. pterygoidea* (Figure 4 a-b). This attachment begins as a slight roughening of the bone but soon consists of a flat plateau which may be marked by two, short bony ridges which run anteroposteriorly. The bony plateau has superior and inferior borders that either converge at their anterior extent or that run a sub-parallel course (Figure 4c). When ridges are present on the plateau they run anteriorly across the plateau and are either parallel or slightly convergent anteriorly (Figure 4c-e). The plateau and its associated ridging is the attachment site for septa 6 and 4 of the *m. pterygoideus medialis*. During growth the main bony attachment sites in this region, the *l. pterygoidea* and that for septa 6 and 4, will separate. The degree of separation varies, with the *l. pterygoidea* maintaining a close relationship to the posterior and, variably, the anterior *s. colli* while the septal attachments become well separated from the sulcus (Figure 4a-f). As separation begins, the area below the *l. pterygoidea*, which is initially at the free edge of the medially projecting ledge forming the inferior *s. colli* border, becomes flat to concave (Figure 4a, c-d). With growth the septal attachments continue to separate from the sulcus, and the ridges, when present, separate from each other. There also appears to be a rate disjunction in the latter process as the septal attachments tend to maintain a close relationship well into the juvenile period whereas the combined septa 6 and 4 attachment site becomes well separated from the sulcus in early childhood (Figures 4a-f and 5a-e). We currently believe that there is a superior repositioning of the *l. pterygoidea* during this process and are in the process of confirming this hypothesis (Richards *et al.*, in prep.). This growth process gives rise to tubercles (or pits) which are isolated from the *s. colli* and which are superoinferiorly and anteroposteriorly short (Figure 4a-f). Documentation of this process in our cross-sectional ontogenetic series of recent *H. sapiens* confirms: (1) the positional synonymy of the *m. pterygoideus medialis* attachment site described in the MPT character state and the *tpi* as observed by Creed-Miles *et al.* (1996) and, resultantly, these authors' *tpi* (= MPT) occurrence rates for recent *H. sapiens* (contra Rak *et al.*, 1996; but see above reservations); and (2) that the MPT in the Amud 7 infant as identified by Rak *et al.* (1996) is, within an ontogenetic context, positionally homologous to the MPT of adults (contra Creed-Miles *et al.*, 1996; see below).

2. Factors influencing tubercle area and projection

Having outlined the basic anatomy and developmental sequence in recent *H. sapiens* it is possible to examine some aspects of the size component of the MPT character state. Note that here we provide only specific details related to the issue of tubercle size; a more broad based discussion of attachment site formation is provided below. We have demonstrated a strong medial shelving of the inferior border of the *s. colli* in recent *H. sapiens*. We have also delineated the nature of the *m. pterygoideus medialis* attachment to this medial shelf and provided a statement regarding positioning of these structures during growth. It is clear that in subadults of developmental age ≤ 4.0 years of age it is necessary to separate the amount of medial extension of this shelf related to the developmental processes outlined and that related specifically to the muscle. Further, it is necessary to delineate the degree to which strong medial shelving of the inferior *s. colli* border is related to tubercle size in developmental ages > 4.0 years of age. We suggest that infants with the greatest degree of medial shelving will have a greater likelihood of having medially projecting tubercles in later development. During separation of the *s. colli* and the tubercle the latter would be remodeled but maintained as an isolate. Given our cross-sectional sample, it appears that the tubercle drifts during modeling growth but in later stages becomes both longer and broader through expansion of neighboring fasciculi and coalescence of the posterior aspect of the tendon bundles.

We have described an idiosyncratically expressed degree of tubercle development in early infancy wherein the septa 6 and 4 attachments range from weakly expressed, roughened plateaus to strongly expressed raised plateaus with septal ridging (Figure 4a-f). We have also described a continuum in adults wherein septa 6 and 4, and sometimes septum 2^{III}, are intimately related to tubercle size and extent (Figure 5a-e). The septum 6 ridge is nearly always the largest and its inferior extent ends at the base of the septum 4 ridge (Figure 5b-c). It is possible to have a large, isolated septum 6 tubercle, our Type 1 (Figure 5b-c). The usual configuration observed, however, is for the septal 6 attachment to increase in size, followed by the attachments for septum 4 and sometimes 2^{III} (= Type 2: Figure 5b-e). Whereas the degree of coalescence of the individual attachments follows this sequence it appears that septa 6 and 4 will reach a maximum medial extent and then merge through bony infilling of the interseptal space prior to coalescence with septum 2^{III} (Figure 5d). Because, in most individuals, tubercle size diminishes inferiorly the impression is given of a superior hypertrophy of the muscle as observed in the Kebara 2 Neanderthal (see below) by Tillier *et al.* (1989), Tillier (1991), and Rak *et al.* (1994, 1996).

What is currently unclear, however, is whether the observed bony tubercle morphology actually documents the processes suggested above. Because we have observed tubercles in young infants that are clearly similar to those in which septa 6 and 4 have coalesced and which have a 'filled' interseptal space it is possible that at least part of the observed developmental 'continuum' results from other factors (Figure 4c-f). Note that an alternative to the 'filling' process would be modeling resorption and lateral drift around the septal attachments as discussed by van der Klaaw (1963). In further support of the latter view we observed substantial variation in muscle septa wherein their insertions range from fully separate to posteriorly conjoined (= septa 6 and 4, sometimes also 2^{III}). The latter was also observed in adults by Schumacher (1962) but not noted by him to occur in subadults. Given Schumacher's (1959, 1962) small fetal-to-newborn sample size ($N = 9, \leq 7^{th}$ month; 3, $\leq 10^{th}$ month) it is quite possible, however, that these 'coalesced' septa also occur in subadults. On the other hand, our observations are consistent with Schumacher's, as we have not observed young infants with tubercles which incorporate the septum 2^{III} insertion, although many show independent development of septum 2^{I-III} tubercles early in development. The tubercle or bony ridge associated with septum 2^{III} may be incorporated into the septa 6 and 4 tubercle in later stages or may remain as a large isolate (cf. Zafarraya: Figure 13f). It appears that there is a more intimate relationship between septa 6 and 4 than between these and septum 2^{III}. We provide further statements regarding these relationships below. Of note is if large tubercles are related to size increase in the individual attachment sites and their resulting coalescence due to this size increase, how are large, individual septal attachments maintained as isolates?

Based on our ontogenetic series of recent *H. sapiens* it is clear that strong medial projection of the mandibular ramus at the *m. pterygoideus medialis* superior-most septal insertion sites is related to several ontogenetic factors. This is also noted by Creed-Miles *et al.* (1996). We have also provided evidence which indicates that maintenance of strong medial projection of the attachment site may be related to idiosyncratic variations (Scott 1954) other than *m. pterygoideus medialis* hypertrophy. This possibility is also supported by our observations on the degree to which intramuscular tendons attach to the underlying bone. We found some large and medially projecting tubercles to be associated with strong tendinous bundles which either had only minor attachments to the bone or only inserted into the fibroperiosteal layer which covers the bone, as the attachment was easily removed from the bone. In other cases, similar tendon bundles possessed entheses which penetrated the fibroperiosteal layer, when one was present, and were firmly embedded in bone. This range of attachment variation is discussed by Symons (1954), Dörfl (1980a), and Hems and Tillmann (2000). In cases where the entheses are directly attached to bone, Dörfl (1980a) observed that the entheses are continuous with the fibrous layer of the periosteum peripheral to the bony attachment. Further, large and medially projecting tubercles tend to have concave borders. These borders are lined with fleshy muscle and with tendon entheses, many of which are embedded in bone. Because tendons which insert into concavities around the periphery of the tubercle do so at varying angles on any given edge, thereby forming a semi-radiate pattern around the tubercle, it is clear that they are only partially related to the individual main septal insertions (= septa 6, 4, 2^{I-III}). This is reinforced by our observation that tendons and muscle attached to the anterior aspect of the tubercles have a different orientation than the main muscle mass. We observed many of these fibers to be part of the anterior head of the *m. pterygoideus medialis*. Observations on the course of these musculotendinous bundles show them to fold at mid-bundle on mandibular closure and to become taut on full extension. It is probable that hypertrophy of muscle related to these insertions of the anterior and posterior parts of the muscle are partially responsible for driving medial expansion of the tubercle. The latter process could be similar to that occurring in the formation of sagittal (Scott, 1957) or nuchal crests. In the latter cases, then, medially projecting tubercles with strongly concave borders may be formed, in part, by hypertrophy of muscle fibers related to either the anterior head fibers or to a broad portion of the posterior head fibers which are the most intimately related to the ramus. Note that in our cadaver dissections and observations on dry bones that we confirmed Antón's (1996) observation of little correspondence between general robusticity and large tubercles. We also found little correspondence between general size and robusticity and tendon entheses which inserted into fibroperiosteum, as opposed to directly into bone.

We have discussed mandibular ramus anatomy directly related to the *s. colli* and superior attachment site of the *m. pterygoideus medialis*. In these discussions we noted that the region interposed between the *s. colli*'s inferior border and the septum 6 attachment varies from flat to highly concave (Figures 4d-f and 5a-e). In some individuals these superior concavities have secondary pits filled with tendons and fleshy muscle fibers (cf. Kebara 2, Roc de Marsal 1, recent *H. sapiens*). We have also noted weak-to-strong concavities along the anterior and sometimes on the inferior border of the septa 6 and 4 tubercles. Creed-Miles *et al.* (1996) observed a disparity between the positive relief of the tubercle and the negative relief of the *f. pterygoidea* in older individuals. This configuration may result from bone loss consequent to reduction of the muscle mass with age (Scott, 1957; Miller, 1991). In this case, Creed-Miles *et al.*'s (1996) observation may only reflect the accentuation of normal variation in late growth stages. In either case the relationship of tubercle to *f. pterygoidea* relief is particularly apparent in an ontogenetic series of *P. troglodytes*. Given these observations and those we presented regarding soft tissue relationships to these surfaces it is clear that a delineated or prominent tubercle can result from: (1) resorption around the tubercle; (2) apposition at the tubercle; or (3) a combination of these factors. Further, development of a tubercle and surrounding depressions may or may not be related to the same process or they may reflect aspects of a single process. Given our observations it appears that multiple, but not necessarily directly related, factors result in tubercle formation and size, *f. pterygoidea* relief, and the relationship of these throughout ontogeny.

Antón (1994a, 1995, 1996) attempted to quantify the degree of MPT prominence in recent *H. sapiens* and Neanderthals. Reference to the same casts employed shows her values to incorporate both the medial projection of the septum 6 insertion site and, when present, the amount of what appears to be laterally directed resorption along its superior concavity. Note that the superior concavity is generally associated with fleshy muscle originating at the bone's surface and attaching to the tendon mass of septum 6 but that it may also be related to the fleshy *origin* of muscle fibers associated with septum 7. With reservations we expressed above regarding the degree of association of tubercles and depressions aside, simple reference to the specimens measured demonstrates the inability of her measurements to accurately describe tubercle prominence. The value provided by Antón (1994a, 1995, 1996) for Amud 1 essentially reflects the depth of the superior concavity as the septum 6 ridge has only a slight medial extent. The lack of tubercle development in Amud 1 is also discussed by Coqueugniot (1999). Antón's value for Régourdou 1 records the medial extent of the septum 6 ridge, as it lacks a superior concavity (Figure 13a-b). Further, comparison of her dimensions for the poorly developed tubercles of Amud 1 (1.6 mm) or Régourdou 1 (1.3 mm) with the strongly developed one in La Quina H5 (1.5 mm) makes it clear that Antón's metric analysis does not usefully quantify MPT prominence in Neanderthals and recent *H. sapiens* (Figure 13a-b, e). Further, given such an analysis it is not possible to distinguish subadults from adults as we have demonstrated that tubercle development is initially medially directed but that in later development both superoinferiorly and anteroposteriorly directed expansion of the tubercle occurs. Incidentally, Antón (1996) observed that 18% of recent *H. sapiens* had 'MPTs' of < 0.7 mm and that the 'MPT' ranged from < 0.3 mm in this group; however, it is clear that 'tubercles' of < 0.3 mm, or even < 0.7 mm, cannot be included within the MPT character state as defined by Rak *et al.* (1994, 1996). It is of interest that this author (Anton, 1993; Antón, 1994a, b, 1995, 1996) while correctly observing a 100% occurrence rate for this aspect of the muscle's attachment site in a presumably detailed cross-taxonomic comparison of the musculotendinous-bone interface (Antón, 1994a) failed to recognize the multiplicity of disparate biological processes underlying observed variation prior to metric analysis. The inappropriateness of pursuing metric analysis of a character state prior to understanding the nature of the character is discussed by Lieberman (1995). Quam and Smith (1998) also observed variation in the 'MPT' of Neanderthals but did not consider its importance in their comparisons.

3. The role of ligaments in producing and maintaining medial ramal morphology

To clarify the roles of the *ll. sphenomandibulare* (*s.l.*) and *stylomandibulare* in the formation of tubercles in the superior aspect of the attachment site, we employ observations from our ontogenetic series of dry bone specimens and recent *H. sapiens* cadaver dissections. The former ligament is a complex, layered, and highly variable structure comprising the *l. sphenomandibulare* (*s.s.*) and thickenings of deep cervical fascia (Testut, 1896; Hovelacque and Virenque, 1913; Patte, 1957; Baker and Davies, 1972; Moss and Moss-Salentijn, 1978: Figure 3a-d). Hovelacque and Virenque (1913) appear to be the only investigators to have evaluated this region in human infants, finding no difference relative to the adult state. Note, however, that Matyas *et al.* (1990) observed significant changes in the structural properties of the medial collateral ligament of rabbits during ontogeny, and it seems unlikely that the *l. sphenomandibulare* (*s.s.*) and its associated deep cervical fascia would not also change during growth. The posterior-most of the deep cervical fascial thickenings (cf. maxillo-glaserien ligament of the interpterygoid aponeurosis of Hovelacque and Virenque, 1913) gives rise to an idiosyncratically expressed tubercle slightly superior to the septal 6 attachment site, the *tsc*. The *l. sphenomandibulare* (*s.l.*) is also related to a series of crests or lines on the medial ramus including the *c. intermedia* (in part, attachment Site 1), the *l. pterygoidea* (in part, Site 2), and the superior insertion of septum 6 of the *m. pterygoideus medialis* (in part, Site 3: Figure 2a-c). In fetal to newborn individuals these attachments form the medial surface of a U-shaped cradle or fascial pouch (Barker and Davies, 1972) which houses neurovascular and related soft tissues of the middle-to-superior aspect of the mandibular ramus. It is due, in part, to this attachment and subsequent expansion of enclosed soft tissue that a strong medial extension of the ramus occurs at the base of the *s. colli*. The *l. sphenomandibulare* (*s.l.*) is, then, intimately involved in the more medial positioning of the *m. pterygoideus medialis* main attachment site and to that bony attachment being inferior to the superior lip of the medial shelf. With growth, ligament attachment Sites 2 and 3 separate as the septal 6 attachment site and *s. colli* separate. The most medial layer of the ligament will continue to play a role in tubercle formation as it is continuous with or comprises a portion of the fibroperiosteal sheet which forms the muscle's ramal attachment, as noted by Hovelacque and Virenque (1913) and Billy and Vallois (1977). The morphology of the attachment region of the *l. sphenomandibulare* (*s.l.*) at Site 3 will vary depending on the degree to which the tendon attaches to bone. With incorporation of entheses into bone the fibroperiosteum is either penetrated or incorporated into the bone with the tendon (Dörfl, 1980a). Whereas attachment Site 3 of the *l. sphenomandibulare* (*s.l.*) may continue to play a role in creating or maintaining medially extended tubercles its role is moderated by attachment Site 2. In some cases, however, this ligament may be more intimately involved in creating medially projecting tubercles and especially those with concave superior borders. This situation will potentially arise when the neurovascular bundle, generally positioned superior to attachment Site 2, is bifurcated. In these instances the inferior bundle will run for a variable distance in the space between Sites 2 and 3. In these cases attachment Site 2 will be minimally or not expressed as a bony ridge. This configuration will result in the *s. colli* extending inferiorly to become coincident with the septal 6 attachment site and may account for some of the superiorly arched (=

hooked or lipped) nature of that tubercle (Figure 4e). Whereas we provide further statements regarding this structure below, it is clear that the role of the *l. sphenomandibulare* (*s.l.*) in tubercle formation, and perhaps maintenance, varies idiosyncratically and through ontogeny.

The *l. stylomandibulare* is thought by some to function (become taut) in extreme mandibular protrusion whereas it is said to fold on extreme opening (Burch, 1970; DuBrul, 1980). Alternatively, given the observed and known (Kaufman and Irish, 1970; Correll *et al.*, 1979) idiosyncratic variation in adult *p. styloideus ossis temporalis* length and in the ligament's attachment to either or both the bony process and associated muscle bundles in recent *H. sapiens*, we agree with Williams and Warwick (1980) who consider its function uncertain. Ontogenetic changes in the ligament's angular relationship to the ramus and its effect on mandibular morphology are also unclear. Further, given that the ligament can originate from muscle bundles attached to the *p. styloideus ossis temporalis* it is unclear what effect, if any, the lack of an ossified process (Hobgood, 1989) and differences in positioning of craniofacial components in fossil taxa would have on ligament function. Little understanding of the ligament's function is gained from literature descriptions of great apes. In *Pongo*, Zuckerman *et al.* (1962) observed a similar origin for the ligament as found in *H. sapiens*, at the tip of the *p. styloideus ossis temporalis*. Winkler (1991) observed, however, that the process in *Pongo* does not ossify and that the *l. stylomandibulare* has a broad insertion onto the ramus, from the posteromedial aspect of the condylar neck to the upper one-third of the ramus. In *P. troglodytes* a strong *l. stylomandibulare* was observed to attach to the *processus vaginalis* of the *pars tympanica* of the *ossis temporalis*. Whereas we concur with Creed-Miles *et al.* (1996) that the *l. stylomandibulare* may play a role in the formation of tubercles in the superior aspect of the muscle's attachment site, we believe that role to be a minimal one but are unable to provide further clarification due to the nature of our samples and available literature descriptions.

4. Summary

In the preceding we have provided evidence to document ontogenetic changes occurring in the medial mandibular ramus of recent *H. sapiens*, along with a discussion of regional anatomy related to these changes. Within this context we have detailed ontogenetic changes in the *s. colli* region and their relationship to the attachment site of *m. pterygoideus medialis*. Further, we have discussed both idiosyncratic and age related variation in the formation of and shape changes in tubercles in the superior aspect of the *m. pterygoideus medialis* attachment area. It is important to note that the insertion for septa 6 and 4 ranges from a slight-to-moderately-deep depression, which may contain septal ridges, bounded by a rampart, to a large tubercle. We have also attempted to account for factors related to the observed variation. Due to the general complexity of the topic we have not, however, provided discussion or resolution of the suggested functional reasons for tubercle formation as presented in Rak *et al.* (1994, 1996). Further discussion of aspects of mandibular ontogeny and ligament, tendon, and muscle development which bear directly on this topic and on the bony anatomy in this region are provided below. We have, however, demonstrated the incorrectness of observations by Rak and Kimbel (1995) that: (1) even the most robust *H. sapiens* individuals have tubercles which are homogeneously distributed throughout the area of muscle insertion; and (2) that large medially projecting tubercles fitting the definition of the MPT character state do not occur in substantial frequencies in either subadult or adult recent *H. sapiens*. These results are consistent with those presented by both Creed-Miles *et al.* (1996) and Coqueugniot (1999).

III. ONTOGENY OF MEDIAL RAMAL ANATOMY IN GREAT APES AND ISSUES IN CHARACTER HOMOLOGY

1. Overview of great ape medial ramal anatomy

Great ape medial ramal anatomy has been shown to differ significantly from that of recent *H. sapiens* (Straus, 1950, 1962; Weidenreich, 1936). This mandibular morphological disparity derives, in part, from significant differences in craniofacial anatomy related to the fact that apes differ from most hominids in locomotion and behavior, minimally. These differences combine to generate unique cranial base, craniofacial, and dentofacial morphologies which are reflected in development, function, and maintenance of muscle-bone relationships. Although these basic differences exist, Rak *et al.* (1994) contend that both *Gorilla* and *Pan troglodytes* individuals share a generalized (symplesiomorphic) morphology of the insertion site for *m. pterygoideus medialis* with modern *H. sapiens* and all non-Neanderthal hominids. To evaluate this contention we examine small ontogenetic samples of *Gorilla gorilla*, *Pan troglodytes*, *P. paniscus* and *Pongo pygmaeus*.

In our sample, excepting *Pongo*, the great ape condition is characterized by isolation of the *s. colli* under a projecting *c. endocondyloidea* (Figure 7a-d). The anterior *s. colli* component is marked by long superior and inferior crests around the *f. mandibulae* in *P. troglodytes* but shorter ones in other great apes. In available subadult *Pongo* and *Gorilla* and in adult great apes the posterior sulcal component is generally weakly marked, although it may attain some prominence in adult *Gorilla*. In both subadult and adult great apes the anterior component is generally separated from the *m. pterygoideus medialis* attachment site, although they may be adjacent to one another in some *Pongo* and *Gorilla* (Figure 7a-d). In subadult *P. troglodytes* the *s. colli* components form a continuous depression which is more linear than in adults. When both components are apparent, a slightly to strongly raised area occurs mid-sulcus in both subadults and adults of *P. troglodytes*, *Pongo*, and *Gorilla* (Figure 7a-d). The latter feature marks a disjunction between the: (1) subvertical orientation of anterior component soft tissue structures; (2) posterior and horizontal orientation of posterior component soft tissue structures; and (3) anteroinferiorly directed and well separated course of the *l. pterygoidea*. This *s. colli* morphology differs generally from the more continuous and superoinferiorly and anteroposteriorly deep concavity seen in recent *H. sapiens* (Figures 5a-e and 7a-d).

In adult and subadult great apes, the posterosuperior aspect of the *l. pterygoidea* is positioned relatively high on the mandibular ramus and it runs a strong anteroinferiorly directed course from the posterior ramal border (Figure 7a-d). The strength of this inclined attachment is less in *P. troglodytes* due to the generally more horizontal orientation of the *m. pterygoideus medialis* insertion. In adults of this taxon, and less frequently in *Pongo* and *Gorilla*, the mylohyoid groove is positioned well posterior to the *f. mandibulae* (Straus, 1950, 1962: Figure 7a-c). Note, however, that Straus (1950) suggests that there is some indication of age related changes in the mylohyoid groove-*f. mandibulae* relationship. In recent *H. sapiens*, the *n. mylohyoideus* branches from the *n. alveolaris inferior* anywhere from 5.0 to 23.0 mm ($\overline{X}$ = 14.7 mm; Wilson *et al.*, 1984) superior to the *f. mandibulae* (contra Barker and Davies, 1972 and Arensburg and Nathan, 1979). In some cases the two nerve branches run a parallel course whereas in others the *n. mylohyoideus* takes a slightly more posterior course prior to arcing back towards the mylohyoid groove. In *Pan*, it appears that the mandibular branch of the *n. trigeminalis* (CN V) is more posteriorly placed in relation to the *f. mandibulae* but not in relation to the mandibular condyle. The nerve-to-condyle positioning is similar to that in humans. Given the nerve-to-mandibular relationship in *Pan* the *nn. alveolaris inferior* and *mylohyoideus* enter the *s. colli* well posterior to the *f. mandibulae* with the nerves having a more extensive relationship to the sulcus. Even with the more posterior course of the mylohyoid neurovascular bundle in *Pan* the *l. pterygoidea* is still generally positioned slightly more posteroinferiorly to the mylohyoid groove as earlier observed by Patte (1957) in prosimians and apes. With growth the *l. pterygoidea* becomes further separated from the anterior component of the *s. colli* whereas the two structures may become coincident in humans and some *Gorilla*.

Given the above and our confirmation of Weidenreich's (1936) observation that a *l. mandibulae* does not occur in great apes, it is clear that the mandibular attachment(s) of the *l. sphenomandibulare* (*s.l.*) in great apes will differ from recent *H. sapiens*. In *P. troglodytes* infants the ligament is here considered to attach to the superior and inferior crests surrounding the *f. mandibulae* (Figure 7a). The inferior crest we consider as homologous with the *c. intermedia* in recent *H. sapiens* (= Site 1: Figures 2a and 7a). Unless the *l. sphenomandibulare* (*s.l.*) is directly coincident with the superior edge of the *m. pterygoideus medialis* attachment (= *l. pterygoidea*) no bony trace of its attachment to the posterior *s. colli* component could be discerned in great apes (Figure 7a-d). Note that in humans we use the single term *l. pterygoidea* to refer to the condition where the two attachments are coincident (Figure 2c1-2). The combined attachment area in adult humans is ca. 1.0-2.0 mm wide and represented by a low, rounded line. In great apes the line is generally more narrow and it is difficult to attribute it to a 'doubled attachment site' as in humans. Further, we were unable to demonstrate a *tsc* in the great apes examined and this would be consistent with the latter observation (Figure 7a-d). Descriptions of soft and hard tissues of this region are extremely limited for great apes (Cave, 1979). Therefore, pending evidence from dissections of great apes, we suggest either differences in or, less likely, the absence of supplementary thickening of the deep cervical fascia which would produce bony crests or lines and tubercles (*tsc*) in this specific region. Absence of this specific aspect of the deep cervical fascial thickenings would potentially result in a functional difference wherein there is a lack of ligament (muscle?) mediated tubercle formation along the posteroinferior *s. colli*.

In subadult *P. troglodytes* the *m. pterygoideus medialis* attachment to the medial shelving of the inferior *s. colli* border is most similar to that in recent *H. sapiens*. In *P. troglodytes* there is, however, little separation of the *l. pterygoidea* and the septum 6 insertion during growth (Figure 7a-d). In adults the muscle's insertion site ranges from a broad roughened area to one with well developed tubercles. In the latter cases the septum 6 attachment site is closely related to the *l. pterygoidea*. This differs from the condition in humans where a variable but wide space develops between the two structures (Figures 5a-e and 7a-c). We observed significant variation in the morphology of the superior-most tubercles of the *m. pterygoideus medialis* in *P. troglodytes* relative to those observed in humans but consider the variants to be singularly related to the development of septum 6. There also appears to be some involvement of minor tendons interposed between septa 6 and 4 and between septum 6 and the *l. pterygoidea* (= septum 8?). Note, however, that it is unclear whether an 8th septum occurs in *P. troglodytes* as Schumacher (1961, 1980) only provided details of septal arrangements for *Pongo*. Schumacher (1961) did find, however, that some recent *H. sapiens* have an 8th septum in the superior-most portion of the muscle's insertion. In most great ape mandibles we examined, large tubercles in the superior portion of the muscle's attachment site did not occurred as isolates but, when present, were associated with tubercles lining the posterior ramal border. Weidenreich (1936) and de Lumley (1972, 1973) discuss the range of variation in tubercle size in both *Pongo* and *P. troglodytes*. In the latter taxon, minimally, tubercle development appears to indicate more evenly spaced septa with emphasis on the posterior-most fibers. This gains support from Schumacher's (1962) figures of septal attachments in *Pongo*; they are depicted as: (1) relatively narrow; (2) evenly spaced along the posterior ramal border; and (3) superoinferiorly long. In recent *H. sapiens* we confirmed Schumacher's depiction of the septal attachments as: (1) being of varying anteroposterior length; (2) having a variable spacing between septa; and (3) being generally oriented anterosuperiorly (Figure 1a-f). The differing distributions of *m. pterygoideus medialis* related tubercles implies a significant difference between these taxa in the: (1) emphasis placed on development of individual intramuscular septa; (2) degree to which septa are spatially separated; and (3) functional constraints placed on these septa. Differing functional constraints would also include variation in function through ontogeny. These observations are consistent with the works of Gaspard *et al.* (1973a, b) on non-pongid anthropoids.

Based on comparisons of medial ramus bony anatomy in our ontogenetic series of recent *H. sapiens* and great apes we consider the *m. pterygoideus medialis* septal attachment sites to be homologous in these taxa. Slight differences in positioning of the attachment sites and, presumably, in the function of specific aspects of the muscle between these taxa are considered to have no effect on tubercle homology. The latter view is consistent with Owen's (1843) definition of homology as discussed in de Beer (1971), Rieppel (1993), and Hall (1995). For a specific application of this concept to muscle insertion sites refer to Lewis (1989). Note that these muscle insertion sites are also potentially consistent with an expanded concept of homology [see Schoch (1986), Rieppel (1993), and Hall (1995)] as presented in Van Valen (1982) and Roth (1988).

2. Discussion of medial ramal tubercle homology in great apes and recent *Homo sapiens*

Whereas we consider the intramuscular septa and their attachment sites to be homologous between great apes and humans, this does not mean they do not differ. As discussed, a variably sized space arises during ontogeny between the septum 6 attachment and the *s. colli* in recent *H. sapiens* but not in great apes and both tubercle morphology and number of septa involved in tubercle formation differ between these groups. We are currently unable to detail the reasons for the development of the intervening space. It may result from the: (1) attachment site in humans drifting inferiorly relative to that of great apes; or (2) *s. colli* drifting superiorly during ontogeny in humans but not in great apes. In the case of tubercle morphology and septa involved, it appears probable that a portion of the difference between great apes and humans results from a reduction in the superoinferior extent of the insertion area available for septa 6 and 4 in humans. It is probable that the septum 6 attachment site is displaced inferiorly in humans, thereby resulting in the space between the *s. colli* and the septal attachment and in the resultant commingling of the posterior fibers of septa 6 and 4. The generally more expansive septa 6 and 4 attachment site in recent *H. sapiens*, relative to those of great apes, may then be the result of changes in either or both the positioning or function of intramuscular septa following changes in craniofacial hafting. Differences in craniofacial hafting could be expressed in the overall higher degree of complexity of the human *m. pterygoideus medialis* relative to that of non-human primates (Gaspard *et al.*, 1973a, b; Van Eijden *et al.*, 1997). The septum 2^{III} site, although many times incorporated into the septa 6 and 4 attachments, would not be involved in this process as its expansion and incorporation with those attachments appears to be related to a different mechanism. These observations are consistent with both our observations and those of Schumacher (1962) and Gaspard *et al.* (1973a, b) on the positioning and arrangement of intramuscular septa in both humans and great apes. We also consider the absence of a *tsc* in great apes to be related to significant differences in the attachment and function of the *l. sphenomandibulare* (*s.l.*). However, because the septum 6 attachment is located in close proximity to the *l. pterygoidea* throughout growth in *P. troglodytes* the lack of a significant *tsc* may be related to this factor (i.e. the muscle's attachment obscures the *tsc*). Also note that in both *Pongo* (Schumacher, 1962) and *Gorilla*

(Raven and Hill, 1950) the *m. pterygoideus medialis* insertion site is extremely large compared to the recent human condition. Further, the anterior aspects of the muscle (= anterior head, in part) comprising Schumacher's (1962) septum 1 and septum 5 have extensive fleshy origins reaching anterosuperiorly into the *f. mandibulae-c. pharyngea* region. In humans, fleshy origins for septa 1, 3, and 5 have similar orientations but these muscle bundles are more variable in their development.

In this context it is important to note that Antón (1996:401) considers the MPT (= septa 6, 4 and, variably, 2^{III}) in macaques and humans to be related to the "...main intramuscular tendon..." of the *m. pterygoideus medialis*. Based on our observations and those of the other authors cited in the above discussion, we do not consider such a structure to exist in the *m. pterygoideus medialis* of great apes, humans, nor probably in macaques. In humans we have noted convergence of the posterior-most aspect of the septa 6 and 4 ridges and their associated intramuscular septa and the variation in the consequent coalescence at that portion of the attachment site. Details of the relationship of the superficial portion of septum 2 (= 2^{III}) and its relationship to septa 6 and 4 are also provided. Further, we have provided observations on bony and soft tissue anatomy of humans which, in conjunction with Schumacher's (1962) descriptions of *m. pterygoideus medialis* anatomy in humans and great apes and those of Gaspard *et al.* (1973a, b) for humans and non-pongid anthropoids, point to significant developmental and phylogenetic differences between these taxa. It is important in this context to note that both Grant *et al.* (1980, 1981) and Benjamin and Ralphs (1995) state that detailed knowledge of the position at which a tendon inserts is of key importance to its function. Given Antón's (1994a, b, 1995, 1996) perfunctory approach to anatomical description, especially in light of detailed prior work (Gaspard *et al.*, 1973a, b; Schumacher, 1959, 1961, 1962, 1976, 1980), we consider her observations to result solely in the obfuscation of both interspecific and intraspecific, functional, and phylogenetically relevant anatomy.

Given these data we cannot support the claim of Hovers *et al.* (1995) and Rak *et al.* (1996) that the septal attachment sites referred to in the MPT character state differ from those defining a *tpi* (= septum 6, septa 6 and 4, or septa 6, 4, and 2^{III}); the septal attachment sites for the *m. pterygoideus medialis* are clearly homologs in great apes and humans. Variation in tubercle placement and shape does, however, reflect phylogenetic and functional differences in the *m. pterygoideus medialis* between these taxa as demonstrated herein and as discussed by Gaspard *et al.* (1973a, b) and Grant *et al.* (1980, 1981). We agree with Rak *et al.* (1996) that the septal attachments observed in subadults are homologous with those of adults (contra Creed-Miles *et al.*, 1996). We concur with Creed-Miles *et al.*'s (1996) observation, however, that numerous developmental factors impinge on ramal anatomy in subadults and that functional differences exist throughout ontogeny. Further, note that we have identified interspecific and intraspecific variation in the relationship of the septa 6 and 4 attachments relative to the *s. colli* and the relative extent of those structures. These potential differences in position or, alternatively, differences in relations to surrounding structures and potential differences in function throughout ontogeny do not, however, bear on the question of tubercle homology. Further, we have identified a variably expressed tubercle, the *tsc*, which is located slightly above the *tpi* in recent *H. sapiens* but which does not occur in great apes and which appears unrelated to *m. pterygoideus medialis* development. Given our observations on this area, we also cannot support the claim of Rak *et al.* (1996) that the *tpi* in recent *H. sapiens* is represented by a tubercle located above the MPT but inferior to or coincident with the *s. colli*. The latter clearly represents the *tsc*.

3. Summary

We have provided evidence to document ontogenetic factors involved in the production of bony anatomy in the region of the *s. colli-m. pterygoideus medialis* attachment site for great apes and recent *H. sapiens*. We consider these data to: (1) clarify issues in *m. pterygoideus medialis* tubercle homology; (2) clarify aspects of the ontogeny of these tubercles; and (3) undermine the functional arguments attached to the MPT character state. Further details related to the last point are provided below. Since the definition of a character state does not rely on ontogenetic or functional statements for validity (Lewis, 1989), it remains to demonstrate the viability of the character state in the absence of these additional statements.

IV. ONTOGENY OF MEDIAL RAMAL ANATOMY IN FOSSIL HOMINIDS

1. Medial ramus morphology of australopithecines

1.1. *Australopithecus afarensis*

In *A. afarensis* the *c. endocondyloidea* is strongly expressed posteriorly but by mid-ramus it becomes broad and flat excepting in AL 333-43b, 333w-52 and Mak VP-1/2 where it remains strongly expressed (Figure 8a-d). Comparison of specimens AL 333-43b and AL 288-1 shows ontogenetically the degree to which the *c. endocondyloidea* appears to be reduced and truncated in response to repositioning of craniofacial structures within early members of the hominid lineage (Figure 8a-b). Depending on ancestral condition employed, placement of the *f. mandibulae* appears to have been substantially (*Gorilla-Pongo*) or relatively unaffected (*P. troglodytes*) in the ramal reconfiguration. Relative to the *P. troglodytes* condition, *A. afarensis* specimens AL 288-1, 333-43b, and 333w-52 and Mak VP-1/2 and 1/12 present with a more vertical orientation of the *f. mandibulae*. In conjunction with this feature the anterior *s. colli* component is more vertically oriented and this results in an angular relationship between the anterior and posterior sulcal components (Figure 8a-d). Only Mak VP-1/83 retains a more posteriorly opening *f. mandibulae* and subvertical and linearly connected sulcal components. In this specimen the superior aspect of the foramen is: (1) positioned on the lower third of the *c. endocondyloidea*; and (2) associated with a small *l. mandibulae* which possesses a minimally developed lingular notch. The medial wall of the *f. mandibulae*-*c. mandibulae* is well formed and reaches to the level of the *s. colli* (Figure 8c). We consider this morphological pattern as consistent with that found in younger material but regard it as minimally meeting the requirements of a true *l. mandibulae*. Of note is that some Hadar and Maka specimens present with a third sulcal component, as a portion of the posterior aspect of the sulcus bends from subvertical to horizontal in the region inferior to the condylar neck (cf. AL 288-1: Figure 8b, d). The mylohyoid groove arises from the anterior-most aspect of the *f. mandibulae* and, although bridged in AL 288-1, is open in AL 128-23 and Mak VP-1/2, 1/12, and 1/83. The degree of prominence of the inferior *s. colli* border varies, with the Hadar specimens AL 288-1 and 333-43b being much more strongly marked than the Maka specimens (Mak VP-1/2, 1/12, and 1/83: Figure 8a-d). In these Hadar specimens the inferior border comprises the *c. intermedia* and *l. pterygoidea* and is continuous from the *c. pharyngea* to near the posterior ramal border. This morphology creates a superiorly open 'trough' for the contained neurovascular bundles in AL 288-1 and 333-43b (Figure 8a-b). This feature is less marked in AL 333w-52. In all Maka specimens the *s. colli* is extremely shallow whereas it ranges from shallow to deep in the Hadar sample (Figure 8a-d). Two factors are responsible for the observed sulcal morphology in *A. afarensis*. Sulcal depth is related to variation in positional relationships of soft and hard tissue primordia and soft tissue packing requirements whereas the strength of the inferior border is related to the latter and to the relationship of the *m. pterygoideus medialis* to the sulcus. The unusual strength of the *s. colli* border in the Hadar specimens AL 288-1 and 333-43b we consider to be related to development of the muscle. Because of the strongly developed inferior *s. colli* border and due to poor preservation of the medial ramus in *A. afarensis*, generally, only Mak VP-1/83 preserves an observable *c. intermedia* (Figure 8c). The *l. pterygoidea* in this specimen is continuous from the posterior ramus to the posterosuperior border of the mylohyoid groove. The *c. intermedia* lies *in* the *s. colli* above the *l. pterygoidea* (Figure 8c). Whereas the morphology of Mak VP-1/83 links it with later hominids this specimen also retains primitive features of the *s. colli*, as discussed. Although the Hadar and Maka samples tend to differ in *c. endocondyloidea* and *s. colli* morphology, these are most probably related to temporal differences and either or both idiosyncratic or sexual variation, as morphological overlap occurs in most mandibular features, as described in White *et al.* (2000).

Attachment sites for the *l. sphenomandibulare* (*s.l.*) are significantly altered in *A. afarensis* in relation to the great ape condition. Great apes present with a *c. intermedia* which: (1) is either long (*P. troglodytes*) or short (*Gorilla, Pongo*); (2) does not enter the *s. colli*; and (3) is only coincident with the *l. pterygoidea* in some individuals (Figure 7a-d). In *A. afarensis* the *c. intermedia* lies within the *s. colli* (Mak VP-1/83) or is incorporated into the *s. colli*'s inferior border with the *l. pterygoidea* (Figure 8a-d). Given these observations, the coincident nature of the *c. intermedia* and *l. pterygoidea* in some great apes is morphologically and functionally distinct from the hominid condition. Differences in the orientation of the *c. intermedia* and *s. colli* appear to reflect a reorientation of neurovascular and related structures and the attachment sites for the *l. sphenomandibulare* (*s.l.*) in hominids. Whereas these changes result in a repositioning, by anterosuperior rotation, of the *l. sphenomandibulare* (*s.l.*) attachment(s), with the exception of Mak VP-1/83 they do not present with a *tsc*. The absence of a *tsc* is especially curious in AL 288-1 and 333-43b as they have a significant Site 2 attachment for the *l. sphenomandibulare* (*s.l.*). Unlike later hominids the especially strong Site 2 attachment in these individuals terminates prior to reaching the posterior ramal border (Figure 8b). This morphology may be the initial resultant of the maintenance of a great ape-like ligament attachment pattern in conjunction with the rotational changes seen in the *f. mandibulae* region.

The relationship of the *m. pterygoideus medialis* attachment to the posterior component of the *s. colli* in *A. afarensis* is derived relative to great apes. Bony insertion sites for *m. pterygoideus medialis* range from weak (Mak VP-1/83, 1/12, and 1/2) to strong (AL 288-1, 333-108: Figure 8a-d). The subadult AL 333-43b presents with a weak septa 6 and 4 tubercle whereas the area is not preserved in AL 288-1 nor in

Mak VP-1/83. Although having weakly marked *m. pterygoideus medialis* insertion site both Mak VP-1/2 and 1/12 present with strong septa 6 and 4 (Mak VP-1/2) and septum 6 (Mak VP-1/12) tubercles, respectively (Figure 8d). Some lipping of the superior aspect of the septum 6 tubercle occurs in the latter specimen. Unlike great apes, this hominid taxon clearly demonstrates convergence and, in part, coalescence of the posterior-most fibers of septa 6 and 4 and the development of a space between the *s. colli* and the insertion site of septum 6 (Figure 8d). Significantly, both Mak VP-1/12 and 1/83 have small tubercles (= septum 8?) located between the septum 6 insertion and the *s. colli* (Figure 8c-d). This feature is present in most *A. robustus* and *A. boisei* but absent in our small and poorly preserved *A. africanus* sample. As noted for AL 288-1 the insertion site for septa 6 and 4 is missing and this is the only specimen which retains the inferior aspects of the attachment site. Under these circumstances, it is not possible to determine the degree of development of more inferiorly placed tubercles (= septum 2^{I-III}) relative to that of septa 6 or 4. With or without reference to the recently described Maka material and given the "...total morphological pattern..." (Le Gros Clark, 1964:16) expressed in *A. afarensis*, we cannot support the observation of Rak *et al.* (1994) that *A. afarensis* presents a generalized recent *H. sapiens* morphology.

1.2. *Australopithecus africanus* and *Australopithecus robustus*

Positioning of structures under discussion is similar in *A. afarensis*, *A. africanus*, and *A. robustus*. In *A. africanus* and *A. robustus* positioning of the *f. mandibulae* relative to the *c. pharyngea* is similar to *A. afarensis*. Although variably developed in the *A. africanus* specimens MLD 40, Sts 52b, and Stw 498 there is clear evidence of a *l. mandibulae*, as indicated by the presence of a medially extended tip and lingular notch (Figure 9a). The lingular region in Sts 36, however, lacks these features (Figure 8e). In *A. robustus* specimens SK 12 and 23 the *f. mandibulae* is positioned within a swelling at the base of the *torus triangularis* and this positioning results in or provides for a very minimal development of the *l. mandibulae*. In the developmentally young SK 64 and SKW 5 specimens a rudimentary *l. mandibulae* appears to be present. Confirmation of this condition in more specimens will clarify whether the *l. mandibulae* in *A. robustus* is: (1) developmentally similar to *A. africanus* but is subject to a different growth trajectory in later postnatal stages; or (2) more similar to the great ape condition. In all *A. africanus* and *A. robustus* specimens the medial wall of the *f. mandibulae-c. mandibulae* is well formed and reaches to the level of the *s. colli*. In *A. africanus* the combined *c. intermedia-l. pterygoidea* is less well developed and superoinferiorly concave, and the superior aspect of this ridge angles into the *f. pterygoidea*. In *A. robustus* (SK 12, 23, 64) the *s. colli* is superoinferiorly narrow and more clearly continuous from the *f. mandibulae* to the posterior ramal border. Further, the combined *c. intermedia-l. pterygoidea* is straight in *A. robustus*, excepting SKW 5. Neither a *tsc* nor a marked septum 6 or 4 insertion are present in either *A. africanus* (Sts 36 and 52b) or *A. robustus* (SK 12, 23, 64) specimens. Positioning of the superior aspect of the *m. pterygoideus medialis* is relatively high in these taxa, being similar to great apes, especially *Gorilla* and *Pongo* (Figure 8e).

The *A. robustus* specimen SKW 5 is similar to other members of this species in the features examined with two exceptions. In this individual a well developed septa 6 and 4 tubercle that is similar to those found in *Homo* is present. Further, the superior attachment site in SKW 5 is sub-triangular and well separated from the *s. colli*. The region between the *l. pterygoidea* and the insertion site is similar to other *Australopithecus*, but differs from *Homo*, by having a small secondary tubercle superior to the septum 6 attachment. This secondary tubercle is not a *tsc*. Further there is a slight separation of the *c. intermedia* and *l. pterygoidea* in this specimen but this configuration may be related to the subadult age of SKW 5.

1.3. *Australopithecus boisei*

The *A. boisei* specimens, Peninj and KNM-ER 729, document a substantial range of idiosyncratic variation in medial ramal structures. Neither specimen differs substantially from *A. robustus* specimens in *c. endocondyloidea* shape whereas only Peninj shares a *s. colli* configuration with this group. The *s. colli* region in KNM-ER 729 is more similar to the Maka *A. afarensis* material. A true *l. mandibulae* is not present in either of these specimens. Both *A. boisei* specimens have weakly developed *tsc*'s and small tubercles located between the *tsc* and the septum 6 insertion. Only Peninj preserves the region of the septa 6 and 4 insertion bilaterally and the region is weakly expressed and differentially developed on the two sides.

Some of the morphological changes observed in the medial ramus of *Australopithecus* are variable but clearly maintained in all later *Homo*. These changes consist of: (1) a reduction in medial extent of the *c. endocondyloidea*; (2) the development of a moderate to strong concavity in the middle of this crest; and (3) the development of a vertical groove at mid-crest, for transmission of neurovascular structures. Whereas we have noted significant intraspecific and interspecific variation in the *c. endocondyloidea* we will only detail specific aspects of this region in the remaining discussion. We consider it important, however, that changes observed in this structure be understood as part of a total morphological pattern which relates to the positional relationship(s) of the: (1) *f. mandibulae* complex (*c. mandibulae*, *l. mandibulae*, and lingular notch); (2) *s. colli* complex (*c. intermedia*, *l. pterygoidea*, and *tsc*); and (3) *m. pterygoideus medialis* (*l. pterygoidea*, intramuscular septal insertions, and general insertion area) on the medial ramus.

2. Medial ramus morphology of *Homo*

2.1. *Homo habilis* (sensu lato)

The *H. habilis* (*s.l.*) sample is limited to OH 13. *Sulcus colli* anatomy differs somewhat from that in *A. africanus* (Figure 9a-b). The *s. colli* is similar in being deep in the anterior component but in this specimen it does not broaden posteriorly. The preserved posterior component also differs as it appears to have been shallow and more horizontally positioned on the ramus. The *f. mandibulae* opens into a superoinferiorly elongate anterior component and when combined with an extreme anterior positioning of the foramen on the ramus results, in part, in the lack of a developed *l. mandibulae* and lingular notch (Figure 9b). It appears that the combination of an extreme anterior positioning of the foramen with an equally extreme vertical orientation results in the medial wall of the *f. mandibulae-c. mandibulae* being positioned below the inferior *s. colli* border in both OH 13 and *A. africanus* specimen STW 498 (also cf. KNM-BK 67: Figure 9a-c). The Olduvai specimens probably also differed from *A. africanus* in the possession of a *c. intermedia* which is not lineally coincident with the *l. pterygoidea*.

2.2. *Homo erectus* (sensu lato)

The medial ramus of *H. erectus* (*s.l.*) individuals reflects significant idiosyncratic variation which is most probably accentuated by geographic and temporal factors. Discussion of specific features in these individuals can best be accommodated in the following two groups: (1) KNM-BK 67, OH 22, and the Zhoukoudian material; and (2) SK 15, Ternifine 2 and 3, and Thomas Quarry 1. Aspects of the morphology of KNM-ER 992 are included in one or more of these groups as appropriate. Further, note that more general aspects of the morphology of these individuals are grouped for brevity.

Whereas the medial ramus is poorly represented in *H. habilis* (*s.l.*), preserved features of OH 13 show distinct similarities to those expressed in KNM-BK 67 and OH 22. Morphology of the anterior *s. colli* component in all these specimens is similar due to a vertical sulcal orientation (Figure 9b-c). The Zhoukoudian specimens, alternatively, have an anterior sulcal component that is less vertical and possess a *f. mandibulae* that opens posterosuperiorly. In general, the *s. colli* pattern is similar in these *H. erectus* specimens. The unique features observed in the *s. colli* of KNM-BK 67 appear to relate to a taller and more vertical ramus in that specimen (Figure 9c). In the Zhoukoudian specimens G1 (Figure 9d) and H1 the ramus is shorter and when combined with the posteriorly rotated *f. mandibulae* eliminates the potential for a secondary attachment of the *l. sphenomandibulare* (*s.l.*) as observed in KNM-BK 67. Whereas the superior aspect of the *s. colli* differs between the Baringo specimen and the Zhoukoudian material, the overall pattern is very similar. All these specimens essentially lack a developed inferior border to the *s. colli*. This results in a broad depression between the *c. endocondyloidea* and septum 6 insertion. The morphology of the *l. pterygoidea* is not clear in KNM-BK 67 but the Zhoukoudian material documents a pattern in which the *l. pterygoidea* is positioned inferiorly, running from the septum 6 attachment to the mylohyoid groove (Figures 9c-d and 10a). This pattern occurs in recent *H. sapiens* where there is a bifurcation of the maxillary artery associated neurovascular bundle. We suggest that the *s. colli* pattern observed in the Zhoukoudian material derives directly from the African pattern as represented by KNM-BK 67 and OH 13 and 22. We also suggest that this pattern is slightly modified by the presence of a simple variant of the normally occurring neurovascular bifurcation pattern which occurs at a high frequency in this population. It is interesting to note that in cases where the neurovascular bundle is bifurcated that the superior-most fleshy fibers of the *m. pterygoideus medialis* insert into ligament and not bone. This fact probably accounts for the strongly developed *c. intermedia* observed by Weidenreich (1936) in all adult Zhoukoudian specimens.

Morphological features of the medial ramus in SK 15, Ternifine 2 and 3, and Thomas Quarry 1 differ from other adults in this group although they are generally similar to those of Zhoukoudian G1 and H1 (Figure 9d-e). The *s. colli* differs between the Zhoukoudian specimens and the SK 15, Ternifine 2 and 3, and Thomas Quarry 1 specimens mainly due to the bifurcated nature of the sulcus in the former specimens. The latter specimens are more similar to the 'normal' pattern with the Zhoukoudian material presenting with a high frequency of a normally occurring variant of the neurovascular pattern and resultant bony morphology (Figure 9d-e). The Ternifine 2 mandible has a morphological pattern in the *s. colli* region which is more similar to earlier material. This specimen possesses a: (1) minimally developed *l. mandibulae* complex; (2) vertical anterior sulcal component with short, horizontal posterior component; and (3) *c. intermedia* which is not separate but which is incorporated into the *l. pterygoidea*, due to the posterosuperior expansion of the *m. pterygoideus medialis* insertion site. Thomas Quarry 1 is more similar to temporally younger specimens in possessing a: (1) more generally horizontal *s. colli* due to a longer posterior sulcal component; (2) clear separation of the *c. intermedia*, although it is still relatively vertically oriented; (3) separation of the septa 6 and 4 insertion site from the inferior border of the *s. colli*; and (4) more developed *l. mandibulae* complex.

A *tsc* is not present in KNM-BK 67 nor in the Zhoukoudian specimens, presumably because the *l. sphenomandibulare's* (*s.l.*) posterior attachment is coincident with the septum 6 insertion (Figure 9c-d). A *tsc* is not present in SK 15 but one is present in KNM-ER 992. Whereas the *m. pterygoideus medialis* insertion area is strongly marked in adult Zhoukoudian specimens they do not possess well developed tubercles. The septa 6 and 4 insertions are marked by slightly developed ridges within a larger depression which is bounded by raised bone (Figures 9d and 10a). On the other hand, both KNM-BK 67 and SK 15 show development of septa 6 and 4 tubercles. Medially directed tubercle expansion ranges from strong to moderate in the latter specimens, respectively. Because of the *s. colli* configuration in KNM-BK 67 and the Zhoukoudian material a separate and delineated space does not occur between the *s. colli* and the septum 6 insertion site (Figure 9c-d). The SK 15 specimen appears to show development of a space between the muscle insertion and the *s. colli* whereas one was clearly present in KNM-ER 992. Given the poor preservation of the inferior ramus in this group it is not possible to determine the degree of development of more inferiorly placed tubercles or depressions (= septum 2^{I-III}) relative to the septa 6 and 4 insertions. A composite of the right and left rami of KNM-ER 992, however, shows this individual to have relatively equally developed *m. pterygoideus medialis* tubercles. Based on our observations, we do not agree with Rak *et al.* (1994) that the *m. pterygoideus medialis* insertion in this specimen displays a typical recent *H. sapiens* pattern. The overall pattern of the *m. pterygoideus medialis* attachment in KNM-ER 992 is most similar to that of *Australopithecus* and early *Homo* excepting that it lacks the secondary tubercle situated between the *tpi* and *tsc* as seen in most *Australopithecus*.

Subadult morphology in *H. erectus* (*s.l.*) is preserved in KNM-ER 820, KNM-WT 15000 and Zhoukoudian B1 and F1. The latter two individuals range in age from 8.0 to 9.0 years. Expression of the *s. colli*'s inferior border ranges from strongly projecting in F1 to a lack of medial projection in B1. Mandible F1 resembles the condition generally seen in much younger human infants. An incipient *c. intermedia* is present in both B1 and F1 and divides the sulcus as in adults G1 and H1. In both mandibles a *l. pterygoidea* is present but only mandible B1 exhibits some prominence of the septa 6 and 4 insertions. As in many recent *H. sapiens* subadults a *tsc* is not present in either B1 or F1. The KNM-WT 15000 individual is developmentally aged at 10.5 years. Even though this individual's developmental age is close to that of the Zhoukoudian subadults, the morphology of the *s. colli* region is significantly different. Features of note are the: (1) strongly expressed *c. endocondyloidea* which lacks a midramal concavity; (2) shallow and anteroinferiorly slanted *s. colli*; and (3) poorly developed medial wall of the *f. mandibulae-c. mandibulae*. In these features KNM-WT 15000 differs significantly from the configuration in *H. habilis* (*s.l.*). Whereas hypertrophy of the *m. pterygoideus medialis* would most certainly result in a slight angular relationship between the anterior and posterior *s. colli* components, it is unlikely to result in morphological similarity to KNM-BK 67, SK 15, or Zhoukoudian specimens. We consider the morphology expressed in KNM-WT 15000 to be, in part, a direct resultant of a more posteriorly extended condylar neck, as noted in *P. troglodytes* and some *A. afarensis*. As in other *H. erectus* (*s.l.*) subadults a *tsc* is not present. The *m. pterygoideus medialis* insertion site is not well marked and the septa 6 and 4 insertions are only slightly developed.

Lingula mandibulae morphology is similar in KNM-BK 67, KNM-ER 820 and 992, KNM-WT 15000, and OH 22. Only minimal development of a lingular notch and posteromedially extended *l. mandibulae* occurs in these individuals (Figure 9c). This adds support to our hypothesis that these features reflect relationships between craniofacial components which are established early in the growth process. In this case, similarity between individuals in this age series indicates the absence in this taxonomic group of craniofacial relationships associated with strong lingular development. There is morphological similarity between the *l. mandibulae* of *A. africanus*, *H. habilis*, and these specimens (Figures 8e and 9a-c). Contrastingly, in both the Zhoukoudian subadult (B1, F1) and adult (G1, H1) mandibles the *l. mandibulae* shows strong medial projection in conjunction with strong expression of the lingular notch (Figure 9d). These specimens are slightly advanced in the morphology of the superior aspect of the *l. mandibulae* but they retain the more primitive morphology of the inferior aspects of the lingula. The general pattern in this and earlier taxa is one in which the *l. mandibulae* has only a minimal posterior extension in its inferior aspect (Figures 9d and 10a). Smith (1978) notes the possibility that mandible H1 possesses a lingular bridge. Considering the morphology of mandibles B1, F1, G1, and H1, it is clear that the *l. mandibulae* of H1 is not bridged. Whereas mandible G1 is slightly more developed, in specimens B1, F1, and H1 the *l. mandibulae* virtually lacks posterior extension and its posterior border is angled strongly anteroinferiorly. The latter morphology leaves a substantial portion of the medial wall of the *c. mandibulae* 'uncovered' by the *l. mandibulae* (Figures 9d and 10a). This morphology has been mistaken for a potential lingular bridge. Ternifine 2 and 3 and Thomas Quarry 1 present with *l. mandibulae* morphology generally consistent with that of the Zhoukoudian material (cf. G1: Figure 9d-e).

2.3. Archaic *Homo sapiens*

2.3.1. Morphology of the medial pterygoid region

In general, adult specimens assigned to our ArHs group (Arago II and XIII, Mauer, and Montmaurin 1) have the anterior *s. colli* component oriented similarly to that of *H. erectus* (*s.l.*), except it is slightly less vertical (Figure 11b-d). With the exception of Arago XIII which has a *l. mandibulae* morphology similar to that in *H. erectus* (*s.l.*), all individuals in this group (Arago II, Ehringsdorf F and G, Mauer, and Montmaurin 1) present with a modern pattern in this region (Figures 10b and 11b-d). This pattern includes: (1) a deep lingular notch; (2) strong medial projection of the lingular tip; and (3) a tendency for the superoinferiorly short lingula to be posteriorly extended at its inferior aspect. The posterior *s. colli* component in Mauer and Montmaurin 1 is generally similar to *H. erectus* (*s.l.*) whereas all others are more distinctly delimited (Figure 11b-d). Generally, the *s. colli* is now shallow but clearly continuous from the *f. mandibulae* to the posterior ramal border and restricted in its superoinferior extent on the ramus. Mauer differs only slightly from the basic configuration found in the Arago specimens due to an anterosuperior extension of the *m. pterygoideus medialis* into the region posterior to the mylohyoid groove (Figure 11b). Note that we differ from de Lumley *et al.* (1982) who consider the *l. pterygoidea*, proper, to be absent in the Arago specimens. Because of the *l. pterygoidea* extension in Mauer the inferior border of the *s. colli* is strongly marked, walled off from the *m. pterygoideus medialis* attachment region anteriorly, and, resultantly, presents as a more narrow and well defined sulcus (Figure 11b). A *c. intermedia* is present in Montmaurin 1 and possibly Arago II but one is not apparent in Arago XIII and Mauer (Figure 11b-d). In the latter two individuals the *c. intermedia* is most probably reduced as a consequence of the *l. pterygoidea* extending anteriorly into the posterosuperior mylohyoid groove region (Figure 10b). This extension probably displaced the function of the Site 1 *l. sphenomandibulare* (*s.l.*) attachment to the Site 2 attachment. This basic mechanism also appear to be present in AmHs and recent *H. sapiens*, although its rate of occurrence is higher in the latter and Neanderthals. Whereas no ArHs in our sample presents with the so-called 'Horizontal-Oval' (H-O) configuration to the *f. mandibulae*, as described in Smith (1976, 1978), its presence is confirmed in the Atapuerca sample. Although the absence of lingular bridging has been noted as an invariant trait of the Sima de los Huesos sample population (Rosas, 1997), it is clearly present in the AT-83 mandible fragment (Rosas, 1987, 1995; Rosas *et al.*, 1991). The overall frequency of this bridging type in the Sima population (Rosas, 1987, 1995, 1997; Rosas *et al.*, 1991) and ArHs in general is, however, currently low.

The *tsc* is variably expressed in the ArHs group, with all but Mauer and Montmaurin 1 having a small tubercle. Further, the attachment site for *m. pterygoideus medialis* extends relatively high on the ramus and we consider this to be related to the superoinferiorly short *s. colli* (Figure 11b-d). The *l. pterygoidea* forms the inferior border of the *s. colli* and is well marked in all specimens (Figure 11b-d). Because the muscle's insertion is superiorly and anterosuperiorly directed the relationship of the inferior *s. colli* border to the septum 6 insertion is such that a relatively broad area exists between the sulcus and the septal insertion site (Figure 11b-c). This intervening space was clearly filled with idiosyncratically expressed fleshy muscle and minor tendons. Expression of a tubercle at the septa 6 and 4 insertion ranges from very slight to strong in the following series: Arago II, Arago XIII, Mauer, and Montmaurin 1 (Figure 11b-d). Tubercle formation in Montmaurin 1 shows unilateral involvement of septum 2^{III} (left) and is at the maximum end of the size range, bilaterally (Figure 11d). Both Mauer and Montmaurin 1 possess developed septa 6 and 4 tubercles as isolates whereas this attachment in Arago XIII is not significantly different from the remainder of the *m. pterygoideus medialis* related tubercles (Figure 11b-d).

2.3.2. Population level variation in the medial pterygoid insertion
Although the Atapuerca, Sima de los Huesos sample population is not included in our observations, reference to figures and descriptions in Rosas (1992, 1995, 1997) demonstrates the range of variation in tubercle formation in a site specific sample of ArHs. In order of increasing tubercle size, specimens AT-604, AT-505, AT-606(?), AT-83, AT-607, AT-605, and AT-721 document a broad range of variation in tubercle formation at the septa 6 and 4 insertion site. This observation is further substantiated by recent observations on the degree of development of the *m. pterygoideus medialis* insertion site, varying from smooth to strongly developed, in the SH sample (Rosas *et al.*, 2002). Further, Lebel *et al.* (2001) observed that nearly 50% of the individuals in this sample possessed large tubercles in the superior aspect of the attachment site. The range of variation observable in this sample population is consistent with that present in ArHs (in general), Neanderthals, AmHs, and recent *H. sapiens*.

2.3.3. Subadult morphology
Ehringsdorf G is the sole subadult in the ArHs series. The anterior *s. colli* component is deep and relatively vertical in orientation (Figure 11a). The *s. colli* shallows markedly at mid-ramus, thereby creating a very shallow posterior component. The *c. intermedia* is not apparent but was probably similar to that considered to have been present in Arago XIII and Mauer. The development of a *l. mandibulae* and lingular notch is minimal. The *l. pterygoidea* has a strong anteroinferior orientation, similar to that in adult ArHs, excepting Mauer. There is a distinct *tsc* and a large, medially projecting septa 6 and 4 tubercle. This tubercle appears similar to those found in recent *H. sapiens* which are associated with strong tendinous attachment to periosteum. The direct insertion of tendon entheses into bone appears to have been minimal. In cases in which tendons insert directly into bone the cortex at the attachment site displays a dispersed series of shallow, eroded pits. The irregular contours of these pits would have been filled with fibrocartilage.

The ArHs group presents with a total morphological pattern which is only slightly modified in later groups. The general pattern is that found in Arago II and XIII and Montmaurin 1 whereas the Mauer mandible documents the beginning of a pattern modification whose components are then accentuated in some Neanderthals, AmHs, and many recent *H. sapiens*. This variant of pattern is related to: (1) *m. pterygoideus medialis* position and development relative to medial ramal bony and soft tissue structures; (2) the degree of development and extent of the insertion site of the *l. sphenomandibulare* (*s.l.*); and (3) the development of the *l. mandibulae* and medial bony wall of the *f. mandibulae-c. mandibulae*.

2.4. Neanderthals

2.4.1. Lingular and mylohyoid groove bridging
Morphological features of the *s. colli* region observed in Mauer are maintained in adult Neanderthal specimens, being only slightly modified in some individuals (Figures 10c-d and 13a-f). These Neanderthal adults differ from the configuration in Mauer due to ossification of that portion of the *l. sphenomandibulare* (*s.l.*) which: (1) extends

superoposteriorly from the *l. mandibulae* (= lingular extension); and (2) bridges the infundibulum of the mylohyoid groove (= lingular bridging). In these individuals this ossification pattern gives rise to the H-O trait (in part?: Table 4: Gorjanović-Kramberger, 1923-1924; Kally, 1955a, b, 1970; Smith 1976, 1978). As discussed by Smith (1978) the extended ossification front modifies lingular morphology but does not imply its absence (contra Creed-Miles *et al.*, 1996). This fact is evidenced by those Neanderthals which have been described as lacking bridging (McCown and Keith, 1939; Sergi and Ascenzi, 1955; Piveteau, 1959; de Lumley, 1972, 1973; Trinkaus, 1983; Goudot,1999 Condemi, 2001: Table 4) and those with bridging which retain a *l. mandibulae* (cf. Kebara 2, Zafarraya: Table 4). We differ slightly from Smith (1978), however, in seeing this process as resulting in modified function. Given the significance and extent of venous drainage positioned between the ramus and the *l. mandibulae-l. sphenomandibulare* (*s.l.*: Deplus *et al.*, 1996) and that the ligament is compressed during *m. pterygoideus medialis* contraction (Bremer, 1952), ossification of the ligament would appear to have a negative impact on venous blood flow, which relies on the contraction of adjacent muscles to promote flow. However, whereas this ligament has been suggested as functioning to: (1) directly (Posselt, 1952; Baragar and Osborn, 1984; Osburn, 1989) or indirectly (Osburn, 1993) maintain condylar head-glenoid cavity relationships; (2) limit mandibular over-closure in cases of high occlusal wear and tooth loss (Burch, 1966); (3) suppress movement of the mandible during jaw opening (Abe *et al.*, 1997c); or (4) have different functions within the spectrum of jaw opening-closing motions (Osburn, 1989) we consider its role in masticatory function insufficiently understood to discuss a possible modified function within that system. Of note, however, is the observation of Alkofide *et al.* (1997) that because the ligament is vascularized one can assume that it is not placed under constant tension as this would reduce blood flow within the ligament.

In part because of the variation in *l. mandibulae* length and bridging in Neanderthals, the observable *s. colli* varies from short to long (Figure 13a-f). Excepting Tabun C2 and Vindija 207, *s. colli* depth is very shallow. This finding is expected as the moderately deep anterior component is covered to a greater or lesser extent by the ossified *l. sphenomandibulare* (*s.l.*: Figure 13c,f Vs. 13b,d-e). In all Neanderthal individuals the *l. pterygoidea* is in linear continuity with the medial wall of the *f. mandibulae-l. mandibulae* and, resultantly, a *c. intermedia* is not apparent (Figure 13a-f). Excepting Régourdou 1 and Saint Césaire, all specimens have a *tsc*. The *l. pterygoidea* is well separated from the septa 6 and 4 attachment sites in all individuals and the overall relationship is similar to that observed in ArHs and recent *H. sapiens* (Figures 5a-e and 14a-f).

Based on our cadaver dissections, dry bone observations, and reference to anatomical dissections of great apes and humans by other authors we consider the mylohyoid groove-*l. mandibulae* bridging pattern observed in some adult Neanderthals the resultant of a single process, ossification of a ligamentous-fascial sheet. This process is brought about by two different mechanisms involving three anatomic regions and, most probably, by the positional relationship of the septa 6 and 4 attachment sites to the *f. mandibulae*.

We concur with other authors (Le Double, 1906; Dodo, 1974; Ossenberg, 1974a, b; Smith, 1976, 1978) that ossification of the *l. sphenomandibulare* (*s.l.*) results in both bridging of the mylohyoid groove (in part, superior aspects) and extension of the *l. mandibulae*. Although we agree with many of Ossenberg's (1974a, b) observations regarding the relationship of the mylohyoid neurovascular bundle to the *l. sphenomandibulare* (*s.s.* / *s.l*), we consider others only partially correct. We confirmed, by dissection, the observations of Alkofide *et al.* (1997) that the *l. sphenomandibulare* (*s.s.* / *s.l*) is organized in sheets and therefore allows transmission of neurovascular elements. Our observations are also consistent with the 'X-arrangement' of the ligament as detailed by Bossy and Gaillard (1963). The combination of these observations eliminates the need for Ossenberg's (1974a, b) arguments regarding the embryology of this ligament and its relations to the neurovascular bundles and Meckel's cartilage; the latter is detailed by Richany *et al.* (1956) and Bossy and Gaillard (1963). Further, the impetus for Ossenberg's (1974a, b) observations on mandibular embryology derive from her attempt to demonstrate that the perichondrium of Meckel's cartilage is the source of osteogenic cells which result in bridging of the mylohyoid groove-*l. mandibulae*. Whereas other authors (Smith, 1978; Lundy, 1980; Arensburg and Nathan, 1979) have not questioned the need for this correlation, we note that it is unnecessary as deep cervical fascia which envelopes the ligament derives from embryonic mesenchyme and, as such, possesses an osteogenic potential. In this context note that Sperber (1981) states that Meckel's cartilage lacks, or does not express, the enzyme phosphatase which is found in ossifying cartilages. He considers the lack of this enzyme to preclude direct ossification of the ligament, which derives from the perichondrium of Meckel's cartilage. This suggestion is supported by the observation of Ishizeki *et al.* (2001) that epidermal growth factor induced inhibition of alkaline phosphatase activity results in prolonged calcification of chondrocytes comprising Meckel's cartilage. However, the process appears more complex as Ishizeki *et al.* (1999) also consider it unlikely that chondrocytes in Meckel's cartilage are transformed directly into bone-related cells in the anterior regions of the cartilage which later becomes ossified. These authors did, however, observe such a transformation in the posterior parts of the intramandibular portion of Meckel's cartilage. Further, Benjamin and Ralphs (1998) observed that fibrocartilage associated with ligament or tendon entheses only develops within them by cellular metaplasia. They note, therefore, that the presence of endochondral bone or chondroprogenitor cells (*sensu* Hall, 1971, 1979) is not necessary for cartilage formation as tendon or ligament entheses can effectively function as 'growth plates' (Benjamin and Ralphs, 1998). Given the above, bone in the *l. mandibulae* region may form from: (1) deep cervical fascia (i.e. the *l. sphenomandibulare*, *s.l.*); (2) ossification of calcified cartilage derived directly from

Meckel's cartilage, its perichondrial remnant, or tendon-ligament entheses; or, most probably, (4) a combination of these sources.

We differ from Ossenberg (1978a, b) but concur with Yamano and Yamaguchi (1976) and Smith (1978) in recognizing two mechanisms which can result in mylohyoid groove bridging. The first bridging mechanism results in bony extensions from either or both the anterior or posterior borders of the mylohyoid groove. Ossification in this case begins in the intermediate layer of the *l. sphenomandibulare* (*s.l.*) and spreads to the medial layer (Figure 3a-d). The resultant of this ossification is initially observable as mediolaterally flattened extensions from the groove's borders. Coalescence of these extensions results in a smooth, flattened surface which can occur in small, isolated patches or result in complete medial closure of the groove (cf. Krapina 63). The second bridging mechanism is differentiated from the first as it comprises bony plaques which are not smooth and which are oriented perpendicular to the groove's long axis. The mechanism which results in the first bridging mechanism is currently unclear but ossification may result from tension induced in the ligament (*s.l.*): (1) during closure from wide gape for incisal function (Baragar and Osborn, 1984); (2) at full opening (DuBrul, 1980; Baragar and Osborn, 1984); or (3) due to idiosyncratic variation in positioning of craniofacial structures. In the first and second cases tension within the ligament may arise by either or both direct (i.e. ligament stretch) or indirect (i.e. *m. pterygoideus medialis* induced stretch) processes. As noted, consensus on *l. sphenomandibulare* (*s.s.* / *s.l.*) function has not been reached (Burch, 1970; Baragar and Osborn, 1984). Confirmation of the third possibility is complicated, in part, due to interspecific differences and intraspecific variation in cranial attachment sites for the *l. sphenomandibulare* (*s.l.*) as detailed by Zuckerman *et al.* (1962) and Burch (1970) and as noted herein for recent *H. sapiens*. The factors which drive the second bridging mechanism appear to be related to: (1) strong tendinous attachments for the anterior head or region of the *m. pterygoideus medialis*; (2) anterosuperior extension of the main mandibular septal attachments (septa 6, 4, and 2^{III}); and (3) fleshy attachments from cranial origins of the muscle. Further, it is probable that the second bridging type induces the former but this remains to be clarified. The second bridging mechanism also results from ossification of or within the intermediate and medial ligamental layers, but is supplemented by fibrocartilage induced by loads exerted on the ligament by overlying, round to ovate tendons and the subsequent ossification of this fibrocartilage. As discussed, we observed some individuals with substantial tendons (ca. ≤ 3.0 mm in diameter) running tangentially across the mylohyoid groove. These ovate tendons are attached along the center of their long axis by strong entheses to the fibroperiosteal layer which lines the *f. pterygoideus* and, variably, to underlying bone. In the latter cases we observed light to strongly marked bony lines in association with these attachments. Ossenberg (1974a, b) also observed these muscular bundles attached to and crossing the mylohyoid groove but placed no special importance on them. Abe *et al.* (1997b) found this to be a common pattern (65.4-69.0%) in their recent human male sample and Jidoi *et al.* (2000) consider these bundles to be involved in groove bridging. We are currently in the process of clarifying relationships of these musculotendinous bundles to the two heads of *m. pterygoideus medialis*, but it seems that many are related specifically to the anterior muscular head or region[1]. Given our observations and the known variation in distribution of the anterior muscular head or region insertion points (Abe *et al.*, 1997a, b) this mechanism can produce bridging throughout the length of the mylohyoid groove.

In the specific case of lingular bridging we believe that there are two processes operating either separately or in combination. The primary cause we consider to be related to: (1) either or both an expanded anterior head/region insertion of the *m. pterygoideus medialis* or a fleshy origin for cranial septa (relative to recent *H. sapiens*, generally) which inserts-originates from or near the septum 4 attachment site and which extends across the *l. mandibulae*; or (2) an anterosuperior extension of septum 4, or (3) an anteriorly conjoined septa 6 and 4 tendon extension which approximates or crosses the *l. mandibulae*. The latter observations are inconsistent with those of Smith (1978) but consistent with those of Barker and Davies (1972) and Ossenberg (1974a, b). Note that the normal situation is for a substantial portion of the *m. pterygoideus medialis* to be positioned over the *l. mandibulae* region but based on modern human dissections it is not generally considered to attach to this area. Positioning of the muscle over this region is not thought to have a direct effect on *l. mandibulae* morphology but it is worth considering bone formation to result, in part, from a response to muscle function (i.e. a bony response to pressure from muscle expansion-contraction). In the current context, we focus only on those tendinous or fleshy bundles directly attaching to fibroperiosteum-bone in the area of the *l. mandibulae*. Whereas attachment of muscular extensions can result in bone apposition at any point within the *f. pterygoidea* or along the mylohyoid groove, in the specific case of lingular bridging we currently consider the positional relationship of the septa 6 and 4 insertion site to the *l. mandibulae-f. mandibulae* as being critical. In cases where the septal insertion is positioned inferiorly relative to the *f. mandibulae* there is a greater likelihood that anterosuperior extension of these attachments will cross the mylohyoid groove inferior to the *l. mandibulae*, resulting in groove but not lingular bridging. This is the general situation found in recent *H. sapiens*, as confirmed by Jidoi *et al.* (2000). We will provide further evidence for this muscle's involvement in producing bridging in the discussion below. Further, note that the orientation of the above structures will also reflect more

---

[1] Further observations of these tendons shows them to be much more complex in strucutre. Tendons running from the anterior head or region of the *m. pterygoideus medialis* are round-to-ovate on their medial aspect but are flat on their lateral aspect. Whether these tendons represent a single 'key-hole' shaped structure or are, in fact, two separate tendons (one round-to-oval and one flat) which become fused (during ontogeny?) is currently unclear. See the Results section for further details.

general craniofacial relationships and that given our current level of understanding of *m. pterygoideus medialis* architecture the degree of importance of septal positioning in this relationship may be more illusion than fact.

In Neanderthals lingular bridging varies from absent to extensive (Table 4: Figure 13a-f). We observed a bony ridge extending the septum 4 insertion site into the *l. mandibulae* region in both bridged and unbridged cases, including Circeo III, Kebara 2, Krapina 53 and 59, La Ferrassie 1, La Quina H5, Tabun C1 and C2, Shanidar 2, Vindija 207, and Zafarraya. Morphology of the ridge extension varies from a relatively linear, triangular-shaped ridge (cf. Zafarraya) to a short, semi-circular arching ridge (cf. Kebara 2, Tabun C2: Figures 10c-d and 13d, f). Other specimens show less clear and more bulbous extensions into the *l. mandibulae* region (cf. La Chapelle, Saint Césaire) or do not show clear extensions (cf. Régourdou, Figure 13b). In the latter case we believe that the extensions were most probably less robust and fibroperiosteally attached. The Neanderthal subadults Teshik Tash and, to a greater extent, Roc de Marsal 1 exhibit well developed septal extensions on the anterior face of the septa 6 and 4 insertion (Figure 12a, c).

Table 4: Presence or absence of lingular bridging on Neanderthal mandibles[1]

Specimen	Lingular bridging	Specimen	Lingular bridging
Amud 1	Absent	La Quina H5[3]	Absent[1a]
Barakaevskaïa	Absent	La Quina H9[4]	Absent[1n]
Bourgeois-Delaunay 1 (La Chaise)	Absent[1p]	Le Moustier	Present[1c]
Circeo III (Guattari)	Absent	Régourdou 1	Absent
Combe Grenal III	Present[1e]	Saint Césaire	Absent
Kebara 2	Present	Scladina 4A-1	Absent[1j,o]
Krapina 53 (mand. C)	Absent	Scladina 9	Absent[1j,o]
Krapina 59 (mand. J)	Present[1c]	Shanidar 1	Absent[1f]
Krapina 63 (ramus 1)	Present[1c]	Shanidar 2	Absent[1f]
Krapina 64 (ramus 2)	Absent[1c]	Shanidar 4	Absent[1f]
Krapina 66 (ramus 4)	Present[1c]	Subalyuk 1	Absent[1a,k]
Krapina 67 (ramus 5)	Absent[1c]	Tabun C1	Absent
Krapina 68 (ramus 6/14)	Present[1c]	Tabun C2[5]	Absent[1h,i] / Present[1m,f]
Krapina 69 (ramus 7)	Absent[1c]	Teshik Tash	Absent
Krapina 70 (ramus 8)	Absent[1b]	Vindija 207	Present
Krapina 71 (ramus 9)	Absent[1b]	Vindija 226	Present[1d]
La Chapelle-aux-Saints	Absent	Vindija 250	Present[1d]
La Fate II[2]	Absent[1g]	Zafarraya	Present
La Ferrassie 1	Present[1c]		

[1] Our observations of *l. mandibulae-g. mylohyoideus* bridging are supplemented by those of the following authors: (a) Szabo, 1935; (b) Kally, 1955a, b; (c) Smith, 1978; (d) Wolpoff *et al.*, 1981; (e) Genet-Varcin, 1982; (f) Trinkaus, 1983; (g) Giacobini *et al.*, 1984; (h) Tillier *et al.*, 1989; (i) Tillier, 1991; (j) Bonjean *et al.*, 1994; (k) Pap *et al.*, 1996; (l) Lioubine, 1998; (m) Quam and Smith, 1998; (n) Stefan and Trinkaus, 1998a, b; (o) Toussaint *et al.*, 1998; and (p) Condemi (2001).
[2] Jidoi *et al.* (2000), citing Giacobini *et al.* (1984), indicate that the La Fate III mandible fragment presents with lingular bridging on the right side. This specimen does not preserve the *l. mandibulae* region (cf. Giacobini *et al.*, 1984; fig. 10). Since they list the La Fate II hemimandible but not the number III mandible fragment in their materials section it is possible that they are referring to La Fate II. However, as noted in Giacobini *et al.* (1984) the La Fate II individual does not possess lingular bridging and is a left hemimandible.
[3] An H-O foramen is noted as bilaterally present in La Quina H5 by Smith (1978) and Jidoi *et al.* (2000). Based on our observations we consider the *l. mandibulae* unbridged in this specimen.
[4] Jidoi *et al.* (2000), citing Martin (1926) and Piveteau (1964), consider La Quina H9 as presenting with a left lingular bridge. However, both Piveteau (1964) and Stefan and Trinkaus (1998a) note only bridging of the *g. mylohyoideus* inferior to the *l. mandibulae* in this specimen.
[5] The *l. mandibulae* is considered to be bridged in Tabun C2 by McCown and Keith (1939), Smith (1978), and Quam and Smith (1998) whereas bridging is considered to be absent or attenuated by Tillier *et al.* (1989) and Tillier (1991). See also Table 1, footnote 6, regarding the taxonomic status of this individual.

The secondary cause of lingular bridging is related to direct ossification of the *l. sphenomandibulare* (*s.l.*) which may or may not be induced by the *m. pterygoideus medialis*. Extension of the *l. mandibulae* varies idiosyncratically but the mechanism producing this variation is unknown. We suggest that lingular length results from a combination of genetic, epigenetic (*sensu* Atchley, 1993), or nonheritable idiosyncratic variation.

In attempting to correlate Neanderthal lingular bridging anatomy with that of recent *H. sapiens* it is necessary to consider the high level of idiosyncratic variation in this area (Patte, 1957; Larnach and Macintosh, 1971; Smith, 1978; Tuli *et al.*, 2000; Richards *et al.*, in prep.) and, specifically, in positioning of the *l. mandibulae-f. mandibulae* on the ramus (Simon and Kömives, 1938). We consider the latter relationship to be at least partially implicated in the documented low incidence of lingular bridging in many populations of recent *H. sapiens* (Ossenberg, 1974a, b; Smith, 1978; Arensburg and Nathan, 1979). It is of interest to note, however, that in a study of bridging in the Khoisan, Lundy (1980) found an extremely high percentage of lingular bridges (68.1%) in individuals with bridging.

In observations of *l. mandibulae* and mylohyoid groove bridging in recent *H. sapiens* subadults: (1) Ossenberg (1974a, b) considered both to be almost universally absent in ages below 11.0 years; (2) Smith (1978) and Lundy (1980) found no occurrences below age 17.0 years; (3) Sawyer *et al.* (1978) observed one case each at 6.0 and 9.0 years of age; and (4) Jidoi *et al.* (2000) found one case in a 9.0 year-old. In the process of other research Richards *et al.* (in prep.) have recently documented a range of lingular bridging, from incipient to complete, in subadults ≥ 8.0-11.5 years of age (Figure 10f-g). The latter pattern is fully consistent with the 'H-O' foramen morphology (Smith 1976, 1978) excepting that the foramen is more round than oval. A similar *f. mandibulae* shape has been observed in Neanderthal infants (Patte, 1957; Ferembach, 1970; Tillier, 1982, 1983b; Coqueugnoit, 1999), excepting in Madre-Dupouy's (1992) assessment of Roc de Marsal 1 where she notes it as being oval-shaped. Also note that Vlček (1993) states that the *f. mandibulae* is oval-shaped in the ArHs subadult Ehringsdorf G. The presence of round foramina is due to the immature status of the individuals and reflects normal development of the *c. mandibulae-f. mandibulae* as discussed by Enlow and Hans (1996). Given this observation it may be necessary to rename this character as the oval-shaped foramen is now applicable only to adults or possibly to immature individuals in the late juvenile period and adults. Of further interest is that horizontally positioned oval foramina are an extension of the morphology seen in vertically oriented oval foramina which occur in the absence of lingular bridging (cf. Amud 1; Suzuki, 1970; and recent *H. sapiens*). Given this fact greater understanding may be attained by examining the individual components of the H-O foramen complex. We do not expect lingular bridging to occur in individuals substantially younger than 8.0 years of age given that the region is undergoing significant posteriorly directed remodeling and because the *m. pterygoideus medialis* is not as developed as in adults. This is consistent with our observations, and those of other authors (Giacobini *et al.*, 1984; Tillier, 1986; Lioubine *et al.* 1986; Bonjean *et al.*, 1994; Lioubine, 1998; Toussaint *et al.*, 1998; Coqueugnoit, 1999), of the lack of mylohyoid groove-*l. mandibulae* bridging in subadult Neanderthals and in recent *H. sapiens* subadults aged < 5.0 years of age. We have, alternatively, observed recent human infants aged > 1.5 years of age to exhibit well developed components of the bridging complex which could give rise to bridging in later age stages.

Because we now have an ontogenetic sequence for lingular bridging we identify three anatomic regions and suggest three factors related to lingular bridges. First, there is high idiosyncratic variation in the extent of the *l. mandibulae* in recent *H. sapiens* (Coqueugnoit, 1999; Tuli *et al.*, 2000). Given this variation in *l. mandibulae* extent it is possible that some lingular bridges form from an expanded or extended *l. sphenomandibulare* (*s.l.*) ossification front. As an isolated process we consider this potential pathway to bridging as unlikely or to occur at very low frequencies. Secondly, a posteroinferiorly directed bony extension from the *l. mandibulae*-anterosuperior mylohyoid groove border may occur. In the overwhelming majority of *Australopithecus*, *H. habilis* (*s.l.*), and *H. erectus* (*s.l.*) this region of the *l. mandibulae*-anterosuperior mylohyoid groove is poorly developed (i.e. lacks posteroinferior expansion: Figure 9a-e). In *A. africanus*, *H. habilis* (*s.l.*), and the *H. erectus* individual OH 22 the anterior *s. colli* is vertically oriented and a narrow distance exists between the *l. mandibulae* and the *l. pterygoidea* which can be bridged by a developed *l. mandibulae*-anterosuperior mylohyoid groove region (cf. OH 22: Figure 9a-b). In all other *H. erectus* and ArHs the anterior *s. colli* component is either: (1) associated with a broad and deep posterior component (KNM-BK 67); or (2) a less vertically oriented anterior component and a broad distance between the *l. mandibulae* and the *l. pterygoidea*. Combining the latter with a *l. mandibulae* which in almost all cases angles strongly anteroinferiorly this results in the medial wall of the *c. mandibulae* being uncovered by the *l. mandibulae* (Figures 9c-e and 10a). The latter condition typifies the "Sinanthropus" material (Figures 9d and 10a). This morphological pattern creates a broad superior entrance to the mylohyoid groove and results in the need for an extreme expansion of the *l. mandibulae*-anterosuperior mylohyoid groove region before bridging can occur. In some ArHs and recent *H. sapiens*, all Neanderthals, and most AmHs the *l. mandibulae*-anterosuperior mylohyoid groove region is more developed and, as such, both covers the *c. mandibulae* and more closely approximates the *l. pterygoidea* (Figures 5a-e, 10b-g, 11b-d, 13b-f, and 14a-c). Extensions of the *l. mandibulae*-anterosuperior mylohyoid groove region can occur in isolation or as part of the bridging process as also observed by Jidoi *et al.* (2000). Thirdly, an anterosuperior extension of the *l. pterygoidea* may occur such that it reduces the distance between the *l. mandibulae*-anterosuperior mylohyoid groove region and the *l. pterygoidea*. Note that our use of the term 'extension' may be in error as it is probable that this is actually a restriction of the muscle's attachment region, as discussed further below.

This 'extended' condition typifies Neanderthals, most AmHs, and many recent *H. sapiens*. Note that many examples of the latter extension occur, however, without involvement of the *l. mandibulae*. It is, therefore, the combination of an expansion of the *l. mandibulae*-anterosuperior mylohyoid groove region and the anterosuperior extension (or superoinferiorly directed redirection) of the *l. pterygoidea* which we now consider to produce the vast majority or totality of lingular bridges. Specimens such as Vindija 207, Zafarraya, and many recent *H. sapiens* mandibles present particularly clear examples of this process (Figure 10c-g). This combination of processes may also occur in individuals with superoposterior *l. mandibulae* extensions, as noted above in some Neanderthals. When present the latter will merely contribute to the overall extent of *l. mandibulae* extension over the *s. colli*. Further, details related to the bridging process are provided in the morphological summary section below.

2.4.2. Morphology of the medial pterygoid region

In evaluating the septa 6, 4 and 2^{III} attachment sites in adult Neanderthals we divided the sample into five categories based on tubercle morphology and areal extent. Overall variation of the insertion sites comprised tubercles which were weakly expressed and indistinguishable from others in the attachment site to large, medially projecting, and isolated tubercles. The range of variation displayed in the Neanderthal sample is significant but well within the confines of that displayed in recent *H. sapiens* (Figures 5a-e and 13a-f). The latter fact was earlier noted by Billy and Vallois (1977) in a sample comprising La Chapelle, La Ferrassie 1, Malarnaud, and Le Moustier. Morphology of the septa 6 and 4 associated tubercles ranges from isolated septum 6 tubercles (Type 1) to more superoinferiorly elongated multiseptal tubercles (Type 2: Figure 13a-f). The most developed tubercles (La Quina H5, Tabun C2, Zafarraya) all show involvement of septum 2^{III}, although note that bilateral differences exist in the degree of septal coalescence (Figure 13e-f). Further, these tubercles all display significant variation in the overall development and degree of bony infilling between the septa (Figure 13c-f). Based on our recent *H. sapiens* data the latter observation means that significant variation was present in the degree of septal coalescence and extent of tendon entheses reaching the tubercle. Relative to Neanderthals, KNM-BK 67 and SK 15 present with septa 6 and 4 insertion morphology and development which lies between that expressed in Tabun C2 and La Quina H5 (Figures 9c and 13e). The ArHs specimens Ehringsdorf G presents with a Group four tubercle whereas Montmaurin 1 has a Group five tubercle which is nearly identical to that in Zafarraya (Figures 11a, d and 13f).

In Neanderthal subadults the anterior and posterior *s. colli* components combine to form a broad depression which encompasses the distance from the *f. mandibulae* to the posterior ramal border in Gibraltar 2 and Krapina 53 (Figure 12b). A more defined sulcus occurs in Roc de Marsal 1, Pech de l'Azé, and Teshik Tash but for different reasons (Figure 12a, c). In Roc de Marsal 1 the *c. endocondyloidea* is strongly expressed and overhangs the *s. colli* whereas in Pech de l'Azé it is the strongly developed *l. pterygoidea* which creates a more defined sulcus (Figure 12a). In Teshik Tash the sulcus is more defined due to developmental age (Figure 12c). The overall level of variation is similar to that found in Zhoukoudian B1 and F1 and recent *H. sapiens* (Figures 4a-f and 12a-c). The *l. pterygoidea* is coincident with the inferior sulcal border. This border varies from slightly to strongly developed in the following sequence: Gibraltar 2, Krapina 53 and Teshik Tash, Pech de l'Azé, and Roc de Marsal 1 (Figure 12a-c). Whereas the *s. colli*-mylohyoid groove pattern in all these infants prestages that described in adult Neanderthals which have bridging there is clear evidence showing that the pattern may be arrested at any point in its development (Figure 13b-f). In no instance is there bridging of the medial border of the *f. mandibulae*-mylohyoid groove region in these subadults (Figure 12a-c). This observation is consistent with the lack of bony attachment sites in the *f. pterygoidea* of these individuals. In these specimens the mylohyoid neurovascular bundle runs in a well defined groove (Figure 12a-c). The *l. pterygoidea* pattern differs from recent *H. sapiens* in being more consistently horizontally oriented. In many recent *H. sapiens* the *l. pterygoidea* tends to angle inferiorly prior to reaching the superior aspect of the posterior border of the mylohyoid groove. Ehringsdorf G presents with a morphology intermediate between Neanderthals and recent *H. sapiens* by extending the *l. pterygoidea* horizontally past mid-ramus prior to taking a steep anteroinferior course to the mylohyoid groove (Figure 11a). Significantly, Gibraltar 2 presents with a *s. colli* morphology (Buxton, 1928) that is unique for the Neanderthal group as it includes a short *c. intermedia* and a very lightly marked *l. pterygoidea* (Figure 12b). Subadults in the Neanderthal group all present with a *tsc* and septa 6 and 4 tubercles. The latter vary significantly in overall development of the tubercle and, resultantly, in the nature of the septal attachments. These insertion sites range from weak to strongly projecting for subadults but vary little in areal extent (Figure 12a-c). As in ArHs and recent *H. sapiens* the septum 6 insertion is well separated from the *l. pterygoidea* (Figures 4a-f and 11a).

2.4.3. Population level variation in the medial pterygoid attachment

Based on our observations, descriptions in Smith (1976), and figures in Radovčić *et al.* (1988), the Krapina mandibles (59, 63, 64, 65-68, and 75) can be shown to exhibit a weak to pronounced attachment site for the *m. pterygoideus medialis* and to present with a broad range of septa 6, 4, and 2^{III} prominence. Alternatively, the Shanidar sample (Shanidar 1, 2, and 3) all show highly developed *m. pterygoideus medialis* attachments (Trinkaus, 1983) with moderate to large, albeit variably independent, septa 6, 4, and 2^{III} tubercles. Whereas we are not currently able to fully document the morphology of the Krapina and Shanidar sample populations we consider these preliminary observations sufficient to demonstrate both septal insertion site variation in these geographically restricted samples and that the observable ranges are generally consistent with that occurring in ArHs to recent *H. sapiens*.

2.4.4. Shape characteristics of medial pterygoid related insertion tubercles

In defining the 'MPT character state' Rak *et al.* (1994, 1996) observed that in Neanderthals the MPT: (1) terminates in a distinct lip at its superior border; and (2) is not only prominent but also reflects a superiorly directed gradual increase in tubercle size. We assessed the first feature in 21 Neanderthal mandibles. We found the septum 6 insertion to: (1) lack superior lipping in 15 (71.4%); (2) have unilateral lipping in 2 (9.5%); and (3) potentially have bilateral lipping in 3 (14.3%) individuals. In the latter case only two specimens fully preserve the attachment site bilaterally (Figures 12a-d and 13a-f). We assessed the second feature in 20 Neanderthal mandibles. In subadults only Gibraltar 2, Pech de l'Azé, and Teshik Tash preserve relevant anatomy. Gibraltar 2 shows greater development of the septum 2^{I-II} tubercles in conjunction with moderate development of the septa 6 and 4 tubercle (Figure 12b). Pech de l'Azé is similar to the latter but lacks the degree of septa 6 and 4 development seen in Gibraltar. In Teshik Tash there is only slight unilateral development of the septum 2^{III} tubercle in conjunction with the developed septa 6 and 4 tubercle (Figure 12c). In adults tubercles inferior to those of septa 6 and 4 are either not significantly different from tubercles related to these septa (Amud 1) or are not developed to any real extent in Krapina 59 and 63, Tabun C1, and Vindija 207 (Figure 13a, d). In La Chapelle, La Ferrassie 1, La Quina H5, and Zafarraya there is variation in both the development of the septum 2^{III} tubercle and the degree of its inclusion in tubercle formation. In the latter cases note that the remainder of the attachment area is not as well marked (Figure 13e-f). Only in Kebara 2 and Tabun C2 is there clear evidence of a continuous but gradual increase in tubercle size from the anteroinferior aspect of the *m. pterygoideus medialis* attachment to the superior aspect of the septum 6 insertion site (Figure 13c). The latter range of variation is fully consistent with that observed in recent *H. sapiens*.

2.5. Anatomically modern *Homo sapiens*

In AmHs *s. colli* morphology follows a general pattern of being: (1) anteriorly deep; (2) shallow to very shallow posteriorly; and (3) relatively horizontal (Figure 14a-c). Only Dar es Soltan 5, Ein Gev I, and Omo-Kibish 1 deviate from this pattern and then only in the latter feature. Ein Gev 1 is the only specimen to present with a *c. intermedia* similar to that found in many modern humans. In all specimens retaining the feature the *l. pterygoidea* varies from weak to relatively strongly expressed and, with the exception of Ein Gev I and Haua Fteah II, is coincident with the *c. intermedia* (Figure 14a-c). The latter specimen is most similar to ArHs. This group differs from the basic configuration observed in most Neanderthals by the lack of bridging of the superior aspect of the mylohyoid groove. Although they lack bridging they present with a *l. pterygoidea*-mylohyoid groove relationship similar in pattern to Mauer, Régourdou 1, Saint Césaire, and Tabun C1 (Figures 11b, 13b, and 14a-c). Given the latter morphology, AmHs (excepting Omo-Kibish 1) differ from all ArHs except Mauer by having the anterosuperior aspect of the *l. pterygoidea* superiorly placed (Figures 11c-d and 14a-c). AmHs are essentially intermediate in the latter relationship between ArHs and Neanderthals. Extension of the *l. pterygoidea* to the mylohyoid groove results in a more linear and horizontal appearance to the *s. colli*. Observations of the *tsc* are limited due to poor specimen preservation but Border Cave 4, Haua Fteah I and II, and Omo-Kibish 1 lack the feature. In AmHs development of the septa 6 and 4 insertion site ranges from very weak septal associated ridging to moderately strong tubercle formation (Figure 14a-c). In general, tubercle expression in this group is less marked than that found in *H. erectus* (*s.l.*), ArHs, and Neanderthals. Relative to the latter group overall development of *m. pterygoideus medialis* tubercles in Skhul 5 is less than that in Amud 1 whereas that in Fish Hoek is similar to those Neanderthals in tubercle Group four. The septum 6 and 4 insertion site in Fish Hoek is generally similar to that observed in Ehringsdorf G and La Chapelle. Of note is that Dar es Soltan 5 presents with a septa 6 and 4 insertion region which is similar to Zafarraya in areal expanse and only slightly smaller that that in Montmaurin 1. Alternatively, in the latter specimens the septa 6, 4, and, variably, 2^{III} tubercles are at the maximum limit for medial extent of the tubercle whereas Dar es Soltan 5 is only slightly extended medially. We consider this example to underscore the complex interaction of soft and hard tissues in this region, as opposed to a species level difference.

Sulcus colli morphology of the subadult Qafzeh XI is similar to adult AmHs. Sulcal morphology differs bilaterally with only the right side showing the pattern arising from anterosuperior extension of the *m. pterygoideus medialis* attachment. Whereas there are differences in the overall configuration the specimen shows clear affinities with phylogenetically earlier sulcal anatomy. Comparison of the perilingual region (*sensu* Balogh and Csiba, 1972) in Qafzeh XI with that of Teshik Tash indicates the degree of similarity, although note that one must consider the developmental trajectory of the septal attachments, as outlined for recent *H. sapiens*, relative to the differing developmental ages of the fossils. The septa 6 and 4 insertions are differentially expressed bilaterally. Specimen preservation precludes confirmation of a *c. intermedia* but preserved portions leave little doubt that one was present.

2.6. *Homo sapiens* ssp. indet.

We have shown that medial ramal anatomy of the Amud 7 infant is consistent with that of Neanderthals and recent *H. sapiens* (Figures 4c-d, 12a-c, and 12d). Given the young developmental age of the Amud 7 infant and lack of similarly aged fossil specimens our comparisons focus on a large sample of recent *H. sapiens*. Based on our assessment of the ontogeny of the bony insertion sites of *m. pterygoideus medialis* we find no differences between the Amud 7 infant and our recent sample. The taxonomic status of the Amud 7 infant currently rests on: (1) the presence of a MPT; (2) the absence of a mental protuberance; (3) the orientation of the *incisura semilunaris*; (4) shape and size details of the foramen magnum; and (5) the presence of a pronounced occipital torus (Rak *et al.*, 1994, 1996; Hovers *et al.*, 1995; Rak and Kimbel, 1995). As an isolated feature, Rak and Kimbel (1995) note that the lack of a chin has little taxonomic value. The orientation of the *incisura semilunaris* in Neanderthals, while displaying frequency differences from other hominid groups, is not autapomorphic for Neanderthals (Jabbour and Richards, 1998; Jabbour *et al.*, 2002). We have earlier established that the foramen magnum of Amud 7 does not differ in size or shape from that of recent *H. sapiens* (Richards and Plourde, 1995). Whereas Creed-Miles *et al.*'s (1996) assessment of the latter feature supports 'aspects of this character state' further data collection supports our earlier findings (unpublished data). One could argue that the total morphological pattern present in the Amud 7 infant indicates a close affinity to Neanderthals. We suggest, however, that indications of close affinities are not sufficient taxonomic markers and that a random series of unrelated or only potentially related morphological 'traits' do not constitute "...component parts of a total morphological pattern of associated parts..." (LeGros Clark, 1964:16-17). Therefore, based on results of our published, current, and recently completed research we consider the taxonomic status of the Amud 7 infant to be *H. sapiens* ssp. indet.

3. Bilateral development of medial ramal features and the value of anomalous development for understanding observed medial ramus morphology

In assessing the septa 6 and 4 insertion site in recent *H. sapiens* we only considered bilateral occurrences to eliminate problems associated with structural asymmetries (Costa, 1986; Türp *et al.*, 1998). For fossil specimens ($N = 75$) this methodology was largely abandoned due to specimen preservation. In the fossil series only 13 (17.3%) individuals preserve relevant anatomy bilaterally. In nine (69%) of these individuals the septa 6 and 4 associated tubercles differed bilaterally in degree of development and number of septa involved. Significantly, tubercle formation restricted to septa 6 and 4 on one ramus was extended on the contralateral side to include septum 2^{III}, in many cases. The latter difference varied as to the side of expression and could be related to functional (masticatory?) or idiosyncratic differences in septal organization.

In their description of the developmentally malformed (hemifacial microsomia) Mamilla mandible, Nagar and Arensburg (2000) suggest that the *m. pterygoideus medialis* attachment is similar to that of Kebara 2, as described by Tillier *et al.* (1989). We agree that assessment of developmental abnormalities provides an important resource in craniofacial studies. Given our observations and those of Vargervik and Miller (1984), Nakata *et al.* (1995), Kane *et al.* (1997), and Vargervik (1997) on similarly affected individuals we do not, however, agree that the muscle attachment site in Mamilla bares a resemblance to that of Neanderthals.

SUMMARY OF MORPHOLOGICAL DIFFERENCES AND EVOLUTIONARY CHANGE IN THE MEDIAL RAMUS FROM *AUSTRALOPITHECUS* TO RECENT *HOMO SAPIENS*

I. DERIVATION OF AUSTRALOPITHECINE MEDIAL RAMAL MORPHOLOGY

1. Evolutionary change and revision of mandibular skeletal units

Assuming a *Pongo-Gorilla-Pan*-like quadrupedal ancestor it is useful to summarize the differences observed between *Australopithecus* and great apes. White *et al.* (2000) observed a significant anteriorly directed adjustment of the ramus on the mandibular body in *A. afarensis* relative to *P. troglodytes*. Our observations of the total morphological pattern in great apes and *Australopithecus* allow further comment on observed changes. White *et al.* (2000) clearly document the more anterior *extent* of the lateral mandibular ramus in *A. afarensis*. We believe this anterior extension to result from an increase in the size of the *mm. temporalis* and *masseter* that occurs in conjunction with a repositioning of the ramus (> vertical placement) relative to the corpus. Alternatively, we consider that the medial ramus was initially little changed in anteroposterior extent. Support for such a differential placement of the anterior extent of *m. masseter* relative to *m. pterygoideus medialis* can be found in Boyer's (1939) observations on *Pongo*. The degree of medial ramal reduction is, however, dependent on the ancestral condition employed as we have noted significant variation in the ramus to corpus relationship in great apes. Given these observations we believe that the skeletal units of the functional matrices which relate to the ramus (Moss, 1960, 1968; Moss and Renkow, 1968; Moss and Simon, 1968), need to be further clarified. We suggest that a distinction be made between the medial and lateral cortical plates which comprise the ramus inferior to the *c. endocondyloidea*. This distinction would require revision of the areas related to the coronoid, angular, condyloid, and basal skeletal units and necessitate further definition of the 'neurovascular triad' skeletal unit(s) (*sensu* Moss and Simons, 1968) related to medial ramal structures of the *s. colli* region. Given the morphology documented by White *et al.* (2000) and our observations of the medial ramus in *A. afarensis* we believe this subdivision and redefinition of skeletal units and related functional matrices will provide greater resolution of evolutionary changes.

2. Change in medial ramal morphology from the presumed ancestral condition

Australopithecus afarensis presents with medial ramal morphology similar to both *P. troglodytes* and to a combined group of *Gorilla*, *Pongo*, and some *P. paniscus*. The latter group has an *m. pterygoideus medialis* attachment area shape which is more similar to *A. afarensis*. We attribute this feature to a more vertical ramus and a shorter condylar neck region in *Gorilla*, *Pongo*, and some *P. paniscus*. The muscle insertion in *P. troglodytes* is more horizontally placed, generally. This arrangement becomes more apparent in *P. troglodytes* as muscle fiber hypertrophy results in a posterior ramal expansion. This expansion is 'allowed' by the presence of, or results in, a posterosuperiorly extended condylar neck region. The *Gorilla-Pongo* group also presents with a mylohyoid groove-*f. mandibulae* relationship (Straus, 1950, 1962) which is, on average, more similar to *A. afarensis*. Most *P. troglodytes* have a unique mylohyoid groove pattern relative to either *Gorilla* or *Pongo*. Alternatively, positioning of the *f. mandibulae* in *P. troglodytes* is more similar to *A. afarensis* than that observed in *Gorilla-Pongo*.

Derivation of *A. afarensis* medial ramus morphology from a *Gorilla-Pongo*-like ancestral condition superficially requires less morphologic change but the changes involve a repositioning of cranial nerve paths and, as such, are here considered more complex. Derivation of the morphology from a *P. troglodytes*-like template requires a reduction in posterosuperiorly directed condylar growth and a redirection of this growth inferiorly. Support for such a redirection is found in a correlation between condylar growth direction and glenoid fossa topography (Kantomaa, 1988, 1989) and evidence from the temporal bone anatomy of *A. afarensis*. Kantomaa's work suggests that a long, posteriorly directed condylar neck is associated with a shallow glenoid fossa whereas a short, vertically directed neck is associated with a deep glenoid fossa. Anatomy of the glenoid fossa in AL 333-45 would be consistent with the condylar-neck anatomy of Mak VP-1/2 as the glenoid cavity is generally flat and the condylar neck is elongated. Alternatively, AL 58-22, 166-9, and 333-105 have glenoid fossa shapes consistent with the less extended condylar necks of the remaining Maka and Hadar specimens. We consider these latter specimens consistent with a condylar to glenoid cavity relationship which reflects modifications in facial hafting in the absence of significant cranial base (*s.s.*) flexion.

Given a *P. troglodytes*-like ancestral morphology the initial changes, brought about by reduced posterosuperior condylar growth, document a significant reduction in the anteroposterior space available for soft tissues structures of the medial ramus. Laterally directed bending of the *c. endocondyloidea*, resulting in the development of a mid-crest concavity, and an anterolateral tilting of the *torus triangularis* all indicate a more superoinferiorly compacted relationship between the ramus and the pterygoid venous plexus, branches of the maxillary arteries and veins, associated neurovascular bundles, buccal fat pad, and parotid gland. This anterolateral expansion of superior ramus functional matrices appears to be in advance of that of the petrotympanic region (i.e. lateral expansion of the cranial base [*s.l.*]) skeletal unit(s). The resultant of the disjunction appears to create, for the first time, a 'splitting apart' of the medial wall of the mandible which gives rise to the *l. mandibulae*. The latter is associated with the more superior placement of the *f. mandibulae* relative to the *c. endocondyloidea* in *A. afarensis* and *A. africanus* relative to that in great apes and to lateral drift of this *crista* relative to the medial mandibular wall. The beginnings of this pattern are: (1) apparent but variable in the available *A. afarensis* sample; (2) more developed in *A. africanus*; and (3) more similar to the great ape (primitive?/derived?) condition in *A. robustus* and *A. boisei*. Development of the now functionally separate medial wall of the *c. mandibulae-f. mandibulae* in *Australopithecus* results in a medial wall which is well formed. The medial wall of the *c. mandibulae-f. mandibulae* in *P. troglodytes* is highly variable with some specimens essentially lacking the structure on the ramus proper. Further, in *A. afarensis* individuals AL 288-1 and 333-43b the posterior-most attachment of the *l. sphenomandibulare* (*s.l.*) is more anteriorly placed and appears to be intermediate between the condition observed in *P. troglodytes* and later hominids.

Changes in the *s. colli* and *m. pterygoideus medialis* insertion site are less marked and variable, ranging from more primitive (Mak VP-1/2) to more derived (AL 288-1). Relative to great apes we observed a greater association of the anterior and posterior *s. colli* components in *A. afarensis*, apparent in Mak VP-1/83 and most derived in AL 288-1. This more intimate relationship between sulcal components is driven by the more superoinferior orientation of the ramus, but not initially by a reduction in medial ramal width. Only AL 288-1 and possibly AL 333-43b are consistent with, but primitive to, the overall pattern seen in later hominids. Superficially the bony morphology of the *m. pterygoideus medialis* attachment site is less derived relative to *Gorilla-Pongo*, but slightly more relative to *P. troglodytes*. Using a *P. troglodytes*-like model, a substantial reduction in the posterior aspect of the muscle's insertion area is necessary but this must occur in conjunction with a presumed increase in, or maintenance of, masticatory muscle size. This reduction is brought about by restriction in extent of the superoposterior aspect of the insertion site and by a superoinferior extension of that insertion. Although the shape change differs, restructuring of the muscle's insertion area consequent to changes in cranial shape is consistent with data for muscle attachment area shape differences in dolichocephalic and brachycephalic humans (Mosolov, 1972). Note that this change requires modification of the corpus-ramus relationship as the inferiorly directed repositioning is not manifested as an elongation of the insertion site below the inferior border of the corpus. That such disjunctions can occur is readily apparent in cases of hemifacial microsomia. In *A. afarensis* the relationship of the superior extent of the *m. pterygoideus medialis* to the *s. colli* is essentially unchanged, but bony evidence for internal muscle architecture shows it to have differed relative to great apes. In *A. afarensis* there is clear documentation of a more inferior and anteriorly extended insertion of septum 6 and, possibly, septum 4 relative to the *s. colli* and a consequent commingling of the posterior-most aspect of these septal attachments. These changes create a space between the *s. colli* and the septum 6 insertion which is occupied by major-minor septa and fleshy muscle fibers.

Many of the changes observed in *A. afarensis* are continued in other *Australopithecus* species whereas other features of later *Australopithecus* appear to be reversals or are newly derived. In *Australopithecus*, exclusive of *A. afarensis*, the most significant development is reduced angular variation in the relationship between the anterior and posterior sulcal components. The general trend is to retain the vertical orientation of the *f. mandibulae* and anterior sulcal component in conjunction with a more consistently subvertical posterior component. Placement of the posterior component relative to the *incisura semilunaris* is also more consistent. Preserved portions of *A. afarensis* rami indicate a less consistent positioning of the sulcus in this group overall. We have also noted what appear to be homoplasies in the muscle attachment site for these taxa.

II. THE AUSTRALOPITHECINE - *HOMO* TRANSITION AND MEDIAL RAMUS EVOLUTION IN *HOMO*

1. Stasis and change in early *Homo*

An understanding of morphological change in the medial ramus inferior to the *c. endocondyloidea* in *Homo habilis* (*s.l.*) to AmHs is complicated by small and poorly preserved samples which are both geographically and temporally diverse. This problem could be exacerbated by the inclusion of multiple taxa in the species or groups examined. Further, an examination of the extensive range of variation present in recent *H. sapiens* suggests that extreme caution be employed in plotting the evolutionary trajectory of this region. Noting these cautions we summarize the basic pattern of change found in *Homo*.

Given the morphology observed in *Australopithecus* it is only *A. africanus* which clearly presents with medial ramal anatomy similar to that of *H. habilis* (Figure 9a-b). The former taxon shares the following with *H. habilis*: (1) weak medial projection and strong laterally directed concavity of the *c. endocondyloidea*; (2) development of a weak *l. mandibulae* and associated lingular notch; (3) positioning of the superior opening of the *f. mandibulae* on the *c. endocondyloidea*, as opposed to beneath it; (4) positioning of the *f. mandibulae* in close proximity to the *c. pharyngea*; (5) a deeply depressed and nearly vertical orientation to the anterior component of the *s. colli* and *c. intermedia*; and (6) a *l. pterygoidea* which extends relatively horizontally from the posterior ramal border to the mylohyoid groove. Although the orientation of the *linea* cannot be fully assessed in *H. habilis*, it is important to note that the superior extent of the *l. pterygoidea* in *Australopithecus* is coincident or superior to the level of the *l. mandibulae*.

2. Early *Homo* to *Homo erectus* (*sensu lato*)

Some of the morphological features seen in these earlier taxa are consistent with those expressed in early African *H. erectus* (*s.l.*) while others are more similar to later *Homo*. As discussed, KNM-BK 67 preserves features 1-5 above but displays a unique configuration of the posterior *s. colli* component (Figure 9c). Whether this pattern was present in earlier members of the genus *Homo* cannot be discerned from available material. Both KNM-WT 15000 and SK 15 share features 2 and 3 with KNM-BK 67. The West Turkana specimen differs from SK 15 in the greater development of the *c. endocondyloidea*, although this level of difference is seen in later taxa (cf. Qafzeh XI Vs. Skhul 5). Both KNM-WT 15000 and SK 15 possess an anterior *s. colli-f. mandibulae* complex which is not as vertically oriented nor as anteriorly positioned as in KNM-BK 67 and OH 13 and 22. The KNM-WT 15000 individual is unique in presenting with a strongly demarcated, linear, and narrow *s. colli*. The *s. colli* is not well preserved in SK 15. The *m. pterygoideus medialis* insertion site is variable, having an extensive attachment to the *l. sphenomandibulare* (*s.l.*) in KNM-BK 67, a more horizontal orientation in KNM-WT 15000, and a superoinferiorly long but anteroposteriorly narrow shape in KNM-ER 992. The condition in KNM-BK 67 and KNM-ER 992 is the most consistent with both earlier and later material. In all these specimens, however, note that the superior extent of the *m. pterygoideus medialis* is at or well above the level of the *l. mandibulae*. Changes observed in the insertion sites for *m. pterygoideus medialis* septa in *A. afarensis* are consistent with this specimen group. These *H. erectus* (*s.l.*) individuals differ from *Australopithecus*, except for SKW 5, in possessing septa 6 and 4 tubercles which obtain a markedly greater anteroposterior and superoinferior extent. Expression of a *c. intermedia* is variable in this group due to variation in the orientation of the *s. colli-f. mandibulae* complex but ranges from clearly present to fully incorporated into the *l. pterygoidea*.

The morphological pattern in the remaining *H. erectus* (*s.l.*) sample (Ternifine 2-3, Thomas Quarry 1, Zhoukoudian B1, F1, G1, and H1) is more similar to later *Homo* than the above specimen group. Changes in orientation and morphology of the *c. endocondyloidea* and position of the *f. mandibulae* relative to it occurred in *Australopithecus* and, although significant differences probably exist, the general pattern is essentially unchanged. It is clear that these modifications arise in relation to soft tissue packing requirements in response to changes in craniofacial hafting and positioning (i.e. anteroposterior shortening and superoinferior height increase). In this group of specimens the *f. mandibulae* and anterior component of the *s. colli* are rotated posteroinferiorly and, as such, open and are positioned more horizontally, respectively. The Zhoukoudian material is less derived in these features, retaining a slightly more vertically opening *f. mandibulae* and broadly open posterior *s. colli*. The latter is probably due, however, to both the retention of a primitive pattern in the posterior *s. colli*, as expressed in KNM-BK 67, and the possession of a normal neurovascular variant. A *c. intermedia* is not unique to the Zhoukoudian material but adults in this population do present with a high frequency (100%: Weidenreich, 1936) of a normally occurring variant of this structure (Figure 10a). The *s. colli* orientation and *f. mandibulae* position in Ternifine 2-3 and Thomas Quarry 1 display some primitive aspects but are within the morphological boundaries of later *Homo*. The morphology of the *l. mandibulae* and lingular notch are relatively unchanged in the above specimens from the *Australopithecus* pattern whereas the Zhoukoudian material presents with a significant medial extension of the lingular tip and a deepening of the notch (Figure 9d-e). In these features they are more similar to recent *H. sapiens* than available ArHs, Neanderthals, and AmHs individuals. It is in this taxonomic group that the *c. mandibulae* 'appears from under' the *l. mandibulae* (Figure 10a). We attribute this feature, in part, to a posteroinferior rotation of the *c. mandibulae-f. mandibulae* complex. This change occurs in conjunction with medial extension of the *l. mandibulae* but we do not necessarily consider them as related events. Features of the *m. pterygoideus medialis* insertion do not differ from other *H. erectus* specimens in our sample and all are essentially similar to the recent *H. sapiens* condition or variants thereof. Two exceptions to the latter are, however, the: (1) apparent drifting of the *l. pterygoidea* posteroinferiorly away from the superior aspect of the mylohyoid groove; and (2) appearance of large septa 6 and 4 tendon bundles which insert into a combination of depressions and ridges. We provide further discussion of this situation below.

3. *Homo erectus* (*sensu lato*) to Archaic *Homo sapiens*

The total morphological pattern expressed in our ArHs sample is little changed from that in the Zhoukoudian, Ternifine, and Thomas Quarry specimens. Of note is that the *l. mandibulae* and its associated notch are not as well developed in Ehringsdorf F and G and Arago XIII as in the Zhoukoudian material. Alternatively, Arago II, Mauer, and Montmaurin 1 do express a modern pattern (Figures 9c-e and 11b-d). The anterior and posterior *s. colli* components are also now, generally, in linear continuity and are shallow. Further, there is the beginning of a trend toward an anterosuperior positioning of the *l. pterygoidea* such that it reduces the infundibulum of the superior mylohyoid groove. Arago XIII presents with an incipient version of this pattern whereas Mauer has a horizontal *l. pterygoidea* in linear continuity with the base of the *f. mandibulae* (Figures 10b and 11b-c). As in earlier groups the expression of a *c. intermedia* is variable and dependant on the relationship of the *l. pterygoidea* to the *f. mandibulae* base. A significant difference occurs in this group relative to earlier ones as the septa 6, 4, and, variably, 2^{III} insertions are generally more strongly marked by tubercles. It is clear that individuals in this group document the beginnings of a pattern wherein the *l. pterygoidea* is positioned anterosuperiorly such as to become coincident with the entire length of the inferior border of the *s. colli* and to eliminate the infundibulum of the mylohyoid groove. Note that it is currently unclear whether this pattern results from an anterosuperior extension of the insertion site or from a posteroinferiorly directed repositioning of the insertion consequent to muscle size reduction. These changes occur as part of a total morphological pattern which includes an increased incidence of developed septa 6, 4, and 2^{III} insertion sites and the shift to a *s. colli* which is shallow and horizontally oriented along the inferior aspect of the *c. endocondyloidea*.

Recently, Lebel *et al.* (2001) determined that a prominent superior medial pterygoid tubercle was present in the Bau de l'Aubesier mandible and in 50% ($N = 8$) of European Middle Pleistocene specimens dating to between 300-500 ka. This sample comprises, in the main, material from the Sima de los Huesos, Atapuerca. Such occurrence rates would appear to support our above suggestions. In our discussion of this sample population we note, however, that there is a broad range of variation in the expression of the septum 6 and 4 insertion sites and in the *m. pterygoideus medialis* insertion site in general. Lebel *et al.* (2001) do not reference a definition of the character they are examining but only indicate that the feature, superior medial pterygoid tubercle, is a prominent tubercle resulting from hypertrophy of the superior *m. pterygoideus medialis* insertion. Given our assessment of photographs of this region for the Sima de los Huesos sample it is clear that Lebel *et al.* (2001) employ criteria for delineation of this character state which differ from those employed by Rak *et al.* (1994, 1996) for definition of the MPT character state. In the absence of a clear definition of the character state/feature under consideration it is not possible to employ the results of Lebel *et al.* (2001) in taxonomic or phylogenetic studies.

4. Archaic *Homo sapiens* and Neanderthals

Morphological features of the medial ramus in Neanderthal specimens are essentially a continuation of processes documented in ArHs. The most significant differences appearing in the Neanderthal medial ramus relate to changes in the *l. mandibulae* and anterior component of the *s. colli* and in the insertion site of the *m. pterygoideus medialis*. In this group, generally, the lingular tip does not strongly project medially and the lingular notch is not well developed. These features combine to give the *f. mandibulae* a compressed oval shape and when combined with extension of the *l. mandibulae* result in the H-O foramen trait. Modifications of the *l. mandibulae* are apparent in both its posterior extent and in the further development and extension of its inferoposterior aspect. The former extension covers the anterior component of the *s. colli* whereas the latter extension covers the medial wall of the *c. mandibulae*, and in some cases extends over the mylohyoid groove (Figure 13a-f). This expanded bone from the anterior *s. colli-l. mandibulae* complex occurs in concert with a higher frequency of anterosuperior positioning of the *l. pterygoidea*. As discussed above, these two components are involved in bridging of the superior aspect of the mylohyoid groove. We have also documented the extension of *m. pterygoideus medialis* related insertion sites into this area (Figures 10c-d, 12a, and 13d, f). That a total morphological pattern which may result in mylohyoid groove-*l. mandibulae* bridging can be present early in postnatal development is demonstrated by the fact that the Ehringsdorf G juvenile, all infant and juvenile Neanderthals, excepting Gibraltar 2, and many recent human infants and juveniles express development of the basic features of this complex (Figures 10g, 11a, 12a-c). Note, however, that the apparent homogeneity of expression of these features in most subadult Neanderthals results in a heterogeneous expression in adults, as discussed above and observed by Coqueugnoit (1999).

Whereas it is tempting to suggest that these features and the known presence of strong septal attachments in Neanderthals (Boule 1911-1913; Boule and Vallois, 1957; Patte, 1958; Heim, 1974, 1976; Trinkaus, 1983; Tillier *et al.*, 1989) documents an anterosuperior expansion of the *m. pterygoideus medialis* into the *l. mandibulae* region and an increase in muscle strength, we believe that other possibilities exist. This results from the potential that KNM-

BK 67 and the Zhoukoudian material possessed a *m. pterygoideus medialis* insertion which was superiorly and anteriorly expanded relative to later *Homo*. This expanded insertion appears to have involved the *l. sphenomandibulare*'s (*s.l.*) mandibular attachment, forcing it superiorly relative to that in recent *H. sapiens*. If such is the case we consider it likely that the pattern observed in Neanderthals is the result of: (1) further changes in craniofacial hafting in these hominids; (2) resultant changes in positioning of soft tissue matrices and their associated medial ramal skeletal units; and (3) a reduction in overall size of the *m. pterygoideus medialis* such that the muscle portions become more intimately related to the *l. mandibulae* region.

Alternatively, one could also suggest that the presence of a MPT in Neanderthals documents the occurrence of muscular hypertrophy. Curiously, however, neither Rak *et al.* (1994, 1996) nor Creed-Miles *et al.* (1996) provide details of variation in expression of the MPT character nor in the frequency at which it occurs in Neanderthals. Antón (1996) provides such values but we have earlier shown these to inaccurately reflect tubercle morphology (size and shape). Quam and Smith (1998) observed that the MPT is variably developed in Neanderthals but 'clearly' present in 70% ($N = 10$) of individuals examined. Coqueugnoit (1999) assessed the range of development of tubercles and crests associated with the *m. pterygoideus medialis* in recent *H. sapiens* and Neanderthals. Frequency values for her subadult series ($N = 8$) indicate that 62.5% of Neanderthal infants present with a MPT whereas 63.6% of recent *H. sapiens* subadults present with a *tpi*. Given our assessment of the medial ramus it is difficult to interpret these results. Lebel *et al.* (2001) suggest that hypertrophy of the superior *m. pterygoideus medialis* insertion occurs in 71.4% ($N = 7$) and 81.3% ($N = 16$) of 'pre-Neanderthals' and 'Neanderthals', respectively. Since these two categories mostly comprise what we have here considered Neanderthals the occurrence rate would be 78.3% ($N = 23$). Based on our observations it is clear that Antón (1996), Quam and Smith (1998), Lebel *et al.* (2001), and, probably, Creed-Miles *et al.* (1996) did not adhere to the definition of the MPT character state (Rak *et al.*, 1994, 1996) in deriving their frequency values. One should note, however, that specimens considered to possess a MPT by Rak *et al.* (1994, 1996) also violate the stated definition of a MPT, as fully detailed above. Alternatively, we have shown that: (1) the range of variation observable in the septa 6, 4, and 2^{lll} insertion sites in Neanderthals is consistent with that seen in recent *H. sapiens*; (2) there is a clear reduction in the overall extent and degree of development in the *m. pterygoideus medialis* insertion site within *Homo* through time; and (3) there is not a clear correlation between the degree of tubercle development and muscle hypertrophy, as shown above and discussed further below.

Creed-Miles *et al.* (1996) suggest that a reduced gonial region and highly excavated *f. pterygoidea* in classic Neanderthals are related to the presence of a MPT in this group. They also suggest that deep excavation of the *f. pterygoidea* can be related to strong "...remodeling activity (resorption)..." of the medial ramus and that the cause of this remodeling activity must be considered prior to proposing functional interpretations of the region (Creed-Miles *et al.*, 1996:152). Because of similarity in *m. pterygoideus medialis* insertion and *f. mandibulae-s. colli* region morphology in Saint Césaire, which has an obtusely oriented gonial angle, and Zafarraya, which has an acute angle, it is apparent that gonial angle shape is not necessarily related to observed tubercle morphology. Further, we do not believe that bony *f. pterygoidea* shape characteristics (topography) result solely from resorptive activity. The complexity of remodeling activities involving the medial ramus is broadly discussed by Enlow (1965), Hoyte and Enlow (1966), and Enlow and Hans (1996). Shape characteristics of bone reflect a combination of associated soft tissue anatomy and biomechanical and phylogenetic constraints under which the bone develops as experimentally demonstrated by Moss and Rankow (1968). We do, however, concur with Creed-Miles *et al.* (1996) that an understanding of remodeling activity is a necessary component of any attempt to delineate features / character states of bone.

We provide new observations with which to evaluate the development of the H-O foramen character state. It is of interest, however, to examine its suggested frequency of occurrence and value as a taxonomic marker (Table 4). Smith (1978) tabulated the percentage occurrence of the H-O foramen, finding it present in 46.2% ($N = 26$) of Neanderthals and in 23.1% ($N = 13$) of European Upper Paleolithic specimens. His samples reflect the total number of observable foramina in both juveniles and adults. Considering only the trait as present or absent in individuals and only sampling adults, it is present in only 36.4% ($N = 8$) of his Neanderthal sample. Trinkaus (1983) found the H-O trait to occur in 61.5 % of adult European Neanderthal individuals ($N = 13$). Frayer (1992) recalculated Smith's (1978) data to eliminate most subadults and determine the number of H-O foramina present per individual. He also applied this method to his determination of the percentage of occurrence of the trait in Early and Late Upper Paleolithic populations. He found the H-O trait to be present in 52.6% ($N = 19$) of Neanderthals and 44.4% ($N = 9$) and 5.3% ($N = 38$) of Early and Late Upper Paleolithic European populations, respectively. An occurrence rate of 41.7% and 26.7% in European late archaic (Neanderthal) and early modern human individuals, respectively, was calculated by Stefan and Trinkaus (1998b; E. Trinkaus, pers. com.). Recently, Jidoi *et al.* (2000) found the H-O trait to occur in 51.7% ($N = 29$) of Neanderthal foramina. The latter value is the percentage occurrence of their 'total bridging pattern' (= presence of *l. mandibulae* and mylohyoid groove bridging). If one only considers the percentage occurrence in individual Neanderthal specimens the value is 48% ($N = 25$). Lebel *et al.* (2001) determined lingular bridging to be present in 50.0% ($N = 11$) of specimens dating to between 300-100 ka and in 42.9% ($N = 21$) of those dating to between 100-28 ka. These groups they designate as 'pre-Neanderthal' and 'Neanderthal', respectively. We observed that 33.3% (12/36: this value does not include Tabun C2; see Table 4, footnote 5) of Neanderthal individuals possess superior mylohyoid groove-*l. mandibulae* bridging (H-O foramen). However, removal of the Krapina (50% occurrence) and Vindija (100% occurrence) specimens from this group results in only five of 23 Neanderthals (21.7%) with such bridging. In this context note that the 'pre-Neanderthal' sample of Lebel *et al.* (2001) comprises mostly Krapina individuals.

The H-O foramen has been variously considered: (1) as a Neanderthal autapomorphy (Stringer, 1982; Stringer *et al.*, 1984); (2) as failing the criteria for a synapomorphy in Neanderthals (*sensu* Habgood, 1989); and (3) as not being an ancestral condition (plesiomorphic: Smith, 1978; Lebel *et al.*, 2001). Lieberman (1995) included the H-O foramen in an assessment of character states, finding it to violate his tests for both homology and character state polarity. As one of his criteria for rejection he notes, however, that the H-O foramen morphology, as described by Smith (1978), is present in 58% of *P. troglodytes* examined. We find this observation curious given our understanding of the processes and morphology which result in the H-O foramen morphology. Specifically we note that his observation is incompatible with: (1) the relationship of the mylohyoid groove to the *f. mandibulae* in *P. troglodytes*, as noted by Straus (1950, 1962) and ourselves; (2) the relationship of the *s. colli-f. mandibulae* to the *m. pterygoideus medialis* insertion in *P. troglodytes*, as discussed herein; and (3) the fact that non-human anthropoids differ from hominids in the *absence* of a *l. mandibulae*, as previously observed by Weidenreich (1936). In a recent assessment of mandibular discrete traits Stefan and Trinkaus (1998b:462-3) determined that only the H-O foramen relative to: (1) *f. mentale* and *incisure* crest position; (2) presence of a retromolar space and angular notch; and (3) *incisure semilunaris* shape can be considered a "...primary biological trait...". Based on our observations we consider mylohyoid groove and *l. mandibulae* bridging the resultant of both isolated and multiple ossification events driven by both related and unrelated idiosyncratic, epigenetic (*sensu* Atchley, 1993), and biomechanical processes. Given this position we differ from Jidoi *et al.* (2000) who consider it acceptable to consider bridging of these structures as a single trait and see only a small effect of environmental factors in producing the H-O morphology. Our multiple origins hypothesis helps explain the broad range of opinions regarding the status of the character and provides a basis for greater resolution of incidence rates.

Further, Smith (1978) observed Upper Pleistocene hominids to possess aspects of a strong masticatory complex and to exhibit a relatively high frequency of *l. mandibulae* bridging (H-O foramen) compared to recent humans. His observations are consistent with the hypothesis of a significant reduction in both heads of the *m. pterygoideus medialis* in Middle Pleistocene to recent *Homo*. Gaspard *et al.* (1973b) determined that reduction of this muscle most likely occurred in the anterior portion and in the superficial layer of the posterior portion (see also below). Such a reduction in muscle mass is also consistent with a reduction in anterior ramus size consequent to *mm. temporalis* and *masseter* reduction as discussed by Trinkaus (1983, 1987) and Franciscus and Trinkaus (1995). Reduced incidence rates of lingular bridging may reflect, in part, reduced levels of muscle fiber hypertrophy and mandibular size (Billy and Vallois, 1977) due to either or both differences in diet or cultural practices and not species-specific differences. It should be noted, however, that the extent of the muscular insertion and the muscle's positioning relative to the mandible are probably as or more important than the degree of force transmitted to the bone. If the extent of *m. pterygoideus medialis* attachment to raised crests and tubercles is an accurate indication of the degree of force transmitted to the bone then force is clearly not of high importance as *l. mandibulae*-mylohyoid groove bridging occurs in both strongly and lightly marked mandibles.

We do not consider the presence of lingular bridging (*s.l.*) to be derived in Middle to Late Pleistocene populations. Such bridging occurs in *A. afarensis* (AL 288-1) and in OH 22 (cf. *H. erectus*). We do, however, consider the *bridging pattern* observed in later Middle Pleistocene to recent *H. sapiens* to be derived. We have shown that development of the inferior aspects of the *l. mandibulae* (*l. mandibulae* to mylohyoid groove transitional region) is only present in specimens here assigned to ArHs and later *Homo*. Whereas the mechanism which results in bridging in hominids may be similar, the developmental or epigenetic events leading to its expression in later *Homo* differs, as detailed above. We currently believe that phenotypic differences observed in this region between ArHs, Neanderthals, and recent *H. sapiens* reflect both the repositioning of functional matrices as a consequence of hafting changes of the craniofacial region and modifications in diet and reduced paramasticatory influences. Given our overall assessment of the *l. mandibulae*-mylohyoid groove region we concur with Lundy (1980) and Kaul and Pathak (1984) that use of the bridging pattern as a genetic marker of demes in recent *H. sapiens* (Ossenberg, 1974a, b; Sawyer *et al.*, 1978; Sawyer *et al.*, 1990; reviewed in Hauser and De Stefano, 1989) may not be entirely tenable. We do, however, consider that available data for Pleistocene *Homo* indicates that this trait may be more useful as a demic marker rather than an indication of species level differences. Further analysis of this region which documents the individual factors which result in mylohyoid groove-*l. mandibulae* bridging should result in the delineation of useful populational and, potentially, taxonomic markers.

5. Neanderthals and anatomically modern *Homo sapiens*

Our sample for AmHs is small and geographically more diverse than either our ArHs or Neanderthal samples. In general, orientation and development of the *c. endocondyloidea* in this group is similar to all earlier *Homo*. A curious pattern emerges, however, wherein the *l. mandibulae* lies inferior to or under this *crista* and shows only very minimal development of the lingular notch. This pattern occurs in the Amud 1 Neanderthal and in the AmHs specimens Dar es Soltan 5, Qafzeh XI and Skhul 5 (Figures 13a and 14b). It also appears to be present in Qafzeh IX and

Skhul 4. This pattern has the appearance of a local (North African - Middle Eastern?) variant and may prove of further interest. The total morphological pattern of the medial ramus expressed in AmHs is one which is clearly linked to the pattern expressed in ArHs and Neanderthals. The relationship of the anterior and posterior *s. colli* components is similar as is the general configuration of the *l. mandibulae-f. mandibulae* complex (Figures 13a-f and 14a-c). The only difference between these two groups is the lack of lingular extension both over the *s. colli* and over the mylohyoid groove in AmHs sampled (Figure 14a-c). None of the individuals in our AmHs sample present with a bridged lingular region but, as discussed, it has been noted in high frequencies in Upper Paleolithic populations (earlier > later: Smith, 1978; Frayer, 1992; Stefan and Trinkaus, 1998b). The AmHs group is also similar to Neanderthals in having an anterosuperiorly positioned *l. pterygoidea* and horizontal orientation to the *s. colli*, generally (Figure 14a-c). Of interest in this context is that the Zhoukoudian Upper Cave 101 individual also displays this morphology (Figures 10e and 14c). This indicates that this pattern is not restricted to Western Europe, as might be implied by our ArHs and Neanderthal samples. Both juvenile and adult AmHs differ from ArHs and Neanderthals, however, in that the insertion site for the *m. pterygoideus medialis* is less strongly marked. Whereas individuals in this group display strong septa 6, 4, and 2^{III} tubercles they do not attain the medial extent seen in some ArHs, Neanderthals, and recent *H. sapiens*. The reasons for this apparent difference are certainly multifactorial. Resolution of the significance of such a difference must await further understanding of the relationship between septa and tubercles and the delineation of ontogenetic events related to the initial appearance of tubercles and their maintenance throughout ontogeny.

6. Anatomically modern *Homo sapiens* to recent *Homo sapiens*

Our recent *H. sapiens* sample population displays significant variation in features under discussion (Figures 4a-f, 5a-e, and 10f-g). Further, quantification of the variation in a series of medial ramal structures will be required to clarify issues of importance to systematics. Of interest, however, is that a similar range of variation in *m. pterygoideus medialis* insertion site morphology to that in ArHs, Neanderthals, and AmHs occurs in this group. Given available data it appears that there has been both: (1) a slight reduction in the overall degree of development of bony crests and tubercles related to the *m. pterygoideus medialis*; and (2) slight shifts in the degree of emphasis placed on individual attachment sites. In both cases it is important to recall that substantial variation occurs in these features and that it is most likely that patterns observed in fossil taxa will reflect differences in Pleistocene demes and not species level differences. We consider that differences observed between Pleistocene populations and recent *H. sapiens* reflect a reduction in masticatory and paramasticatory factors which occur in conjunction with shifts in the repositioning of related functional matrices.

III. SUMMARY

We have conclusively demonstrated that *m. pterygoideus medialis* insertion site morphology is significantly altered during growth in recent *H. sapiens*. These differences reflect both changes in muscle function and orientation and in soft tissue packing requirements during growth. Such requirements are, of course, tied to more complex functional matrix-skeletal unit relationships. We believe that fossil taxa observed also conform to these growth pattern changes. On this basis, studies which directly equate adult muscle origin-insertion site morphologies with those of subadults but which do not account for functional differences and changing relationships between functional matrices should be rejected. For the above reasons, we do not provide a direct comparison of our occurrence values for the MPT character state with those for fossil taxa. We consider our values as only useful in demonstrating that the 'MPT character state' (as defined by Rak *et al.*, 1994, 1996) occurs in high frequencies in recent *H. sapiens* populations and is not, therefore, autapomorphic for Neanderthals. Any other usage of these data is of no value, as we have demonstrated the complexities of the region which render the simple assessment of 'MPT present or absent' to be of no value to systematics.

Although the data is somewhat conflicting, current evidence does not indicate high frequencies of the 'H-O' character state in recent *H. sapiens* populations. We have demonstrated, however, that elements of the 'bridging complex' phenotype are likely influenced by both muscle function and idiosyncratic and population level variations in positioning of functional matrices. Also, based on preliminary observations we have shown that recent humans express all elements of the bridging complex. Since the character state has been considered in discrete terms (present / absent) the more important observation of variation in structures which are involved in the 'bridging phenotype' has been overlooked. These data can be combined with the facts that: (1) Middle to Late Pleistocene populations exhibit a gradual reduction in occurrence rates for the H-O character state; and (2) the character state has a variable rate of occurrence in Pleistocene population level samples. Given these data we consider the bridging phenotype to be a better marker of Pleistocene demes than species. This observation may, upon further quantification, be extended to recent *H. sapiens* populations. Lacking such analyses it is not now possible to delineate populations which show a significant reduction in the complex from those which retain the more primitive condition or the extent of idiosyncratic variation within populations or recent *H. sapiens*, generally. Without such data we are left to compare samples (and individuals) on the basis of end-points in the range of variation. This is clearly an undesirable situation for phylogenetic analysis of closely related populations and species.

ROLE OF TENDONS, LIGAMENTS, AND MUSCLES IN CRANIOFACIAL GROWTH

I. TENDON AND LIGAMENT DEVELOPMENT AND FUNCTION

1. Introduction

We have brought a wide array of direct observational data to bear on the validity of the MPT, H-O foramen, and *c. intermedia* features/character states and on discussion of evolutionary change in medial ramal anatomy. Our intent has not, however, been to simply address the validity of these character states. We noted earlier that the original and subsequent publications, discussions, and usage of the MPT character state have raised broader issues (Rak *et al.*, 1994, 1996; Antón, 1995, 1996; Creed-Miles *et al.*, 1996; Quam and Smith, 1998; Tillier, 1998; Nagar and Arensburg, 2000; Lebel *et al.*, 2001) of import to evolutionary biology in general. Further, in the preceding text a number of important aspects of medial ramal anatomy have either not been addressed or have been presented as queries, as more in-depth treatment would have unnecessarily complicated prior discussion. Therefore, here we build on our observational data to address broader issues related to: (1) the role of tendon, ligament, and muscle in creating and maintaining bony ramal morphology; (2) mandibular ontogeny; (3) functional matrix-skeletal unit relationships; and (4) application of ontogenetic data to questions of evolutionary history.

2. Tendon and ligament development and mechanics in craniofacial growth

In assessing the role of tendons and ligaments in tubercle formation it is important to recall that they are passive structures which are metabolically relatively inert (Elliott, 1965). Tendon functions to eliminate the need for any unnecessary muscle length between origin and insertion and enables convenient muscle placement relative to the joint over which it acts while allowing for concentration of its pull onto a relatively small area of bone (Jones, 1941; Elliott, 1965; Gans and Brock, 1965). Ligaments generally function to restrict movement. The functional role(s) of many craniomandibular ligaments are complicated, however, by their association with fascial thickenings, whose development and effect on function is obscure at best. Both tendons and ligaments are structurally elastic only within narrow limits and are protected from excessive loading by direct and indirect reflexive muscular contraction, respectively (Haines, 1932; Smith, 1954). Tendon elasticity decreases with age, however, and may be related to or results from a decrease in water content of from 80-85% in infants to about 70% in adults, with mature tendon varying in content from 58-70% (Elliott, 1965; Matyas *et al.*, 1990). Due to the effects of tendon aging there is a change in the stress-strain curve as tendon ages (Elliott, 1965) and this is reflected in the morphology of the attachment sites (Moss and Moss-Salentijn, 1978). The effects of aging, coupled with variation in tendon-ligament attachment anatomy, translate into higher tendon avulsion rates in young individual but higher tendon rupture rates in older individuals (Steindler, 1955). Although earlier considered to lack the ability for interstitial growth (Haines, 1932), tendons are now known to increase in length interstitially, particularly at the musculotendinous junction (Williams and Warwick, 1980; Benjamin and Ralphs, 2000). A decreasing growth gradient has been observed from their junction with the muscle towards their osseous attachment (Williams and Warwick, 1980). Because an increase in tendon substance can be effected at the musculotendinous junction it is more difficult to posit an increase in bony tubercle size as related to the need to increase musculotendon length.

It has been demonstrated by Symons (1954) that some muscles in *H. sapiens* develop a definitive collagenous attachment to bone by the third month *in utero*. In the main, however, most muscles are considered to be attached to bone via the periosteum (Amorino and Cattaneo, 1937; Lacroix, 1951; Rayne and Crawford, 1971; Moss and Moss-Salentijn, 1978; Hurov, 1986). Note that in young animals Amprino and Cattaneo (1937) observed that the periosteum differed from its mature state both structurally and in its method of attachment. Prior to tendons inserting into bone or periosteum the tendon primordia arise independently of the muscle primordia (Christ *et al.*, 1977; Chevallier *et al.*, 1977) and in the absence of functional constraints (Shellswell and Wolpert, 1977). Given the latter it is, therefore, most probable that, in areas where major tendons arise in the *m. pterygoideus medialis*, specific regions of muscle are attached via tendinous tissue and not directly to periosteum. This observation implies either: (1) the synchronous origin of all major pretendinous or tendinous primordia with variation in rate of regional tendon formation; or (2) that there are primary and secondary tendon primordia. This is of interest as the former implies synchronous genetic induction with subsequent genetic-epigenetic interaction whereas the latter implies either disjunct diachronic genetic induction with subsequent genetic-epigenetic interaction or genetic induction of some primordia with others appearing later due to subsequent genetic-epigenetic interactions.

Recently, work on the avian limb by Kardon (1998) provides some insights into resolution of these issues in attachment development. In avian limb buds she observed that the relationship between developing tendon primordia and the bone rudiment depends on their relationship within the developing limb bud. In the proximal part of the limb bud, she found that tendon primordia form as a single unit and then subdivide to form individual tendons in the proximal portion of the limb. These primordia can be traced directly to the skeleton from their first appearance (Kardon, 1998). As such, the development of tendon entheses occurs simultaneously with the rest of the tendons (Benjamin and Ralphs, 2000). Alternatively, tendon primordia in the intermediate and distal limb segments are not initially attached to the skeleton (Kardon, 1998). In this case, the primordia combine with tendinous outcroppings from the bone which appear to arise from the periosteum or perichondrium. Thus, in these cases, tendon entheses and their primordia are initially separate but later fuse. Further development of the tendinous attachment varies according to the type of enthesis developed (Benjamin and Ralphs, 2000).

Although a few histological studies on tendinous and ligamentous attachments to bone in human fetuses have been available (Symons, 1954; Hems and Tillmann, 2000) systematic study of infant entheses are not available and those for juveniles and adults have only recently become available (Vogel, 1995; Hems and Tillmann, 2000). On the basis of studies of limb bones it has been demonstrated that the development of tendon and ligament entheses is dependent on the mode of osteogenesis (Knese and Biermann, 1958; Benjamin and Ralphs, 2000; Hems and Tillmann, 2000). Tendons or ligaments that are attached to epiphyses of long bones or to carpal and tarsal bones have been shown to develop zones of fibrocartilage at their entheses early in postnatal life (Benjamin and Ralphs, 1995, 2000). In all other sites entheses remain fibrous (= periosteal or bony attachments: Benjamin and Ralphs, 2000). Of note is that the time when fibrocartilaginous entheses (as determined from the medial collateral ligament) lose their original cartilaginous attachment (i.e. tissue sequence changes from: bone ⇨ cartilage ⇨ fibrocartilage ⇨ ligament; to bone ⇨ fibrocartilage ⇨ ligament) corresponds to the time when the mechanical strength of the ligament-to-bone complex increases substantially (Benjamin and Ralphs, 2000). Further, these two attachment variants, periosteal and fibrocartilaginous, have been equated with their ability to migrate on developing bone. Fibrous or periosteal attachments, inclusive of entheses inserting directly into bone, are associated with regions where substantial migration of the developing tendon or ligament attachment occurs whereas fibrocartilaginous attachments associate with less mobile attachment regions (Knese and Biermann, 1958; Benjamin and Ralphs, 2000).

To determine whether observed variations in the method of tendon or ligament attachments are controlled by the method of bone formation, Hems and Tillmann (2000) analyzed masticatory muscle insertion sites in adult humans as these muscles originate or insert into bone formed from intramembranous, endochondral, and secondary cartilaginous sources. Rather than showing the expected site specific and uniform fibrocartilaginous or fibrous attachment method, masticatory muscle tendons had entheses which differed structurally within a single attachment region. Hems and Tillmann (2000) found that the *m. pterygoideus medialis* insertion area comprised three different methods of tendon attachment. These attachment types include: (1) short tendon fibers interwoven with collagen fibers of the periosteum; (2) long tendon fibers inserting directly into bone; and (3) long tendons attaching by way of fibrocartilaginous tissue, which is calcified close to the bone, at the pterygoid tuberosity (septa 6, 4, 2^{III} attachment sites). In their assessment of *mm. masseter* and *pterygoideus medialis* entheses, Hems and Tillmann (2000) only observed a tidemark (line of separation between uncalcified and calcified cartilage above the bone's surface) at the attachment site of the *m. pterygoideus medialis*. Combining these data with the earlier work of Fischer and Tillmann (1991), Hems and Tillmann (2000) conclude that tendon and ligament attachment methods for masticatory and anterolateral thyroid cartilage (Fischer and Tillmann, 1991) musculature are not controlled by the mode of osteogenesis. Note, however, that in avian embryos: (1) attempts to develop fate maps for the laryngeal cartilages, traditionally thought of as branchial arch derivatives, by following neural crest transplantations have been unsuccessful; and (2) that the embryonic origin of the tracheal cartilages is unclear, as avians lack these cartilages (Noden, 1982, 1986). It has been determined, however, that the arytenocricoid and all of the tracheal ring cartilages are labeled following the transplantation of lateral plate mesoderm (Noden and de Lahunta, 1985). Given these results it would be of interest to better understand the developmental origin of cartilages examined by Fischer and Tillmann (1991). This type of information may undermine supporting data for the lack of correlation between entheses type and the mode of osteogenesis. This results from the fact that primary and secondary cartilages differ in their developmental origins and, resultantly, in their overall development (reviewed in Richards, in prep.). In the limbs, carpals, and tarsals the method of attachment, as noted above, maps well with the mode of osteogenesis.

Given the work of Hems and Tillmann (2000) it would appear that alternative explanations for the origin and development of attachment site variation in masticatory muscles must be considered. Any such work will be complicated by the fact that the *mm. pterygoideus lateralis* and *medialis* and *m. masseter*: (1) are initially associated with Meckel's cartilage (Lee *et al.*, 2001); (2) ultimately associate with bone derived from a combination of primary and secondary cartilaginous and intramembranous sources; and (3) lack an influence imposed by functional constraints on the initial development of tendon and ligament attachments. The role of the initial attachment of specific regions of the *mm. pterygoideus medialis* and *lateralis* to Meckel's cartilage and their subsequent detachment and reattachment to intramembranous bone and secondary cartilage of the ramus (Lee *et al.*, 2001) will need to be clarified as it is known from studies of long bones that cartilage in fibrocartilaginous attachments derives, in part, from their association with bone of endochondral origins (Benjamin and Ralphs, 2000).

Although not useful for understanding the earliest stages of attachment site development, once function impacts the site it is possible to understand the maintenance or origin of variation in attachment methods. Benjamin *et al.* (1986) observed in adults that fleshy muscular insertions produce smooth, featureless surfaces, indistinguishable from areas of bone covered by periosteum alone. Alternatively, attachments of tendons and aponeuroses produce distinct markings (e.g. lines, tubercles, pits, *fossae*, etc.). In dry bone the quantity of fibrocartilage formerly present is reflected in the attachment site morphology. Rough markings indicate little fibrocartilage was present whereas smooth, circumscribed areas which are devoid of vascular foramina (resembling articular regions) indicate areas of more extensive fibrocartilaginous entheses (Benjamin *et al.*, 1986; Benjamin and Ralphs, 1998, 2000). On inspection, surfaces between uncalcified and calcified fibrocartilage and those between calcified fibrocartilage and bone are highly irregular and this complex interlocking of tendon and bone is likely to be a major factor in securing their attachment (Cooper and Misol, 1970; Benjamin and Ralphs, 1998, 2000). Gao and Messner (1996) have shown that the complex interdigitation observed at the interface between calcified cartilage and bone only forms around puberty and within a relatively short time frame. This is consistent with our observation that *m. pterygoideus medialis* septa 6, 4, and 2^{III} tubercles are similar from early infancy into the juvenile period. Gao and Messner (1996) observed that the shape of the soft tissue interface and the thickness of the calcified fibrocartilage at a ligament attachment may reflect two different kinds of physiological adaptations. One reflects a response to tensile loading of ligaments around puberty whereas the other reflects a response to loads applied at the interface in later (adult) growth stages and is an adaptation to both the amount of tensile loads and motion at the interface.

The presence and quantity of fibrocartilage has been shown in studies of limb bones to be highly correlated with the extent of movement between tendon and bone (Benjamin and Ralphs, 1998; Hems and Tillmann, 2000). It is known that the incompressibility of chondrocytes in uncalcified fibrocartilage reduces the amount of transverse stress on the tendon resulting from compression and, thus longitudinal strain on the tendon fibers (Vogel, 1995; Benjamin and Ralphs, 1998; Hems and Tillmann, 2000). The presence of calcified fibrocartilage between the uncalcified fibrocartilage and bone, as uniquely observed for masticatory muscles in superior tubercles of the *m. pterygoideus medialis*, may protect the bone from either or both excessive sheer (Hems and Tillmann, 2000) or compressive stress (Matyas *et al.*, 1995; Benjamin and Ralphs, 2000). Further, Gao and Messner (1996) suggest that the thickness of the zone of calcified fibrocartilage may be related to tendon strength and the degree of loading it experiences. It is unclear whether the fibrocartilaginous enthesis insertion method for *m. pterygoideus medialis*, with its uniquely developed tidemark, indicates an adaptation to withstand such increased levels of sheer or compressive loading throughout development (Cooper and Misol, 1970). The presence of fibrocartilage may indicate, alternatively, a growth plate-like function (Cooper and Misol, 1970) in which the cartilaginous component permits rapid lengthening of the attachment region during bone growth. In later developmental stages this fibrocartilaginous region may subsequently function to mitigate the effects of increased sheer and compressive loading at the tendon-bone interface. Periosteal attachments of the *m. pterygoideus medialis* differ from the fibrocartilaginous ones as fibroblasts associated with these attachments are thought to be associated with greater levels of tensile stress (Matyas *et al.*, 1995).

Whereas muscle and tendon are developmentally autonomous once the tendon-bone interface is established, tendon is acted upon during muscle function (Rayne and Crawford, 1971). Note, however, that in early stages of attachment, when only minimal force transmission can be expected, bone morphology related to the insertion of tendon is not necessarily oriented in line with the direction of muscle force (Rayne and Crawford, 1971). In this context, 'early stages' are functional component specific and some may last well into the early postnatal period as observed by Kardon (1998) and as discussed further below. Subsequent growth of tendon will depend on an increased or decreased distance between origin and insertion and on any alteration in muscle architecture due to changes in the relative range of movement (Elliott, 1965). This observation is supported by the work of Mollier (1937) and Elliott (1965) as they found that, in larger tendons where joint movement changes the angle of insertion into bone, the arrangement of tendon fibers is more complex. Further, these larger tendon bundles have cross-branches and are plaited such that loads are transmitted equally throughout the tendons insertion in all positions of the joint. Whereas fiber orientation within the tendon supports the hypothesis of a mechanical influence upon their growth, strain is not necessarily the sole factor that determines connective tissue growth (Elliott, 1965). Furthermore, whereas larger muscles tend to have larger tendons a strict correlation does not exist between tendon thickness and muscle size or the maximum strength which the muscle can exert. Comer (1956) observed nearly identical growth curves and rates for length of the tibia, muscle belly, and tendon. The latter observation implies that tendon growth is related, in part, to the amount (Haines, 1932; Comer, 1956; Elliott, 1965) and duration (Elliott, 1965) of strain applied to the tendon. Contrastingly, work by Skerry (2000) suggests that the duration of strain is a relatively unimportant variable. Within an evolutionary context we must caution that the amount of tendon at any individual site, as represented by the areal expanse of its associated bony surrogate, may reflect repositioning via coalescence or lack of separation of individual tendon primordia and not necessarily a change in muscle function.

Whereas adult attachment morphology has received some recent attention, van der Klaauws' (1963) observation that only minimal work on the ontogeny of the projections, deepenings, and undulations of the surface of the skull in relation to the attachment of muscles is still current. He also noted that such was the case with the ontogeny of tendons and aponeuroses relative to muscle ontogeny. It is clear that an understanding of the origin of attachment site variation in the *m. pterygoideus medialis* must be sought in early stages of growth. Separation of factors related to the timing of the development and the continued maintenance of fibrocartilaginous attachment sites can only result from examination of individuals aged between 8th months *in utero* and circa 2.0 years of age. In this period the muscle becomes detached from Meckel's cartilage, reattaches to the developing bony ramus (Öğütcen-Toller and Keskin, 2000; Lee *et al.*, 2001), functions in early masticatory movements, and only subsequently begins its development of adult functional characteristics (see below). It is in this time frame that an understanding of factors related to the initial development of the muscles attachment and those related to its function can be sought.

3. Correlation of primary and literature-derived data

Given our results and those available from literature sources, development of tendinous tissue in the *m. pterygoideus medialis* appears to show development of 'primary' and 'secondary' tendons, although note that the term 'secondary' may only refer to the gross expression of tendon matrix and not time of origin. On gross examination of human fetal-to-newborn muscle insertions, Schumacher (1962) observed well defined tendons in the inferior aspect of the *m. pterygoideus medialis* (= septum 2^{I-III}) but only a musculoperiosteal attachment in the superior muscle. This observation is consistent with that of Haines (1932) on late fetal musculature; it is similar to adults, except that there is relatively more muscle and less tendon. Symons (1954), alternatively, found the muscle to be attached to bone by collagenous fibers in the posterosuperior aspect of the insertion site in the same time period. We are inclined to agree with Symons' observation (1954) as in both our work and that of Schumacher (1962) sites reflecting a bony (fibrocartilaginous?) attachment for superior septa can be observed. As discussed and based on Schumacher (1962), the septum 4 attachment site is generally present in the newborn whereas that for septum 6 is more variable. Within this context it is important to recognize that the septa 6 and 4 primordium are either co-incident, or nearly so, at this stage or that a bony septum 6 insertion site only appears around the pre-to-post-partum junction. Based on the work of Kardon (1998) we suggest that a single tendon primordium for septum 6 and 4 of the *m. pterygoideus medialis* develops and then splits into a 'primary' and 'secondary' tendon. Septum 2^{III} may also be involved in this process but this is unclear (see below). As discussed, we believe that a clear separation of these specific tendon primordia is more common in great apes whereas the degree of separation is less clear in hominids. In recent *H. sapiens* the result of this process is a wide range of variation in the configuration of tendon entheses for septa 6, 4, and 2^{III} as noted above. Clarification of the developmental origins of tendon primordia will be necessary to allow some resolution of the evolutionary changes observed in the quadruped-biped transition.

Based on our earlier observations and given the above it is possible to examine the role of both ligamentous attachments and tendinous insertions in creating medial ramal morphology. In considering the *l. sphenomandibulare* (*s.s.* / *s.l.*) we suggest multiple functions that vary ontogenetically. We consider the *l. sphenomandibulare* (*s.s.*) to function during early ontogenetic stages to maintain mandibular-cranial base relationships. Following birth this structure continues to function in maintaining structural relations and, in so doing, may become tensed during extreme protrusive movements (see below). These activities reflect high idiosyncratic variation and may be a factor in the observed variation in *l. mandibulae* morphology. Further, the *l. sphenomandibulare* (*s.s.*) is co-opted to function as the superior boundary of a potential space. The smooth fusiform shape of this ligament is well suited for this application as it is in close contact with the *nn. alveolaris inferior* and *mylohyoideus* and numerous vessels. Deep cervical fascia envelopes and is suspended from this ligament. As discussed, the latter fascia acquires numerous bony attachments within and around the *s. colli*, mylohyoid groove, and *f. mandibulae*. The apparent degree and duration of transmitted force reflected in the associated fascial thickenings and bony attachments is highly variable. Given our observations on the inferior *s. colli* border, however, it does not appear that there is a significant change in the degree of *l. sphenomandibulare* (*s.s.* / *s.l.*) mediated bone formation throughout ontogeny. We consider the prolonged and medially arching nature of the *s. colli*'s inferior border to reflect soft tissue packing requirements, as opposed to a ligament mediated extension. In fact, recent observations (Richards *et al.*, in prep.) indicate that the inferior *s. colli* border is significantly reduced and may migrate superiorly or remain stationary as other structures migrate inferiorly during growth. The only *l. sphenomandibulare*-related structure that appears to be increased or become more defined in adults is the *tsc*. The *tsc* is highly variable, however, as is the degree of ligament (fascial) thickenings reaching this tubercle. Whether the ligamentous-fascial thickenings reflect an increase in and duration of loads applied to the ligament is unclear. Variations resulting in the latter could reflect slight differences in positioning of related structures, both ontogenetic and idiosyncratic, or slight differences in degree and extent of protrusive movements, with moderate thickenings of the cervical fascia reflecting the increases. In this context, however, note that deep cervical fascia extending from the *l. sphenomandibulare* (*s.s.*) and attaching to the *tsc* forms the posterior boundary of this fascial space and, thusly, may become thickened solely by association with neurovascular structures as implied by DuBrul (1980). In sum, we currently do not consider the *l. sphenomandibulare* (*s.s.* or *s.l.*) as playing a significant role(s) in mandibular biomechanics, excepting possibly in late prenatal and early postnatal stages. Further, in the later stages we consider the ligament to function primarily as a surrogate bony wall which maintains neurovascular relationships during mandibular function. Because of the observed degree of structural variations and in the absence of a more complete analysis we are unable to clarify the role, if any, of the *l. stylomandibulare* in mandibular function or in its relationship to tubercle formation on the posterior ramal border.

We have discussed bony morphology of the mandibular insertion of *m. pterygoideus medialis* in early subadult stages and shown how this site is affected more by the organization of functional matrices relative to their associated skeletal units than by factors mediated by musculotendinous development or muscle function. Within this context we have observed that there is a high degree of variation in medial extent of the insertion sites in infants. In this context, note that the degree of development of the insertion site (in rats) has been demonstrated to be greater than that of the origin in early stages of growth (Rayne and Crawford, 1971). We currently believe this variation in medial extent of the septa 6 and 4 attachment is maintained in later stages. As in all structures, there is a range of tendon lengths derived from variation in the positioning and quantity of precursor mesenchymal cells at the site of tendon development and in the onset and duration of induction of tendon primordia (see Atchley, 1993). Developmentally 'shorter' tendons could attach to more medially extended tubercles as a result of either or a combination of: (1) low precursor cell counts; (2) a more medial positioning of the primordia; or (3) late onset of or a shortened period of induction of precursor cells. We noted above that during growth bone will extend ≤ 3.0 mm in the adult to reach an isolated musculotendinous mass (Chierici and Miller, 1984). During growth, and given the mosaic nature of the various related primordia, a medially projecting tubercle could supplement tendon length and be maintained during lateral cortical drift. Since growth of tendon is interstitial and occurs at the musculotendinous junction (Williams and Warwick, 1980) we can see little reason to replace a bony 'tendon-supplement' once it is established.

Development and maintenance of a medially projecting superior insertion site for *m. pterygoideus medialis* may also be affected by the type of enthesis. It has not yet been established that a fibrocartilaginous enthesis is present at the superior attachment site (septum 6 and 4) of the *m. pterygoideus medialis* in early growth stages. We do consider, however, that such an attachment may develop in this region early in growth and that it may be traced to the muscle's early association with Meckel's cartilage. In conjunction with the above mechanisms which result in medially projecting insertion sites for the muscle, must be added the potential that this site has a growth plate-like function. Given the potential for the rapid deposition of cartilaginous tissue, relative to the rate of bone deposition, and the fact that this is a region of extensive tendinous attachment for the muscle, it is probable that the fibrocartilage provides for greater flexibility during times of rapid repositioning of the attachment site(s). Within this context note that the resultant of the mosaic development of structures in this region may be accentuated by the high level of lateral cranial growth (> 40% increase) in the newborn to one-year-old age range (Tillier,1998; and GDR unpublished data). In this context the use of cross-sectional dry bone samples could be misleading as tubercle size may be being sampled in some individuals at these periods of rapid growth. Such issues complicate the determination of whether tubercle size is related to muscle function or to more complex growth differentials between functional components.

To the above mechanism(s) which produce and maintain tubercle variation must be added that derived from the coalescence or lack of separation of tendon primordia. We noted the close association of septa 6 and 4 tubercles in hominids and the commingling of the posterior-most portions of their related septa. We have also discussed the association of septa 6 and 4 with septum 2^{III}. Given only the bony anatomy in young age stages, it appears that there is a substantial range of posterior convergence or lack of separation of septa 6 and 4 in humans. Clearly, a decreased distance between septa results in a more compacted insertion site. The commingling of tendons may result in tubercles with a greater medial extent simply as a way of providing for a larger tendon mass in a more restricted space. We noted instances in humans where the septa 6 and 4 epitendons are so highly interwoven in their posterior aspect that they have the *appearance* of a single tendon. The latter would, by necessity, reflect both variation in positioning of tendon primordia and their overall development in later age stages. During growth the greater association of septa would result in the tubercle becoming more broad but without clear elevations for the individual septa; this is consistent with our observations on tubercle form in some individuals. It is currently unknown whether superior septa (= 6, 4, 2^{III}) of the *m. pterygoideus medialis* arise from three individual, two separate, or a single primordium. As discussed above, we believe that septa 6 and 4 derive from closely related primordia or one individual primordium whereas that for septum 2^{III} arises from a separate primordium. By example, we observed that the septum 2^{III} tubercle may be well developed and separate from the septa 6 and 4 tubercle (cf. Zafarraya; Figure 13f) or it may be incorporated into it (cf. La Quina H5; Figure 13e). In the latter cases boundaries between these main septal attachments can usually be discerned but many times no clear boundaries exist. The latter leads to the conclusion that it is not necessarily only the developmental origin of the septum 2^{III} tubercle primordium which leads to its association with the septa 6 and 4 tubercle but also its later development in a functioning masticatory system. This minimal range of mechanisms indicates some of the complex interactions which we consider to result in the high idiosyncratic variation observed in the medial projection of the newborn-infant *s. colli*-septa 6 and 4 insertion region in recent *H. sapiens*.

Developmental events which might result initially in relatively large and 'medially projecting' tubercles for septa 6 and 4 of the *m. pterygoideus medialis* are many. Once formed, however, the resulting tubercle is then further acted on by muscle force and ontogenetic changes in muscle tissue and orientation. As discussed the septa 6 and 4 tubercle is restricted in its superoinferior and anteroinferior extent throughout the subadult range but increases in both dimensions in late juvenile and adult stages. The latter observation is consistent with the growth curves of masticatory muscles and tendons which occur during development of the adult dentition and face. Note also that septa 6 and 4 attachment ridges separate from one another during growth and that this is probably a reflection of the maturation by hypertrophy of intervening fetal muscle fibers with aging. We have also noted that the degree of development of muscle bundles, particularly those of the anterior head, attaching at the tubercle base probably also drives or causes maintenance of medially extended tubercles. In the more inferiorly placed septa $2^{\text{I-III}}$ tubercles we also believe that their morphology is consistent with the mechanisms discussed above.

In Neanderthals the MPT has been suggested to simply result from loads applied to this insertion site by hypertrophy of the superior-most fibers (Rak et al., 1994) or fibers of the upper part of the insertion site (Rak et al., 1996) of the m. pterygoideus medialis. These authors also suggest that there is a gradual intensification in tubercle size as the ramus is ascended. In a response, Antón (1996) states that the MPT receives forces from muscle fibers located in all sections of the muscle, not just from the posterosuperior regions. Whereas we do not agree with this Antón's subdivision of the complex septal system (Gaspard et al., 1973a, b) into a main (? septa 6, 4, 2^{III}) and subsidiary (? septa $2^{\text{I-II}}$) grouping, we do concur with her observation, previously made by Schumacher (1959, 1961, 1962) and Gaspard et al. (1973a, b), that tendons attaching at the septa 6 and 4 insertion site receive fibers from a broad portion of the muscle. Based on Antón's (1996) perspective, wherever such complex interweaving of tendons occurs, it negates our ability to delineate individual functional differences in specific regions of muscle from bony anatomy. Although we have herein demonstrated that a gradual intensification of the m. pterygoideus medialis attachment site is not a feature specific to Neanderthals or other groups examined, the more important question which these studies have generated regards the relationship of m. pterygoideus medialis anatomy to the formation of simple and complex bony tubercles at its insertion site and how these structures are modified during growth and muscle function.

II. MUSCLE PHYSIOLOGY AND ARCHITECTURE AND THEIR EFFECTS ON MEDIAL RAMAL MORPHOLOGY

1. Muscle structure and physiology

To address issues of muscle mediated tubercle formation and any ensuing modifications they undergo during ontogeny it is necessary to examine the: (1) effects of the physiological properties of muscle fibers; and (2) architectural arrangement of the fibers upon the property of the entire muscle (Gans and Brock, 1965). Both properties are noted to differ: (1) among species; (2) among the muscles of species; (3) during ontogeny and function (Scott, 1957; Bowden and Goyer, 1960; Burleigh, 1974; Ringqvist, 1971, 1973, 1974; Herring, 1977; Gans and Gorniak, 1978; Strickland, 1981, 1983; Eriksson and Thornell, 1983; Van Eijden et al., 1997; Foucart et al., 1998; Korfage and Van Eijden, 1999; Goldspink, 1999); and, in the former case, (4) within a single muscle fiber (Ennion et al., 1995).

Craniomandibular muscles have different proportions of fiber types (Baker and Laskin, 1969; Burleigh, 1974; Ringqvist, 1974; Eriksson and Thornell, 1983; Soussi-Yanicostas et al., 1990; Mao et al., 1992; Hannam and McMillan, 1994; Ennion et al., 1995; Van Eijden et al., 1997; Korfage and Van Eijden, 1999, 2000; Goldspink, 1999; Sciote et al., 2000). These variant muscle fiber types express myosin isoform genes which encode different molecular motors (Goldspink, 1999). During ontogeny muscles fibers express three myosin heavy chains (MyHC), an embryonic, fetal, and an adult isoform (Soussi-Yanicostas et al., 1990; Mao et al., 1992; Sciote et al., 2000). Although MyHC-fetal is a slow form it is converted into a range of adult isoforms of two basic types. Type I refers to slow-oxidative fibers which have a molecular motor that has a long cycle time and uses ATPase at a slow rate. Type I fibers are adapted for the economical maintenance of isometric force or for the efficient repetition of slow isotonic contractions (Goldspink, 1999). The latter are generally referred to as fatigue resistant fibers. Subtypes of Type II fibers are known and these are all faster but generally more readily fatigued relative to Type I fibers. Fast muscle fiber subtypes express molecular motors that produce more rapid myosin cross bridge cycling rates (Goldspink, 1999). In the *m. pterygoideus medialis* Type II fibers are only recruited when more powerful movements are required or the isometric force produced by the slow fibers is insufficient (Goldspink, 1999). Type II fiber isoforms include: (1) Type IIA-MyHC fibers, which are reasonably fast and adapted for producing sustained power; (2) Type IIM-MyHC fibers, which are very fast, masticatory muscle specific, and appear to function in very rapid mandibular movements; and (3) Type IIX-MyHC fibers, which are faster than Type IIA-MyHC fibers but are non-oxidative, so they fatigue rapidly. The Type IIA-MyHC and IIX-MyHC isoforms are the fast fiber types in human muscles. The relatively faster Type IIB-MyHC fibers found in small herbivorous mammals are not found in human masticatory muscles (Ennion et al., 1995; Goldspink, 1999). The very fast Type IIM-MyHC fibers are only present in masticatory muscles of carnivores and primates, excepting the lesser panda (*Ailurus fulgens*) among carnivores and humans among primates (Rowlerson et al., 1983).

Soussi-Yanicostas et al. (1990) observed that adult muscles predominately composed of slow fibers, such as the *m. masseter*, have a prolonged period of development in which only portions of the MyHC-fetal fibers are converted into adult MyHC isoforms. Contrastingly, adult muscles containing predominantly fast MyHC isoforms develop more rapidly and the MyHC-fetal fibers are converted into adult myosin isoforms. In an assessment of adult *m. temporalis* fibers, Korfage and Van Eijden (1999) found a small proportion of MyHC-fetal and MyHC-cardiac α fibers. The MyHC-cardiac α fibers express molecular motors that produce very slow myosin cross bridge cycling rates.

It is of interest to note that Ennion et al. (1995) observed that rather than every adult fiber falling distinctly into a specific type (I, IIA-B, M, X) there is a continuum of hybrid fibers between these main fiber types. Further they observed the co-expression of multiple MyHC isoforms within the same muscle fiber (Ennion et al., 1995). This level of complexity is indicated in the work of Goldspink (1999) as he found that soleus muscle which does not normally express fast Type IIB-MyHC genes begins gene transcription for very fast fibers after a single day if the muscle fibers are not subjected to stretch or are not producing force. Goldspink (1999) concluded that all muscle fibers will stay phenotypically fast unless subjected to stretch and isometric force development. The latter author further suggests that stimulation frequency itself is not the primary cause of muscle phenotype determination. Instead, he considers the signal for fast to slow fiber change as from mechanical strain rather than stimulation frequency per se. Therefore, the duration as well as the intensity of the mechanical signals is important.

In a major ATPase histochemical study of human masticatory muscles Eriksson and Thornell (1983) found Type IIB fibers. More recently, however, in an immunohistochemical study that employed a comprehensive panel of monoclonal antibodies against different MyHC isoforms, Korfage and Van Eijden (1999) found few Type IIB fibers in masticatory muscles. These authors consider that the finding of Type IIB fibers by Eriksson and Thornell (1983) may result from an inability of standard ATPase histochemistry (at pH 4.6) to differentiate between Type IIB-MyHC and IIX-MyHC fibers (Korfage and Van Eijden, 1999) and, therefore, IIX-MyHC fibers could have been mistaken for Type IIB fibers with ATPase. Korfage and Van Eijden (1999) consider the possibility that the older age range of their sample may have resulted in down regulation of Type IIB-MyHC to IIX-MyHC or even IIA-MyHC fibers. Whereas this suggestion is based on the notion that hybrid fibers are generally considered to arise when there is an alteration from one fiber type to another (Ennion et al., 1995), the absence of Type IIB-MyHC fibers in human masticatory muscles is supported by the work of Ennion et al. (1995) and Goldspink (1999). Further, recent work indicates that human masticatory muscle fibers identified with ATPase histochemistry as Type IIB actually contain a MyHC that is the homologue to the Type IIX-MyHC found in rodents (Schiaffino et al., 1989; Smerdu et al., 1994). The Type IIB fiber type identified in ATPase based studies of humans is currently considered to represent fibers of Type IIX-MyHC (Korfage and Van Eijden, 2000).

The histochemical ATPase work on masticatory muscles by Eriksson and Thornell (1983) is one of the most important of those dealing with m. pterygoideus medialis fiber composition. Details of fiber types in their work appears to differ from that of Korfage and Van Eijden (1999) only in the designation of Type IIX-MyHC fibers as Type IIB and in a slight difference in percent occurrence of intermediate fibers. The latter is probably related to the finding by Korfage and Van Eijden (1999) of MyHC-fetal and MyHC-cardiac α fibers which were not found in muscles examined by Eriksson and Thornell (1983). Given these differences and the potential that there is not an exact correlation of Type IIB fibers with those of Type IIX-MyHC, the percentage occurrence and cross-sectional area of fibers in the study of Eriksson and Thornell (1983) can be used by considering the percentage occurrence of Type IIB-MyHC fibers as equivalent to that of Type IIX-MyHC, as indicated by Schiaffino et al. (1989) and Smerdu et al. (1994). Eriksson and Thornell (1983) found the anterior portion (head?) of the m. pterygoideus medialis to comprise 64% Type I and 27.5% Type IIB fibers while the posterior portion (head?) comprises nearly equal proportions of Type I (43.9%) and Type IIB (44.8%) fibers. The remainder of the fibers were classified as of both an intermediate type and Type IIC, amounting to about 9.9% (Eriksson and Thornell, 1983). The estimated physiological cross-sectional area (p-csa) for Type I fibers comprises 78.6% of the muscle in the anterior portion of m. pterygoideus medialis as compared to 52.3% in the posterior portion. Corresponding values for Type IIB (= Type IIX-MyHC) fibers are 15.9% in the anterior and 41.5% in the posterior portion. These authors observed similar proportions of fibers in the superficial but not deep portion of m. masseter. A predominance of Type I fibers in the anterior part of the m. pterygoideus medialis was recently confirmed by Korfage and Van Eijden (2000). The latter work also demonstrated, however, that the lateral muscle portion contained more Type I fibers than the medial portion. Further, Van Eijden et al. (1997) found the m. pterygoideus medialis to have the shortest fibers and smallest p-csa of the mandibular elevators. The p-csa of the anterior portion (2.47 cm^2) of this muscle was found to be significantly smaller (ca. 50%) than the posterior portion (3.53 cm^2). Further, they observed that the m. pterygoideus medialis has the least mass of contractile fibers of the mandibular closers and largest percentage of tendinous tissue (24%) of both the mandibular elevators and depressors. A similar observation was made by Gaspard et al. (1973a, b).

As discussed the gross subdivisions of a muscle (heads, layers) demonstrate mixed proportions of fiber types. The latter is also the case for fasciculi, although Eriksson and Thornell (1983) have demonstrated that some fasciculi can be completely composed of only Type I or IIB (= Type IIX-MyHC) fibers. The latter authors suggest that as muscle fiber differentiation is considered to be influenced by motoneuron function, it can be assumed that any variability in fiber composition is related to unequal neural influences. Thus the complex fiber pattern of the mandibular elevators must be related to their unique function and this suggests a specialization to provide optimum precision in the control of jaw position and movement (Eriksson and Thornell, 1983). Predominance of Type I fibers (high fatigue resistance, generally lowest activation threshold) in the m. pterygoideus medialis in conjunction with its multipennate structure suggests that it is equipped to regulate the magnitude of the bite force produced (Eriksson and Thornell, 1983; Korfage and Van Eijden, 1999). In the anterior muscle portion Type I fibers are larger than those of Type II. The posterior portion of this muscle is characterized by a relatively high frequency (ca. 45%) of Type IIB (= Type IIX-MyHC) fibers which are of larger diameter than those of the anterior portion. The Type IIB (= Type IIX-MyHC) fibers (sensitive to fatigue, high activation threshold) generate large forces and are best suited for bursts of intense, intermittent activity (Eriksson and Thornell, 1983). The presence of Type IIB (= Type IIX-MyHC) fibers with large cross-sectional diameters in the posterior m. pterygoideus medialis indicates a capacity in the molar region for intermittent high muscular tension. Ringqvist (1974) described a positive correlation in rats between Type II fiber diameter from the m. masseter and maximum bite force. Given these data, Eriksson and Thornell (1983) concur with Ringqvist's (1974) suggestion that the marked differences between Type I (generally larger: Eriksson and Thornell, 1983; Korfage and Van Eijden, 1999) and Type II (generally smaller) fiber diameters represents a functional adaptation of the masticatory muscles of recent H. sapiens (Ringqvust, 1974). They suggest that refined and soft foods might induce inactivity and as a consequence an under-development of Type II fibers (Eriksson and Thornell, 1983; Soussi-Yanicostas et al., 1990). The latter is further supported by results of studies of animals fed a soft diet (Moore, 1965; Moore and Lavelle, 1974). All reports indicate decreased mandibular growth in animals fed a soft diet with the most prominent changes occurring in the ramus (reviewed in Yamada and Kimmel, 1991). These authors note that the decline in bone formation results from a reduction in localized strain and that the change in function affects periosteal more than endosteal cells.

2. Impact of cultural behaviors on masticatory muscles

Understanding the known size reduction in the hominid craniodental complex is complicated by the coincident increase in cultural behaviors relating to food acquisition and preparation (Greene, 1970). Whereas the consistency of foods ingested by recent H. sapiens are, in general, probably softer than those ingested by the earliest hominids, the timing of effects on the craniodental complex which result are less clear. Some indication of the speed of morphological change following dietary change can, however, be gleaned from the work of Armelagos *et al.* (1984). Further, any assessment of the potential effects of dietary changes on the craniodental complex of hominids must account for the fact that the masticatory apparatus is not used exclusively for feeding but functions in a variety of behavioral events (Gans and Gorniak, 1978). It is of interest to note, however, that the above data for modern humans, while not directly paralleling dietary changes in earlier hominids, appears to reflect the same general tendency toward reduced stress on the masticatory apparatus. Of further interest is the lack of Type IIM-MyHC fibers in the masticatory muscles of humans but their presence in *P. troglodytes*. Rowlerson et al. (1983) suggest that the absence of this fiber type in humans and the lesser panda can be explained by dietary and behavioral shifts in both these taxa. They consider the presence of Type IIM-MyHC fibers to be related to an aggressive bite in carnivores and primates, excepting the latter two taxa. Clearly, any attempt to employ non-human primates, particularly *Gorilla* and *Pan*, in assessments of medial ramal evolution will need to clarify the effects of differences observed in muscle fiber composition as noted by Van Eijden and Turkawski (2001). In this context recall that Gaspard *et al.* (1973b) indicated that the *m. pterygoideus medialis* shows a reduction in the superficial aspects of the posterior region of the muscle. Recent work by Van Eijden and Turkawski (2001) on the distribution of masticatory muscle motor units shows that the more superficial and posterior regions contain relatively large numbers of fast fiber types. It is possible that the reduction in muscle size suggested by Gaspard *et al.* (1973b) correlates with the loss of Type IIM-MyHC fibers consequent on canine size reduction in the hominid lineage. Whereas further work will be need to clarify their affect on ramal development, ontogenetic studies will also need to account for the apparent difference in muscle fiber MyHC isoforms in embryonic and fetal muscles. Further, it would be of interest to determine the relative amounts and rates of change of MyHC-fetal into adult MyHC isoforms in both humans and great apes. Such data would greatly enhance our understanding of evolutionary change in masticatory muscles and their affect on craniofacial development.

3. Gross structure and function of masticatory muscles

The gross structural arrangement of masticatory muscles (Parsons, 1896; Sonntag, 1923, 1924; Boyer, 1939; Avis, 1961; Schumacher, 1961; Gans and Brock, 1965; O'Dell *et al.*, 1970; Gaspard, 1972; Gaspard *et al.*, 1973a, b; Herring, 1977; Eriksson and Thornell, 1983; Friedman, 1988) and nerve supply which helps define these components (Schumacher, 1989; Foucart *et al.*, 1998; Van Eijden and Turkawski, 2001) has been the subject of numerous works. Gaspard *et al.* (1973a, b) observed in recent *H. sapiens*, relative to other primates, that the *m. pterygoideus medialis* exhibits the highest level of macroscopic structural complexity and discusses aspects of the phylogenetic transformation of the pterygomaxillary region which led to this complexity. Of note here is the high level of tendinous tissue observed in the muscle and the suggestion that unnecessary muscle tissue will be converted to tendinous tissue. The latter is of import in understanding the transformation of the muscle in the quadruped-biped transition. Further, given the complexity of the *m. pterygoideus medialis*, some confusion has arisen regarding its gross structural architecture. Mosolov (1972) considers it to possess a single head but notes that there are between 3 and 6 intramuscular connective tissue spaces. Alternatively, Honée (1972), Gaspard *et al.* (1973a, b), Van Eijden *et al.* (1995), and Korfage and Van Eijden (2000) consider the anterior and posterior fibers of *m. pterygoideus medialis* to have distinct origins but that a division into two heads is not clear. Further, Gaspard *et al.* (1973a, b) consider the posterior region as comprising superficial and deep sections. The posterior region is usually noted as having slightly more obliquely oriented fibers relative to the anterior region in adults.

Based on fiber orientation in the sagittal plane the *m. pterygoideus medialis* is considered to function as a mandibular elevator whereas fiber orientation in the coronal plane indicates involvement in mediolateral shifts of the mandible. It has also been demonstrated to function in protrusive movements (Moyers, 1950; O'Dell *et al.*, 1970; Miller, 1991; Friedman, 1995; Van Eijden *et al.*, 1995) and to demonstrate strong activity during clenching of the teeth in a position anterior to intercuspation (Hannam and Wood, 1981). As noted above, it is these movements which appear to also result in stimulation (functional activity?) of the *l. sphenomandibulare* (s.l.). The *m. pterygoideus medialis* might best be described as being selectively coactivated with the mandibular closers during mandibular elevation and in lateral and protrusive movements, as opposed to the view that it is a simple synergist of other elevators (Hannam and Wood, 1981). The latter suggestion is important as muscles function as groups (Friel, 1926; Moyers, 1950; Last, 1954; Scott, 1967) and, as such, it is difficult to discuss *m. pterygoideus medialis* function and its resultant on bone morphology in the absence of an understanding of coactivated masticatory muscles. Such an holistic approach was employed by Moss and Simon (1968) to interpret ramal morphology but the work still relies heavily on the correlation of bony morphology with simple synergistic activity.

Van Eijden *et al.* (1995) observed that the *m. pterygoideus medialis* in recent *H. sapiens* has a relatively large attachment area and that the different muscle regions have dissimilar moment arm lengths. During jaw movement fibers in various muscle regions will, therefore, undergo different length changes. Because the muscle has short fibers compared to its moment arm there will be significant length change in the sarcomeres and, resultantly, muscle force change (Van Eijden *et al.*, 1995). Further, as they did not find a significant intramuscular difference in fiber length, different sarcomere excursions within the muscle are considered as primarily due to different moment arm lengths. Following jaw opening, positions of sarcomeres on the length-force curve are, therefore, not similar for the anterior and posterior portions (minimally) of *m. pterygoideus medialis*. This means that during jaw movement, the distribution of active tension is not uniform but will vary continuously throughout the muscle, due to differential lengthening or shortening of sarcomeres (Van Eijden et al., 1995). Many authors have recognized this ability of different regions of the adult *m. pterygoideus medialis* to be recruited for certain specialized functions and that the muscle can exert different mechanical actions (Herring and Wineski, 1986; Van Eijden et al., 1997; Foucart et al., 1998; Korfage and Van Eijden, 1999; Goto et al., 2001; Van Eijden and Turkawski, 2001). Although subject to complications due to needle placement, electromyographic recording of the adult *m. pterygoideus medialis* also show different patterns of activity in different mandibular movements and positions for the anterior and posterior regions (Gans and Gorniak, 1978; Moyers, 1950; Hannam and Wood, 1981; Eriksson and Thornell, 1983; Basmajian and DeLuca, 1985; Miller, 1991). Van Eijden and Turkawski (2001) suggest that the selective activation of muscle regions introduces the potential for a muscle to have numerous lines of action that differ in orientation and position, especially in the case of architecturally complex muscles like the *m. pterygoideus medialis*. Of interest, however, is that Herring and Wineski (1986) observed that contraction patterns become more heterogeneous with age. Van Eijden and Turkawski (2001) believe that this might imply that infant muscles are less capable of differential contraction, which might be due to larger and overlapping motor units in younger muscles, which, in turn, might be the result of polyneural innervation. Glyogen-depletion experiments on the pig *m. masseter* demonstrate, however, that motor unit territories had already become very restricted in younger animals (Herring et al., 1991). Data for human infants is not currently available. In sum, the capability of the *m. pterygoideus medialis* to produce different mechanical actions is enhanced by a task-dependent regional contraction of muscle portions and by the heterogeneous distribution of motor units and their associated fiber types (Van Eijden et al., 1997; Eijden and Turkawski, 2001). These facts lend support to observations of Parsons (1896) and Avis (1961), in rodents and humans, respectively, of functional hypertrophy of different layers within multipennated masticatory muscles.

It is currently recognized that the detailed shape of any bone is, in part, a result of the morphogenetic primacy of muscle in producing and regulating corresponding extrinsic responses in bone growth and shape change (Washburn, 1947; Last, 1954; Scott, 1957; Geiser, 1958; Avis, 1959, 1961; van der Klaaw, 1963; Enlow, 1965; Epker and Frost, 1966; Hoyte and Enlow, 1966; Nada et al., 1967; Burdi and Spyropulos, 1978; Gans and Gorniak, 1978; Moss and Moss-Salentijn, 1978; Herring and Lakars, 1981; Atchley et al., 1984; Chierici and Miller, 1984; Atchely and Hall, 1991; Atchley, 1993; Herring, 1993; Sato et al., 1994; Vargervik, 1997). Of note, however, is van der Klaaw's (1963) observation that the determination of bone shape is mainly dependent on the relation between the positions of the different elements with shape being determined both by mechanical and spatial factors. The exact role musculature plays in the process of bone formation is not well understood, although it is clearly more than a pressure-tension relationship (Moore and Lavelle, 1974). Further, tensile loading produced by a single muscle can be associated with both subperiosteal deposition and resorption at the same time (Enlow, 1965). To state that muscle tension is directly involved only in subperiosteal deposition on any given surface, to the exclusion of all other remodeling changes, is not warranted (Baume, 1955; Enlow, 1965; Hoyte and Enlow, 1966; Moss and Simon, 1968). Clearly, bony elevations (tubercles, crests, etc.) and depressions (*sulci, fossae*, etc.) are continuously moved and relocated in order to maintain their relative positions on growing bone (Hoyte and Enlow, 1966). Such movements often require subperiosteal resorption of bone from one slope of a tubercle with progressive and simultaneous, subperiosteal deposition on the other. During skeletal growth the *m. pterygoideus medialis* insertion, and to a lesser degree its origin, is continually being readjusted, especially by posterior ramal growth (Kurihara et al., 1980; Hans et al., 1995). This adjustment is essential if the muscle is to maintain a constant spatial relationship to other muscles and bones throughout growth (Scott, 1954; Symons, 1954; Sperber, 1981). In observations on the *m. pterygoideus medialis*, Symons (1954) notes that, in general, only minimal shifting of the insertion site must occur relative to a continual expansion of the site as the ramus increases in area by bone apposition along the posterior border.

4. Summary

Whereas we have indicated numerous ontogenetic factors which are potentially involved in tubercle formation and maintenance it is clear from the preceding that muscle physiology, gross architecture, and activation properties are interacting with muscle origin-insertion sites at any given age stage to produce the observed bony morphology. To this list must be added variation in entheses as observed by Hems and Tillmann (2000). Rak et al.'s (1994, 1996) suggestion of a simple hypertrophy, or lack thereof, of the superior fibers of the *m. pterygoideus medialis* as responsible for observed tubercle morphology is, in this context, not sufficiently explanatory. Similarly, Antón's (1994a, 1995, 1996) recurrent restatement that tendon fibers of the inferior aspects of the muscle are intertwined with those of the superior portions of the muscle and, thereby, redirect forces from the inferior to the superior muscle regions adds little to our understanding. The latter does serve, however, to imply: (1) the lack of functional units within masticatory muscles and their selective activation; and (2) the inability of the superior aspect of the multipennated *m. pterygoideus medialis* to induce an areally restricted bony response. Working from Antón's (1994a, 1995, 1996) stated perspective we are unable to explain the distribution of tubercles in the insertion site of the *m. pterygoideus medialis* and, by extension, to understand the evolution of individual regions in muscles.

Given the above it is clear that the *m. pterygoideus medialis* is a highly complex muscle whose components are selectively activated to produce a range of: (1) movements; (2) stabilization events; and (3) bite force requirements. We recognize that muscle force may be spread over a broad portion of the bone-musculotendinous interface due to the arrangement of intramuscular septa and by the broad distribution of forces in solely periosteal attachment sites (Elliott, 1965; Dörlf, 1980a, b). These facts will have some effect on our ability to fully delineate specific changes in regionally restricted portions of muscle origin and insertion sites.

Whereas the above will have a limiting effect on the delineation of specific muscle functions from dry bone samples, of greater import is the wealth of information available from such sites. It is known that attachment sites for the *m. pterygoideus medialis* are complex and comprise: (1) solely muscle to periosteum; (2) enthesis to periosteum; (3) enthesis to bone; and (4) enthesis to fibrocartilage. We have demonstrated, herein, that significant progress can be made in understanding attachment site development and evolution based on an understanding of this variation.

Further, we have shown the value of understanding muscle region heterogeneity and its effect on bone morphology. In the absence of such an understanding we are unable to explain the complex morphology and distribution of bony features related to the insertion of the *m. pterygoideus medialis*. Further, in attempting to understand the intertaxonomic distribution and development of muscle related tubercles we must factor in the presence and distribution of muscle fiber types and their isoforms and the impact of these on bony morphology. By example; we have provided evidence that the posterior head/portion of the *m. pterygoideus medialis* comprises a high percentage of Type IIX-MyHC fibers and that these fibers produce short bouts of intense activity. Given their high activation threshold and ability to produce powerful movements it would be expected that their tendinous attachment would reflect that function. We have shown that, with some variation, hominid taxa from *Australopithecus* to recent *H. sapiens* have tubercle morphology that reflects this muscular anatomy and function.

MUSCULAR FUNCTION, CRANIOFACIAL ONTOGENY, AND MODELING MANDIBULAR GROWTH

I. MUSCULAR FUNCTION AND CRANIOFACIAL MORPHOLOGY

1. Introduction

In defining the MPT character state Rak et al. (1994) and Rak and Kimbel (1995) suggest that the appearance of the *m. pterygoideus medialis* markings in the form of the MPT in a young, still-suckling individual (Amud 7) attests to the genetic nature of the trait and eliminates consideration of it having been acquired during growth as the result of some specific habitual activity. Recall that these authors believe the adult MPT results from hypertrophy of the superior portion of the *m. pterygoideus medialis*. Given this assertion Rak et al. (1994, 1996) suggest that the presence of a MPT has profound functional implications which are potentially related to masticatory adaptations and the unique architecture of the Neanderthal face. Creed-Miles et al. (1996) support the suggestion of a MPT-facial architecture relationship in Neanderthals but prefer a non-masticatory explanation for tubercle formation. Antón (1996) considers that her observation of a greater development of the MPT in Neanderthals is the result of masticatory forces of a long-vaulted hominid. To clarify the functional significance of the MPT (= septa 6, 4, and 2^{III} insertion), and by extension masticatory muscle attachments in general, throughout ontogeny it is necessary to explore the: (1) interrelated development of the mandible and masticatory function; and (2) role of the masticatory musculature in shaping craniofacial architecture.

2. Mandibulofacial development in relation to the ontogeny of masticatory function

Craniomandibular muscles change in size, complexity, and orientation with postnatal growth (Haines, 1932; Scott, 1957; Bowden and Goyer, 1960; Schumacher, 1962; Moss and Simons, 1968; Rayne and Crawford, 1972; Burleigh, 1974; Herring and Wineski, 1986; German and Myers, 1989; Miller, 1991; Goldspink, 1999; Lee et al., 2001). Maturation of the motor end-plates and commencement of normal muscular function which results in hypertrophy of fetal muscle fibers, does not begin until circa > 7th month *in utero* and is not complete in the limbs until after birth (Scott, 1957; Bowden and Goyer, 1960). The growth rate of muscle fibers in humans is regulated by growth factors, including those induced by mechanical signals, and fiber growth lasts for at least 12.0 years after birth (Burleigh, 1974; Goldspink, 1999). Note, however, that Goldspink (1999) determined that even mature muscles have the capacity of adapting to new functional lengths by adding or removing sarcomeres in series. Scott (1954) observed that between the ages of 1.0 year and adulthood the *m. masseter* increased in thickness and p-csa by about four and eight times, respectively. The latter reflects, in part, an increase in fibrous tissue and tendon substance but mainly reflects hypertrophy of fetal muscle fibers (Scott, 1954). Using Friel's (1926) bite force data Scott (1957) determined that muscle development is not a constant process but that it shows steady, slight, and rapid periods of growth. During this period of muscle size increase new closure patterns are generated in the muscles with eruption of the deciduous dentition, especially in the *mm. pterygoideus medialis* and *temporalis* (Moyers, 1950; Scott, 1967). The establishment of occluso-muscular relationships marks the onset of normal occlusion which occurs with eruption of dM1/1 (Scott, 1967).

Further, these increases in muscle size are supplemented by significant changes in muscle fiber orientation. Whereas Herring et al. (1993) note that detailed observations on growth alterations in the angulation of human masticatory muscles are generally not available, some data exist for *mm. masseter* and *pterygoideus medialis* (Schumacher, 1961, 1962; Scott, 1967; Moss and Simon, 1968; Sperber, 1981; Herring et al., 1993). Changes in fiber orientation starts with eruption of dM1/1 with adult orientations being attained with establishment of occlusal relations in dM2/2 (Schumacher, 1962; Scott, 1967; Moss and Simons, 1968: but contra Burdi, 1978). Similar changes in *m. masseter* fiber direction have been observed in pigs (*Sus scrofa*: Herring, 1977; Herring et al., 1993) but note that in rats angular change in this muscle occurred in the anterior but not in the posterior fibers (Covell and Herring, 1995). In the latter case, Rayne and Crawford (1971) observed that muscle fiber arrangement is simple and parallel until muscle function outstrips the ability of this arrangement to accommodate an increasing range of tensions. This variation in muscle growth patterns, coupled with that discussed for tendon insertions, helps account, in part, for our observation that during growth tubercle morphology does not appear to be significantly altered during broad ranges of postnatal growth.

Mandibular growth reflects this development of muscle from an early stage (Sato et al., 1994). In the 11th *intra uteran* week Meckel's cartilage becomes transformed and the condylar process begins to contribute to mandibular growth (Bareggi et al., 1995; Lee et al. 2001). By the 16th *intra uteran* week the mandibular corpus and ramus have assumed distinct angular variations and exhibit different rates of growth; the former increases more rapidly than the latter in both length and height (Rabkin, 1952; Lavelle and Moore, 1970; Burdi, 1978; Trenouth, 1984; Mandarim-de-Lacerda and Alves, 1992; Sato et al., 1994; Lee et al., 2001). Rabkin (1952) considered this variation as evidence of the existence of a predetermined pattern for the growth and shaping of distinct, individual morphologic characteristics. Alternatively, Humphrey (1971) observed reflexive responses in masticatory musculature by 8.0-8.5 weeks *in utero* and Diewart (1983) observed that *mm. masseter* and *temporalis* are interacting with ramus growth by the 16th week. Recently, Lee *et al.* (2001) suggested that this early muscle function (8th week) may be implicated in the transition of masticatory muscles from their attachment to Meckel's cartilage to one on the developing intramembranous bone-secondary cartilages of the mandible. The size of fetal muscle fibers appears sufficient to carry out these initial pseudo-masticatory tasks, however, as the selective process of fetal fiber hypertrophy does not begin until ca. > 7th month *in utero* (Scott, 1957; Bowden and Goyer, 1960).

Whereas there is clear evidence that prenatal masticatory muscle action is involved in mandibular development the movements produced differ from those documented postnatally. This situation arises because visceral (branchial) arch musculature comprising them is developmentally and behaviorally intermediate between somatic and true visceral muscle of the gut (Scott, 1967). Given normal development and maturation the later developing somatic-voluntary characteristics will begin to predominate over the earlier visceral-involuntary characteristics associated with these muscles. From the 10th week *in utero* onwards, mouth-opening reflexes become progressively less associated with a total lateral body reflex-response to a stimulus, indicating the development of inhibitory nerve pathways (Sperber, 1981; Moyers and Carlson, 1996). However, head movements remain strongly associated with mouth movements even into the postnatal period, accounting for the 'rooting reflex', whereby perioral stimulation leads to ipsilateral head rotation, which is associated with suckling in the infant. At birth, the suckling muscles of the lips (*m. orbicularis oris*) and cheeks (*m. buccinator*) are relatively more developed than the muscles of mastication with *mm. masseter* and *pterygoideus medialis* being more developed than *mm. temporalis* and *pterygoideus lateralis* (Sperber, 1981).

Prior to eruption of dM1/1 infants swallow with the mandible and maxilla separated and with the tongue thrust forward (Sperber, 1981). Infants swallow predominantly by using the facial muscles (Moyers, 1964; Moyers and Carlson, 1996) which are innervated by cranial nerve (CN) seven (*n. facialis*). This pattern is known as the 'infantile swallow' and is a non-conditioned congenital reflex (Sperber, 1981). Following eruption of dM1/1 (ca. 1.5 years), infants tend to swallow with the teeth approximated by masticatory muscle action. The 'mature swallow' is, then, an acquired conditioned reflex which is intermingled with the infantile swallow during a transitional period, until swallowing is controlled solely by CN V (*n. trigeminus*: Sperber, 1981; Moyers and Carlson, 1996). Mastication, then, involves a learning process wherein arises a greater plasticity and individuality than the earlier established non-conditioned process (Scott, 1967; Sperber, 1981). Wickwire *et al.* (1981) have shown that an increase in control over masticatory muscles is a process which extends well into juvenile age stages. Further, not only must the various reflex mechanisms become adapted to such superimposed activities as chewing and the initial stages of swallowing, they must also adapt themselves to the growth of the craniofacial skeleton. Stingl (1972) observed abrupt changes in postnatal development of masticatory muscles in the rat (hyperplasia and hypertrophy of fibers, internal muscular reconstruction) at circa three weeks. He considers these changes as attributable to the abrupt changes in general motor activity at weaning.

Whereas the mandible and maxilla may approximate each other in size in the newborn the mandible tends to be retrognathic to the maxilla (Sperber, 1981). At this stage the condylar head is rounded and positioned at approximately the same level as the gum pads. The glenoid fossa is flattened and lacks a distinct articular eminence (Clinch, 1934; Scott, 1967). The fibers of *mm. masseter* and *pterygoideus medialis* are more horizontally oriented than in the adult and produce mandibular movements characteristic of suckling (Clinch, 1934). Ligaments of the mandibular joint are relatively lax and muscular movements are much less limited by the conformation of the joint structures and dentition (Clinch, 1934). Given this configuration of the temporomandibular articulation, joint stability in infants depends on the strength of ligaments surrounding the joint to prevent dislocation (Clinch, 1934). This anatomy allows for approximation of the gums in the incisor region as the molar segments act as a fulcrum around which the jaw rotates, causing the condyle to be withdrawn from the shallow glenoid fossa. It is probable that the greater development of the *m. pterygoideus medialis* is related to maintaining condylar relations in this developmental stage. Scott (1967) notes that at birth only a limited amount of anteroposterior mandibular movement is possible. Movement in the anteroposterior direction becomes more developed with eruption of dI1/1 whereas side-to-side lateral movements develop with eruption of the dM1/1. Prior to eruption of dM1/1, mandibular growth is relatively greater than maxillary growth whereas following their eruption the relatively equal anteroposterior relationship of the dental arches is established (Clinch, 1934; Sillman, 1948; Humphrey, 1971; Sperber, 1981; Moyers and Carlson, 1996). Ligament strength and muscle fiber orientation also starts to change with eruption of dM1/1 and they reach a more adult-like configuration contemporaneously with establishment of dM2/2 occlusal relationships.

Mandibular growth rates vary with the age of the individual with one characteristic growth pattern never being established (Brodie, 1946; Scott, 1954, 1967; Björk, 1963; Tracy and Savara, 1966; Moss and Salentijn, 1970; Ricketts, 1972; Hans *et al.*, 1995). Whereas details vary by author, clear differences have been observed between the mean growth rate for the juvenile and pubertal periods (Nanda, 1955; Björk, 1963; Tracy and Savara, 1966; Scott, 1967; Woodside, 1973; Baughan *et al.*, 1979; Ekström, 1982; Krieg, 1987; Pirinen, 1995). The developmental age at which these growth spurts occur varies widely, however, as does the intensity of the increase (Björk, 1963; Hans *et al.*, 1995). The mechanism(s) responsible for this variation is unknown (Hans *et al.*, 1995). This rapid degree of growth results, however, in high remodeling rates which produce a significant degree of morphological variability in the mandible (Moore and Lavelle, 1974; Sperber, 1981; Hans *et al.*, 1995) in general, and the gonial region specifically (Björk, 1963). Further, in subadults changes in form occur in conjunction with spatial relocation of the mandible whereas in adults changes in mandibular form occur without necessarily being associated with positional changes (Moss, 1968).

3. Masticatory muscles and craniofacial shape

Various studies are available which examine the relationship between masticatory muscles and craniofacial shape in adults (Spyropoulos, 1977; Ingervall and Helkimo, 1978; Corruccini, 1984; Shaughnessy *et al.*, 1989; Weijs, 1989; Van Spronsen *et al.*, 1991, 1992, 1997; Varrela, 1992; Kilaridis, 1995; Raadsheer *et al.*, 1999; Katsaros, 2001; Watanabe and Watanabe, 2001). There is general agreement that craniofacial shape differences are associated with masticatory-functional demands. Ingervall and Helkimo (1978) found reduced inter-individual variation of facial form in persons with strong muscles relative to those with weak muscles. These differences were especially marked for vertical facial dimensions with short anterior and long posterior facial heights in the weak muscled group. The dimensional difference between the anterior and posterior facial heights results from an anterior growth rotation of the mandible as confirmed by Kilaridis (1995). This study also correlated well-developed angular, coronoid, and condylar processes with increased muscular development. In an initial study employing serial MRI scans, Van Spronsen *et al.* (1991) found no correlation between anterior or posterior facial heights in normal *H. sapiens* males and the p-csa of masticatory muscles. They concluded that only a limited correlation exists between muscle p-csa and craniofacial form in normal male humans. Subsequently, Van Spronsen *et al.* (1992) found significant differences between long-faced and normal adults with the former having significantly reduced masticatory muscles, which they consider may be related to a reduced bite force in these individuals. In the long face group the *mm. masseter, pterygoideus medialis,* and anterior *temporalis* had p-csa which were 30%, 22%, and 15% smaller than in controls, respectively. Significant differences in the functional performance of short versus long faced individuals, as measured by the range of bite force directions and magnitude and joint loads, have also been documented by Weijs (1989). Note, however, that Hannam and Wood (1981) consider that there are so many combinations of biomechanically relevant variables relating to bite force efficiency that similar bite-force efficiencies can be found in subjects with disparate facial features. This result appears to be confirmed by the finding of Raadsheer *et al.* (1999). For masticatory muscles they only found a significant result for the *m. masseter* and in this muscle the p-csa was found to contribute more to bite-force magnitude than variation in craniofacial variables. Shaughnessy *et al.*'s (1989) investigation of fiber-type distribution and craniofacial form found one significant negative correlation, that between the percentage occurrence of Type I fibers in *m. pterygoideus medialis* and ramus height (condylion-gonion). However, in reviewing his results and those of prior work, he could not support the hypothesis that a relationship exists between facial type and selected histochemical characteristics of muscles. We believe that differences in fiber types will have a more limited affect on craniofacial variables and that a useful direction of research will be to evaluate fiber type distribution relative to specific aspects of bony morphology (i.e. origin-insertion sites, tubercles, ridges, etc.).

4. Summary

Given the above we can examine the suggested relationships of the MPT to masticatory and non-masticatory factors and the organization of craniofacial functional matrices. It is clear that masticatory muscles are interacting with ramal growth beginning in the early prenatal period. Further, it has been demonstrated that the *m. pterygoideus medialis* not only has a relatively greater role in late prenatal and postnatal stages (ca. < 2.0 - 3.0 years of age) but has a significantly changed function over this period. We have demonstrated that attachment sites for septa of the *m. pterygoideus medialis* are present in newborns and throughout postnatal growth. We have also detailed how large tubercles related specifically to septa 6 and 4 of this muscle may appear during this and later growth stages. In this assessment, however, we have noted the extensive idiosyncratic variation in these attachment site(s). We have also detailed potential reasons for how this variation arises during growth which includes both masticatory and non-masticatory factors. Based on the ontogenetic studies discussed above it is clear that: (1) pseudo-masticatory function is impacting the *m. pterygoideus medialis* insertion site from early prenatal stages; (2) significant differences are present in the architecture, orientation, and function of muscles throughout growth; and (3) mandibular function is sufficiently variable during these periods to produce significantly different bony architecture both between and within developmental age groups. Because of the observed muscle-to-septal attachment site relationship throughout this complex period of development, we find it difficult to suggest that a MPT develops in Neanderthal infants in the absence of masticatory muscle function as suggested by Rak *et al.* (1994) and Rak and Kimbel (1995). Although, note that 'masticatory' muscle function comprises both pseudo-masticatory and masticatory functions in these early growth stages. Indeed, we have shown Neanderthals to be morphologically similar and to have a similar range of variation to that seen in recent *H. sapiens*. The slight differences observed between these taxa for these features can best be ascribed to demic, clinal, and temporal factors. Further, we consider it unlikely that a large, genetically induced tubercle with no apparent function develops and is maintained not only during a period of complex growth and shape changes but during a time when space for packaging soft tissues into the infratemporal fossa is at a premium. We have also shown how medial ramus morphology reflects differences in timing of the growth of related soft tissues and how these relationships change during growth. Further, given our brief review of the relationship between craniofacial shape and size characteristics and the development of masticatory musculature in humans it is difficult to support suggestions that the development of a MPT is directly related to either or both masticatory adaptations or architecture of the Neanderthal face (Rak *et al.*, 1994, 1996) or cranial vault shape (Antón, 1996). We also disagree with the suggestion that development of a MPT results from non-masticatory forces as suggested by Creed-Miles *et al.* (1996). It is clear that both craniofacial size and shape characteristics, the function of masticatory muscles, and the complex changes they undergo during ontogeny interact to produce medial ramal anatomy.

II. IMPACT OF CURRENT WORK ON MODEL OF MANDIBULAR GROWTH

1. Migration of musculotendinous attachments

We believe that further assessments of medial ramal anatomy and evolution will contribute much to our understanding of craniofacial evolution in hominoids. Advances will be restricted, in the short term, by the lack of detailed comparative histological and anatomical descriptions of these regions for modern hominoids. Further, our understanding of ramal growth processes and models derived therefrom are in need of revision. To this end we provide a short discussion of potential revisions to the current model of mandibular ramus growth based on the above data. Such issues and numerous others, as alluded to above, will need clarification in order to properly evaluate new comparative studies of this region.

Histological studies, employing tetracycline labeling, demonstrate that during growth in length of a bone that ligament and tendon migrations are controlled by a set of conditions that are specific to the different attachment methods (Epker and Frost, 1966; Dörfl, 1980a). Although muscular traction was initially thought to have a role in the migration of tendons and ligaments (Lacroix, 1949; Dörfl, 1980a) further research has shown that role to be minimal or entirely lacking (Grant, 1978; Dörfl, 1980b; Grant et al., 1980, 1981). Grant (1978) concluded from analysis of long bones that bone growth is the controlling factor in soft tissue migration. With growth, soft tissue structures are simply transported to new locations as the periosteum slides over the bone's surface (Grant 1978; Dörfl, 1980a-b; Grant et al., 1980, 1981; Weijs et al., 1987; Herring et al., 1993; Covell and Herring, 1995). Movement of tissues along a bone is allowed as structures (muscles, tendons, and ligaments) associated with the growing long bone diaphyses are attached to periosteum; entheses are generally not considered to penetrate into bone during this process (Amprino and Cattaneo, 1937; Grant et al., 1981; Benjamin and Ralphs, 2000; Hems and Tillmann, 2000). Note that work by Hurov (1986) indicates, however, that the periosteum is attached to the bone's surface during early development by an extensive collagen fiber framework. Maturation of this framework was found to vary with age and by region within specific muscle and ligament attachments (Hurov, 1986). In the generally accepted view, as the periosteum expands interstitially during growth it carries attached structures along with it. In adults diaphyseal entheses ultimately attach: (1) to periosteum; (2) directly to bone with or without an intervening periosteum; or (3) by a combination of these attachment methods. A third category of attachment exists in long bones in which tendons and ligaments attach to epiphyses via fibrocartilaginous entheses. As discussed above, individual masticatory muscles have now been shown to possess most variants of this attachment continuum (Hems and Tillmann, 2001).

The timing and degree to which septal and ligament entheses penetrate into and become embedded in bone raises a number of questions regarding our assessment of medial ramal ontogeny and, specifically, the bony morphology of the septa 6, 4, and 2^{III} insertions. In our assessment we have *tentatively* correlated aspects of bony medial ramal morphology with the attachment of these specific septa of the m. pterygoideus medialis. We have also done this with bony attachment sites for the l. sphenomandibulare (s.s. / s.l.). We noted that there are specific bony ridges in the insertion site of newborn and later infants which we tentatively correlate with septa of the muscle. At a gross level, such sites show strong similarity to those occurring in adults. We have also asserted that aspects of the insertion site morphology are related to the degree of coalescence or lack of separation of the intramuscular septa, specifically that of septa 6 and 4. Further, we have noted differences in attachment site morphology which differentiate periosteal entheses (cf. recent H. sapiens, Gibraltar 2) from those comprising bony or fibrocartilaginous attachments. The latter attachments were identified in literature descriptions, confirmed in our adult cadaver series, and used to identify such attachments in our dry bone growth series. Given the presence of soft tissues attaching directly to bone at mid-ramus in still-growing individuals, a model of mandibular growth in which structures attached to the ramus-condylar neck region (i.e. below the condylar growth plate cartilage) are periosteally attached and are passively translocated with periosteal growth does not account for observed variation in attachment morphology.

Grant et al. (1980, 1981) have suggested, however, that models of soft tissue migrations in long bones may not be applicable to the skull. Current research indicates that the basic mechanisms for soft tissue migrations in cranial and postcranial regions are similar, but that mandibular enthesis variation within individual muscles creates a more complex system (Benjamin and Ralphs, 2000; Hems and Tillmann, 2000). In the case of the mandible our working hypothesis is that the region of the f. mandibulae-s. colli is relatively stable during growth, as noted earlier by Symons (1954). If this region, inclusive of the septa 6 and 4 insertions, is reasonably stable the insertion sites may also be more stable and, therefore, more similar to those of adults. Further, more developed attachments should occur in periods of relative stability whereas less developed attachments should result during periods of high remodeling activity. Both our recent and fossil Homo samples suggest that such a mosaic pattern of variation is present. Of further note is that this attachment site has been shown to include fibrocartilaginous entheses. Given this attachment type it might be expected that the attachment would be more similar to that seen in adults. What is currently unclear, however, is when this fibrocartilaginous attachment develops and what the effect of function is on the attachment site. Note that Matyas et al. (1995) suggest that mechanical factors might be primarily responsible for the development and maintenance of the fibrocartilaginous phenotype in ligament attachments. This fibrocartilage may be present from early fetal stages and later acted upon by muscle function, but this remains to be confirmed.

2. Suggested revision to mandibular growth model

Given the work of Hems and Tillmann (2000) and the possibility that portions of the medial ramus are relatively stable during growth, revision of the current model of mandibular growth is indicated. In the current model, ramus growth occurs in a periosteal sleeve which is loosely attached to the ramus and firmly attached only at the base of the condylar growth plate. Because it would be positioned between the condylar growth region and the ramal growth region, stability of the *f. mandibulae-s. colli* region could constitute a neutral zone. Such a zone was documented in long bones by Lacroix (1949) and discussed by Grant *et al.* (1980) to be a place where periosteum does not slide over the bone's surface. A neutral zone will have its position determined by the relative contribution of each end of the long bone to total bone growth (Lacroix, 1949; Grant *et al.*, 1980). Results of work on mandibular growth in guinea pigs have demonstrated differential migration of the periosteum and its attached musculature along the inferior border of the mandibular ramus (Covell and Herring, 1995). In this taxon a neutral zone results at approximately the center of the tooth row (Covell and Herring, 1995) whereas in humans a neutral zone occurs just posterior to the *f. mentale*. This pattern supports earlier indications of a differential anteroposterior periosteal migration in the mandibles of rabbits (Weijs *et al.*, 1987) and pigs (Herring *et al.*, 1993). Based on recent preliminary results (Moore *et al.*, 2003) and on the work of Hans *et al.* (1995), we consider it likely that a neutral zone is present on the mandibular corpus of recent *H. sapiens*. Note here also the possibility of a difference in periosteal migration patterns for the medial and lateral cortical plates of the ramus. Differential migration along these plates is consistent with our suggestion that the mandible comprises more skeletal units than currently recognized. Recent work on the fate of Meckel's cartilage during mandibular development (Merida-Velasco *et al.*, 1993; Harada and Ishizeki, 1998; Ishizeki *et al.*, 1999, 2001) adds further support for the recognition of such a level of complexity.

Clarification of the development in this region is significant as Grant *et al.* (1981) consider that the periosteal sleeve model implies that in functional and comparative anatomical studies in which the relative positions of muscles or ligaments are used, the ages of the animals used should not affect the results. Further, the model implies that differences in relative positions of muscles and ligaments (on long bones) are expressions of underlying genetic differences rather than of differential developmental conditions (Grant *et al.*, 1980, 1981). These authors state that minor differences in closely related taxa must be considered as expressions of evolutionary adaptations resulting from differences in selection pressures due to differences in habitat and behavior, rather than as developmental plasticity or even reversible physiological adaptations (see Lasker, 1969). In sum, small differences between closely related animals should provide important clues to the functional adaptations related to various behavioral tendencies (Grant *et al.*, 1981). We are currently working to delineate the anatomy of the *s. colli* and *f. mentale* region in dry bone samples (Moore *et al.*, 2003; Richards *et al.*, in prep.) as a first step in establishing an appropriate model which can be tested in a longitudinal growth series. Note however, that the statements of Grant *et al.* (1981) refer to soft tissues and, ultimately rely on detailed descriptions of attachment site variation. We have shown that the presence of soft tissue attachments to bone during growth are variable, minimally developed, and, when present, are continuously being modified. The latter facts will result in significant, but not insurmountable, difficulties for interpreting idiosyncratic, geographic, ontogenetic, and interspecific differences in bony attachment sites in recent dry bone samples and in remains of fossil species.

ONTOGENY AND VARIATION IN SYSTEMATICS

I. ONTOGENETIC AND PHYLOGENETIC ISSUES RELATED TO THE MEDIAL PTERYGOID TUBERCLE

In concluding their analysis of the MPT, Rak and Kimbel (1995:177-178) state that the "...obscuring of derived morphology is a common effect of early ontogenetic stages" and that "[t]he discovery of derived adult skeletal characters in such a very young individual is significant because their appearance must be ascribed to genetic origins". Subsequently, Hovers *et al.* (1996:50) stated that "It has been suggested that some Neandertal traits were not genetic, but developed through the individual's life" and that the occurrence of a MPT in an individual as young as Amud 7 refutes such claims for this character state. A number of important issues are raised in determining the validity of such statements. Of overwhelming importance is the recognition that the vast majority of bony features within a species cannot be singularly ascribed to strictly genetic origins (Scott, 1957; Lieberman, 1995). Bony morphology is a reflection of genetics, epigenetics (*sensu* Atchley, 1993), and nonheritable idiosyncratic variations. Dullemeijer (1974) notes that this interplay of genetic and epigenetic factors differs through ontogeny. More specifically, Spyropoulos (1977) observed that, because the functioning musculotendinous-bone complex is always present, this produces a situation wherein it is extremely difficult to determine the relative role(s) of intrinsic factors and of functional (epigenetic) influences in bone development.

We have shown significant similarities and differences to be present in the *m. pterygoideus medialis* and *l. mandibulae* (*s.l.*) insertion sites of great apes and hominids and discussed changes in these insertions within the evolving hominid lineage. Whereas some of the observed morphology may have a strictly genetic basis we believe that it is not possible to postulate any such correspondence given currently available data. Knowledge of the genetic basis of a feature is not, however, a requirement for use of the feature in systematics. Given this fact, we believe that with sufficient further clarification of the developmental constraints under which these features arise and the range of variation present in some aspects of these insertion sites that they will prove to be useful in hominid systematics.

Rak and Kimbel (1995) indicate further that derived morphology is obscured in young individuals. Therefore, when a derived adult character is found in a subadult it is even more significant in indicating the degree of divergence of two lineages. We consider such statements and their recent application (Golovanova, 1994; Golovanova and Romanova, 1995; Golovanova *et al.*, 1999; Zollikofer *et al.*, 1995) to underscore the need for clarification of the equation of characters defined in adults with characteristics of subadults. First, we do not consider adult morphologies to be obscured in subadults; they are either not present, present, or only in the process of developing to the adult state. As observed by Herring (1993), tissues change with age and in the postnatal period dramatic alterations in cellularity, extracellular matrix, and growth potential occur. She also notes that equivalent changes must occur during the embryonic and fetal periods. Features observed in subadults display substantial variation in their timing of appearance and duration of growth (heterochrony) toward the adult state and in their shape (Heim, 1982; Tillier, 1982, 1983a, b, 1986, 1988,1992; Madre-Dupouy, 1991). Although some features will obviously be *nearing* the adult condition prior to the adult state being reached, with few exceptions (e.g. shape characteristics of dentin, tooth crown morphology, etc.) adult features of hard tissues only occur in adults. Features of subadult anatomy must be considered on their own terms as each ontogenetic stage presents a unique series of demands which are then reflected in observable bony morphology (Dullemeijer, 1974; Thilander, 1995; Jabbour *et al.*, 2002). To fully utilize available subadult remains in assessing phylogenetic relationships it is imperative that: (1) the ontogenetic trajectories of bony features be delineated as fully as possible; (2) the functional constraints under which these morphologies are being produced be delineated and compared; and (3) species definitions should include ontogenetic details of features used in defining the species, as noted by Tillier (1998). Such definitions should also include reference to features of subadult states which are unique to such stages and which are not represented in the adult state, as observed by Schwartz and Tattersall (1996a). Further, ontogenetic studies must be based on samples which allow delineation of the degree of variation present in any age stage and the number of stages employed must be sufficient to allow delineation of the timing of morphological change and to reduce the effects of sampling error (Clark, 2000).

Subsequent to its definition as a Neanderthal autapomorphy, the MPT character state, or a similar character, has been employed in taxonomic and phylogenetic assessments as either an autapomorphy, a synapomorphy, or a character which occurs most frequently in Neanderthals (Rak *et al.*, 1996; Hublin, 1998; Quam and Smith, 1998; Rak, 1998a; Tillier, 1998; Lebel *et al.*, 2001). It was noted some forty years ago, however, that "[t]here is a real, practical, and biological difference between a character that sharply and unambiguously differentiates two groups and one which differs only on the average between them" (Simpson *et al.*, 1960:81). Whereas a definition of the MPT character state has been provided by Rak *et al.* (1994), the only available reassessments of this character state deal specifically with its autapomorphic status. We are of the opinion that a full reassessment of a character's usefulness must precede any attempt to apply the character to systematics in any capacity other then that for which it was originally defined.

II. MORPHOLOGICAL VARIATION AND SYSTEMATICS

Variation in morphology provides the foundation for speciation (Darwin, 1859). All morphological features vary to some extent and an understanding of this variation and its underlying causes is critical to delineating species and speciation events. A complication of delineating variation in characters is, however, that when it is taken into account in closely related groups the ultimate implications of the character are generally inconclusive in cladistic analyses (Trinkaus, 1990, 1995b; Lieberman, 1995; Stefan and Trinkaus, 1998b; Franciscus,1999). For this reason, Wiley (1981), Lieberman (1995), and Wolpoff and Crummett (1995) all suggest that characters which show broad ranges of variation within a species should be avoided in phylogenetic analyses. Highly variable characters, such as some muscle attachment sites, can be employed in phylogenetic analyses, however, "... *as long as the character states vary more between taxa than within taxa*" (itls. in orig.; Lieberman, 1995:189). Such characters should be rigorously defined and accompanied by detailed scoring methods (Lahr, 1995). Delineating variation in adults is complex and the situation is exacerbated when the ontogeny of a character state is considered (Presley, 1993). This situation is driven not only by variation in the development of a character but by the increased sample sizes necessary to delineate developmental stages.

Although investigators differ in how they employ the MPT, or similar, character in taxonomic and phylogenetic analyses, it is only in the works of Antón (1995, 1996), Richards and Plourde (1995), and Coqueugnoit (1999) that a description of morphological variation has been attempted. This includes the original description by Rak *et al.* (1994). We have demonstrated, however, that Antón's (1995, 1996) results best serve to underscore the need to understand the anatomy prior to the application of metric techniques. We find this general lack of attention to morphological variation curious as Turner and Chamberlain (1989), Trinkaus (1990, 1995b), Franciscus and Trinkaus (1995), Lieberman (1995), Richards and Plourde (1995), Wolpoff and Crummett (1995), Arensburg and Belfer-Cohen (1998), Stefan and Trinkaus (1998b), Franciscus (1999), Jabbour and Richards (1998), and Jabbour *et al.* (2002) have all discussed the need to understand variation in character states in Middle to Late Pleistocene *Homo* prior to their usage in taxonomic and phylogenetic reconstructions. In sum, we consider the delineation of morphological variation in a feature or character state to be an obligatory initial step in systematics, no matter which methodological approach to taken to reconstructing relationships between taxa. Given our investigation of features and character states of the medial ramus, we believe that the following comment by Lewis (1989:5) succinctly summarizes our point of view: "At the end of the day, cladistic analysis is only as good as the quality of and sophistication of the functional morphological markers utilized."

CONCLUSIONS

Atchley (1993) notes that the various developmental and skeletal components related to the mandible do not exist as isolates, but rather during embryological development they become integrated into a single functioning skeletal structure. Thus, mandibular embryological heterogeneity results in postnatal morphological heterogeneity (Atchley and Hall, 1991). In this context it is important to recall that the evolution of morphological diversity is nothing more than the evolution of those underlying developmental processes that produced the morphology (Atchley and Hall, 1991; Atchley, 1993). In assessing the origins of the heterogeneity of mandibular bony morphology and its relationship to soft tissues it is important to note the complexity of these relationships. Relevant discussion could include details of: (1) muscle fiber orientation and physiology; (2) muscle heads and layers; (3) the musculotendinous interface; (4) tendon physiology; (5) the tendon-periosteum interface; (6) the tendon-periosteum-bone interface; (7) the ligament-bone interface; (8) bone physiology; and (9) both ontogenetic and functional changes in these relationships. Scott (1967) cautions that it is against such a developmental background that we must seek to understand the functional development of the oral cavity.

Trinkaus (1995b) observed, however, that paleoanthropologists have been reluctant to examine fully the genetic, developmental, and functional bases for features or character states they employ in phylogenetic analyses. More specifically, this fact has been echoed by many authors who note the lack of detailed ontogenetic and functional studies related to character states of Neanderthals (Lieberman, 1995; Rightmire, 1995; Schwartz and Tattersall, 1995; Laitman et al., 1996; Mann and Vandermeersch, 1997; Minugh-Purvis, 1998). This fact is clearly demonstrated in our review of studies related to the medial ramus. Further, Atchley (1993) cautions that resolution of evolutionary questions regarding the origin and diversity of craniomandibular form will require a focus on the biological population. Population level analyses by their very nature employ large samples. Ontogenetic studies require even larger samples as the population comprises numerous developmental age groups which must represent the population at that age stage. We earlier noted the detrimental effects of a reliance on single individuals to represent developmental stages (see Golovanova, 1994; Golovanova and Romanova, 1995; Zollikofer et al., 1995; Golovanova et al., 1999) and note here that the continued reliance on such analyses (Ponce de León and Zollikofer, 2001) adds little to our understanding of the ontogeny of recent or fossil *Homo*. Such problems are accentuated by comparisons made between fossil specimens which are not at similar stages in the life cycle, as discussed by Hennig (1966), Gould (1977), and Roth (1988). Further, Presley (1993) notes that it is important that ontogenetic development be understood as a process and not as an imperative for functional components to arrive at an adult morphology. Important differences may be overlooked by a tendency to describe developing structures in quasi-adult terms (Presley, 1993).

Herein we have attempted to address a broad series of issues raised in conjunction with a proposed autapomorphic character state in Neanderthals, the 'medial pterygoid tubercle' (MPT). To this end we employ evidence from: (1) dry bone samples of recent *H. sapiens* and great apes and fossil representatives of the Hominidae; (2) soft tissue dissections of adult recent humans; and (3) a broad review of literature pertaining to both these samples and to aspects of bone, muscle, and tendon physiology and architecture, and craniofacial growth and development. Our point has not been to simply assess the MPT character state but to evaluate the complexities of the ontogeny of functional matrices and their associated medial mandibular ramal skeletal unit(s) in an effort to investigate the kinds of data available for validation of such a character. Within this context we have provided extensive documentation of the relationship of developing craniofacial functional matrices to the development and evolution of the bony medial mandibular ramus. From these data we provide preliminary suggestions regarding the evolutionary trajectories of the *c. endocondyloidea*, *s. colli*, *f. mandibulae-c. mandibulae*, *l. mandibulae*, mylohyoid groove, and *m. pterygoideus medialis* insertion site. We have also provided preliminary data on evolutionary changes in the *m. pterygoideus medialis*, *l. sphenomandibulare* (*s.s. / s.l.*), and neurovascular bundles of the medial ramus region. These data are evaluated in light of the extensive literature available on relevant soft tissue physiology, anatomy, function, and craniofacial ontogeny.

In conjunction with these more broad-based observations and conclusions we made a number of specific conclusions. Regarding the MPT character state we conclude that, as defined, it is not autapomorphic for Neanderthals as it occurs at a high frequency in recent *H. sapiens*. Further, we demonstrate that a broad range of ontogenetic factors, deriving from genetic, epigenetic, and nonheritable idiosyncratic sources, interact during growth to produce the observed morphology of the *m. pterygoideus medialis* insertion site in hominoids. Given this disparate series of influences we consider it premature to attempt redefinition of the MPT character. Furthermore, we conclude that the *tpi* is also not sufficiently defined for use in comparative anatomy. It is further demonstrated that the MPT and the *tpi*, while referring to homologous muscle regions in hominoids, are not synonymous terms. The MPT character state includes multiple statements regarding its ontogeny, shape, and function which the *tpi* feature lacks. Based on our observations we conclude that both the MPT character state and the *tpi*, as a feature or character state, should be rejected for use in taxonomic reconstructions and phylogenetic analyses. Given these data and this position, we recommend that published frequency values for the MPT character state not be used in further work, as they either incorrectly quantify (Antón, 1996) or do not specifically address (Quam and Smith, 1998; Lebel *et al.*, 2001) the extent of variation in the character. This recommendation applies also to our recent *H. sapiens* data as it is only useful for the limited purpose of demonstrating that this proposed autapomorphy is invalid.

Further, in our assessment of the MPT character we described how: (1) the *m. pterygoideus medialis* impacts the lingular region of hominids; and (2) this influence combines with bony lingular region morphology and *l. sphenomandibulare* (s.l.) development and insertion pattern to produce bony bridging of the superior-most aspect of the mylohyoid groove and extension of the *l. mandibulae*. We conclude that these factors, driven by genetic, epigenetic, and nonheritable idiosyncratic factors combine to produce a portion of the H-O foramen phenotype in middle-to-late Pleistocene populations. Bridging of the *f. mandibulae* is not, however, restricted to populations in this time range. As demonstrated herein, the mechanism(s) underlying bridging appear to be similar in the hominid taxa examined whereas the anatomical foundation for bridging (i.e. spatial and functional relationships) differs significantly in hominids. We conclude that: (1) a more detailed assessment of factors involved in producing the bridging phenotype could result in useful features or character states; (2) the feature is currently a better indicator of demic variation in Pleistocene taxa than a species indicator; and (3) as currently defined the feature does not appear to be useful as a demic indicator for recent *H. sapiens*.

We demonstrate how the *c. intermedia*, a feature noted by Weidenreich (1936) as an invariant characteristic of "Sinanthropus", evolves in hominids and how it is related to the insertion of the *l. sphenomandibulare* (s.s. / s.l.) and *m. pterygoideus medialis* (by way of the *l. pterygoidea*). The possession of a *c. intermedia* is normal for hominids but not great apes. We conclude, however, that the frequency of occurrence of a specific variation of the crest appears to represent a demic marker in "Sinanthropus". Frequency data for this feature was not tabulated by us for recent *H. sapiens*. Whereas such data may be of interest for nonmetric studies, we suggest caution in assessment of the feature given the medial ramal morphology delineated for this group and some African *H. erectus* (s.l.).

Of equal import to the above conclusions is the fact that we provide a tentative correlative scheme for septa and tubercles of the insertion site of the *m. pterygoideus medialis*. Further, we provide new details of the range of variation in this muscle's insertion and how this variation impacts tubercle formation and the creation of both mylohyoid groove bridging and lingular extension. Details of the form and attachment variation of the *ll. sphenomandibulare* (s.s. / s.l.) and *stylomandibulare* are also provided. Within this context we also delineate the development and evolution of the *l. mandibulae* within the hominid lineage.

Whereas our observations result in some clarification of the ontogeny of the medial ramus in an evolutionary context and on currently defined features and character states of this region, many unanswered questions have been raised by our work. Substantial effort will be required to shed light on most of these areas. We believe that our work does demonstrate that a significant quantity of relevant data can be brought to bear on the identification of new and clarification or rejection of previously proposed character states. We also believe that because the delineation of features or character states represents such a critical first step in systematics that all features/characters should be subjected to rigorous evaluation. It is important that any new *feature* being proposed for taxonomic use be presented with reference to: (1) a large comparative sample(s); (2) details of the sample(s) used; (3) a clear and detailed definition; and (4) a full discussion of variation in the feature for each taxon employed in the comparison. In defining *character states* additional criteria, including a discussion of character homology and homoplasy, are necessary. We also recommend the inclusion of an hypothesis of the developmental and functional constraints under which the character arose for each of the taxa examined (see Lovejoy *et al.*, 1999). Although it is possible to define features and character states in the absence of developmental and functional arguments, we believe that a consideration of these greatly enhances the delineation of both taxonomic and phylogenetically useful characters. We urge all investigators to adopt these standards.

BIBLIOGRAPHY

Abe, S., Iida, T., Ide, Y. and Saitoh, C. (1997a). An anatomical study of a muscle bundle separated from the medial pterygoid muscle. *J. Craniomand. Pract.*, 15:341-344.

Abe, S., Orihara, K., Kitamura, S., Takizawa, M., Okada, M. and Ide, Y. (1997b). Anatomical study of arrangement and attachment of the medial pterygoid muscle in Japanese men. *Bull. Tokyo Dent. Coll.*, 38:217-221.

Abe, S., Ouchi, Y., Ide, Y. and Yonezu, H. (1997c). Perspectives on the role of the lateral pterygoid muscle and the sphenomandibular ligament in temporomandibular joint function. *J. Craniomand. Pract.*, 15:203-207.

Akazawa, T., Muhesen, S., Dodo, Y., Kondo, O. and Mizoguchi, Y. (1995a). Neanderthal infant burial. *Nature*, 377:585-586.

Akazawa, T., Muhesen, S., Dodo, Y., Kondo, O., Mizoguchi, Y., Abe, Y., Nishiaki, Y., Ohta, S., Oguchi, T. and Haydal, J. (1995b). Neanderthal infant burial from the Dederiyeh Cave in Syria. *Paléorient*, 21:77-86.

Alkofide, E. A., Clark, E., El-Bermani, W., Kronman, J. H. and Mehta, N. (1997). The incidence and nature of fibrous continuity between the sphenomandibular ligament and the anterior malleolar ligament of the middle ear. *J. Orofac. Pain*, 11:7-13.

Amorino, R. and Cattaneo, R. (1937). Il substrato istologico delle varie modaità di inserzioni tendinee alle ossa nell'uomo: ricerche su individui di varia età. *Z. Anat. Entw-Gesch.*, 107:680-705.

Anderson, J. Y. (2000). Regional cranial stability: constancy of the mid-mandibulo-facial region as defined by foraminal determinants. *Am. J. phys. Anthrop.*, 30 (Suppl.):96.

Anton, S. C. (1993). Internal masticatory muscle architecture in the Japanese macaque and its influence on bony morphology. *Am. J. phys. Anthrop.*, 16 (Suppl.):50.

Antón, S. C. (1994a). Masticatory muscle architecture and bone morphology in Primates. Ph. D. Dissertation, University of California, Berkeley.

Antón, S. C. (1994b). Masseter muscle architecture, bony morphology, and activity. *Am. J. phys. Anthrop.*, 18 (Suppl.):49-50.

Antón, S. C. (1995). Tendon-associated bone features of the masticatory system in Neanderthals. *Am. J. phys. Anthrop.*, 20 (Suppl.):59.

Antón, S. C. (1996). Tendon-associated bone features of the masticatory system in Neanderthals. *J. hum. Evol.*, 31:391-408.

Arambourg, C. (1963). Le gisement de Ternifine, II: l'Atlanthropus mauritanicus. *Arch. Inst. Paléontol. Humaine, Mém.*, 32:37-190.

Arensburg, B. and Bar-Yosef, O. (1973). Human remains from Ein Gev I, Jordan Valley, Israël. *Paléorient*, 1:201-206.

Arensburg, B. and Belfer-Cohen, A. (1998). Sapiens and Neandertals: rethinking the Levantine Middle Paleolithic hominids. In (T. Akazawa, K. Aoki and O. Bar-Yosef, Eds) *Neanderthals and modern humans in Western Asia*, pp. 311-322. New York: Plenum.

Arensburg, B. and Nathan, H. (1979). Anatomical observations on the mylohyoid groove and the course of the mylohyoid nerve and vessels. *J. Oral Surg.*, 37:93-96.

Armelagos, G. J., Van Gerven, D. P., Martin, D. L. and Huss-Ashmore, R. (1984). Effects of nutritional change on the skeletal biology of Northeast African (Sudanese Nubian) populations. In (J. D. Clark and S. A. Brandt, Eds) *From hunters to farmers: the causes and consequences of food production in Africa*, pp. 132-146. Berkeley: University of California Press.

Atchley, W. R. (1993). Genetic and developmental aspects of variability in the mammalian mandible. In (J. Hanken and B. K. Hall, Eds) *The skull.* Vol. 1: Development, pp. 207-247. Chicago: University of Chicago Press.

Atchley, W. R. and Hall, B. K. (1991). A model for development and evolution of complex morphological structures. *Bio. Rev.*, 66:101-157.

Atchley, W. R., Herring, S. W., Riska, B. and Plummer, A. A. (1984). Effects of the muscular dysgenesis gene on developmental stability in the mouse mandible. *J. Craniof. Gen. Dev. Biol.*, 4:179-189.

Avis, V. (1959). The relation of the temporal muscle to the form of the coronoid process. *Am. J. phys. Anthrop.*, 17:99-104.

Avis, V. (1961). The significance of the angle of the mandible: An experimental and comparative study. *Am. J. phys. Anthrop.*, 19:55-61.

Baker, G. I. and Laskin, D. M. (1969). Histochemical characterization of the muscles of mastication. *J. Dent. Res.*, 48:97-104.

Balogh, K. and Csiba, Á. (1972). Topographical-anatomical variation of the lingula and of the foramen mandibulae. In (G-H. Schumacher, Ed) *Morphology of the maxillo-mandibular apparatus*, pp. 200-204. Leipzig: Veb Georg Thieme.

Baragar, F. A. and Osborn, J. W. (1984). A model relating patterns of human jaw movement to biomechanical constraints. *J. Biomech.*, 17:757-767.

Bareggi, R., Sandrucci, A. A., Baldini, G., Grill, V., Zweyer, M. and Narducci, P. (1995). Mandibular growth rates in human fetal development. *Archs. Oral Bio.*, 40:119-125.

Barker, B. C. W. and Davies, P. L. (1972). The applied anatomy of the pterygomandibular space. *Brit. J. Oral Surg.*, 10:43-53.

Basmajian, J. V. and DeLuca, C. J. (1985). *Muscles alive: Their function revealed by electromyography.* Baltimore: Williams and Warwick.

Baughan, B., Demirjian, A., Levesque, G. Y. and La Palme-Chaput, L. (1979). The pattern of facial growth before and during puberty as shown by French-Canadian girls. *Annls. Hum. Biol.*, 6:59-76.

de Beer, G. (1971). Homology: An unsolved problem. *Oxford Bio. Readers*, No. 11:3-16.

Benjamin, M. and Ralphs, J. R. (1995). Functional and developmental anatomy of tendons and ligaments. In (S. L. Gordon, S. J. Blair and L. J. Fine, Eds) *Repetitive motion disorders of the upper extremity*, pp. 185-203. Rosemont IL: Am. Acad. Orthopaedic. Surg.

Benjamin, M. and Ralphs, J. R. (1998). Fibrocartilage in tendons and ligaments: an adaptation to compressive load. *J. Anat.*, 193:81-494.

Benjamin, M. and Ralphs, J. R. (2000). The cell and developmental biology of tendons and ligaments. *Int. Rev. Cytol.*, 196:85-130.

Benjamin, M., Evans, E. J. and Copp, L. (1986). The histology of tendon attachments to bone in man. *J. Anat.*, 149:89-100.

Berns, J. M and Sadove, M. S. (1962). Mandibular block injection: a method of study using an injected radiopaque material. *J. Am. Dent. Assoc.*, 65:736-745.

Billy, G. and Vallois, H. V. (1977). La mandibule pré-Rissienne de Montmaurin. *L'Anthropologie*, 81:273-312, 411-458.

Björk, A. (1963). Variations in the growth pattern of the human mandible: longitudinal radiographic study by the implant method. *J. Dent. Res.*, 42:400-4011.

Bluntschli, H. (1929). Die Kaumuskulatur des orang-utan und ihre Bedeutung für die Formung des Schädels. *Gegenbaur's Morphol. Jahrb.*, 63:531-606.

Bonjean, D., Otte, M., and Toussaint, M. (1994). L'homme de Sclayn. *Archeologia*, 299:26-30.

Bossy, J. and Gaillard, L. (1963). Les vestiges ligamentaires du cartilage de Meckel. *Acta Anat.*, 52:282-290.

Boule, M. (1911-1913). L'homme fossile de La Chapelle-aux-Saints. *Annls. Paléont.*, 6:111-173; 7:21-193; 8:1-70.

Boule, M. and Vallois, H. V. (1957). *Fossil man: A textbook of human palaeontology.* London: Thames and Hudson.

Bowden, D. H. and Goyer, R. A. (1960). The size of muscle fibers in infants and children. *Arch. Path.*, 69:188-189.

Boyer, E. L. (1939). The cranio-mandibular musculature of the orang-utan, *Simia satyrus*. *Am. J. phys. Anthrop.*, 24:417-426.

Brauer, J. A. and Bahador, M. A. (1942). Variations in calcification and eruption of the deciduous and the permanent teeth. *J. Am. Dent. Assoc.*, 29:1373-1387.

Bremer, G. (1952). Measurements of special significance in connection with anesthesia of the inferior alveolar nerve. *Oral Surg. Oral Med. Oral Pathol.*, 5:966-988.

Brodie, A. G. (1946). Facial patterns: a theme on variations. *Angle Orthod.*, 16:75-87.

Bromage, T. G. and Dean, M. C. (1985). Re-evaluation of the age at death of immature fossil hominids. *Nature*, 317:525-527.

Burch, J. G. (1966). The cranial attachment of the sphenomandibular (tympanomandibular) ligament. *Anat. Rec.*, 156:433-438.

Burch, J. G. (1970). Activity of the accessory ligaments of the temporomandibular joint. *J. Prosthetic Dent.*, 24:621-628.

Burdi, A. R. and Spyropulos, M. N. (1978). Prenatal growth patterns of the human mandible and masseter muscle complex. *Am. J. Orthod.*, 74:380-38.

Burleigh, I. G. (1974). On the cellular regulation of growth and development in skeletal muscle. *Biol. Rev.*, 49:267-320.

Buxton, L. H. D. (1928). Human remains. In (D. A. E. Garrod, L. H. D. Buxton, G. E. Smith and D. M. A. Bate, Eds) Excavation of a Mousterian rock-shelter at Devil's Tower, Gibraltar. *Roy. Anthrop. Inst. Gr. Brit. Ireland.*, 58:57-91.

Cameron, J. (1914-1915). The cranial attachment of the internal lateral ligament of the lower jaw: with an investigation into the fibrogenesis of this structure. *J. Anat. Physiol.*, 49:210-215.

Caramelli, D., Lalueza-Fox, C., Vernesi, C., Lari, M., Casoli, A., Mallegni, F., Chiarelli, B., Dupanloup, I., Bertranpetit, J., Barbujani, G., and Bertorelle, G. (2003). Evidence for a genetic discontinuity between Neandertals and 24,000-year-old anatomically modern Europeans. *Proc. Nat. Acad. Sci.*, 100:6593-6597.

Carter, R. B and Keen, E. N. (1971). The intramandibular course of the inferior alveolar nerve. *J. Anat.*, 108:433-440.

Cave, A. J. E. (1979). The mammalian temporo-pterygoid ligament. *J. Zool.*, 188:517-532.

Chávez-Lomelí, M. E., Lory, J. M. and Kjær, I. (1996). The human mandibular canal arises from three separate canals innervating different tooth groups. *J. Dent. Res.*, 75:1540-1544.

Chevallier, A., Kieny, M. and Mauger, A. (1977). Limb-somite relationship: origin of the limb musculature. *J. Embryol. Exp. Morphol.*, 41:245-258.

Chierici, G. and Miller, A. J. (1984). Experimental study of muscle reattachment following surgical detachment. *J. Oral Maxillofac. Surg.*, 42:485-490.

Christ, B., Jacob, H. J. and Jacob, M. (1977). Experimental analysis of the origin of the wing musculature in avian embryos. *Anat. Embryol.*, 150:171-186.

Churchill, S. E. and Smith, F. H. (2000). Makers of the Early Aurignacian of Europe. *Yrbk. phys. Anthrop.*, 43 (Suppl.):61-116.

Clark, G. A. (2000). Spurious species? *Sci. Am.*, 282:12.

Clark, W. E. Le Gros. (1964). *The fossil evidence for human evolution.* Chicago: University of Chicago.

Clemente, C. D. (1987). *Anatomy: A regional atlas of the human body*, 3rd ed. Baltimore: Urban and Schwarzenberg.

Clinch, L. (1934). Variations in the mutual relationships of the maxillary and mandibular gum pads in the newborn child. *Int. J. Orthod. Dent. Childr.*, 20:359-374.

Comer, R. D. (1956). An experimental study of the "laws" of muscle and tendon growth. *Anat. Rec.*, 125:665-681.

Condemi, S. (2001). Les Neandertaliens de La Chaise (abri Bourgeois-Delaunay). Paris: Comité des Travaux Historiques et Scientifiques, Société Préhistorique Française.

Cooper, R. R. and Misol, S. (1970). Tendon and ligament insertion. *J. Bone Joint Surg.*, 52-A:1-20, 170.

Coqueugniot, H. (1999). Le crâne d'*Homo sapiens* en Eurasie: croissance et variation depuis 100,000 ans. *Brit. Archaeol. Rep., Internat. Ser.*, 822:1-197.

Corell, R. W., Jensen, J. L., Taylor, J. B. and Rhyme, R. R. (1979). Mineralization of the stylohyoid-stylomandibular ligament complex. *Oral Surg. Oral Med. Oral Pathol.*, 48:286-291.

Corruccini, R. S. (1984). An epidemiologic transition in dental occlusion in world populations. *Am. J. Orthod.*, 86:419-426.

Costa, R. L. (1986). Asymmetry of the mandibular condyle in Haida Indians. *Am. J. phys. Anthrop.*, 70:119-124.

Covell, D. A. Jr. and Herring, S. W. (1995). Periosteal migration in the growing mandible: an animal model. *Am. J. Orthod. Dentofac. Orthop.*, 108:22-29.

Creed-Miles, M., Rosas, A. and Kruszynski, R. (1996). Issues in the identification of Neanderthal derivative traits at early post-natal stages. *J. hum. Evol.*, 30:147-154.

Darwin, C. (1859). On the origin of species. A facsimile of the first edition. Cambridge: Harvard Univ. Press (1964).

Dean, M. C. and Wood, B. A. (1981). Developing pongid dentition and its use for aging individual crania in comparative cross-sectional growth studies. *Folia Primatol.*, 36:111-127.

Dean, M. C., Stringer, C. B. and Bromage, T. G. (1986). Age at death of the Neanderthal child from Devil's Tower, Gibraltar and the implications for studies of general growth and development in Neanderthals. *Am. J. phys. Anthrop.*, 70:301-309.

Deplus, S., Brémond-Gignac, D., Gillot, C. and Lassau, J. P. (1996). The pterygoid venous plexuses. *Surg. Radiol. Anat.*, 18:23-27.

Demirjian, A. (1986). Dentition. In (F. Falkner and J. M. Tanner, Eds) *Human growth: a comprehensive treatise; Vol. 2., Postnatal growth and neurobiology*, pp. 269-298. New York: Plenum.

Demirjian, A., Buschang, P. H., Tanguay, R. and Kingnorth-Patterson, D. (1985). Interrelationships among measures of somatic, skeletal, dental, and sexual maturity. *Am. J. Orthod.*, 88:433-438.

Diewert, V. M. (1983). A morphometric analysis of craniofacial growth and changes in spatial relations during secondary palatal development in human embryos and fetuses. *Am. J. Anat.*, 167:495-522.

Dodo, Y. (1974). Non-metrical cranial traits in the Hokkaido Ainu and the Northern Japanese of recent times. *J. Anthrop. Soc., Nippon*, 82:31-51.

Dodo, Y., Kondo, O., Muhesen, S. and Akazawa, T. (1998). Anatomy of the Neandertal infant skeleton from Dederiyeh Cave, Syria. In (T. Akazawa, K. Aoki and O. Bar-Yosef, Eds) *Neanderthals and modern humans in Western Asia*, pp. 323-338. New York: Plenum.

Dörlf, J. (1980a). Migration of tendinous insertions: I. cause and mechanism. *J. Anat.*, 131:179-195.

Dörlf, J. (1980b). Migration of tendinous insertions: II. experimental modification. *J. Anat.*, 131:229-237.

DuBrul, E. L. (1980). *Sicher's Oral Anatomy*, 7th ed. St. Louis: CV Mosby.

Dullemeijer, P. (1974). *Concepts and approaches in animal morphology*. Assen: Van Gorcum.

Dwight, T. (1907). Stylo-hyoid ossification. *Annls. Surg.*, 46:721-735.

Eckhardt, R. B. (1989). Matching molecular and morphological evolution. *Hum. Evol.*, 4:317-319.

Edgeworth, F. H. (1935). *The cranial muscles of vertebrates*. London: Cambridge University Press.

Ekström, C. (1982). Facial growth rate and its relation to somatic maturation in healthy children. *Swed. Dent. J.*, 11 (Suppl.):1-99.

Elliott, D. H. (1965). Structure and function of mammalian tendon. *Biol. Rev.*, 40:392-421.

El-Nofely, A. A. and Isçan, M. Y. (1989). Assessment of age from the dentition in children. In (M. Y. Isçan, Ed) *Age markers in the human skeleton*, pp. 237-254. Springfield: CC Thomas.

Enlow, D. H. (1965). The problem of muscle tension and the stimulation of bone growth. *Anat. Rec.*, 151:451(abstract).

Enlow, D. H. (1968). *The human face: an account of the postnatal growth and development of the craniofacial skeleton*. New York: Harper and Row.

Enlow, D. H. and Hans, M. G. (1996). *Essentials of Facial Growth*. Philadelphia: WB Saunders.

Ennion, S., Sant'Ana Pereira, J., Sargeant, A. J., Young, A. and Goldspink, G. (1995). Characterization of human skeletal muscle fibres according to the myosin heavy chains they express. *J. Muscle Res. Cell Motil.*, 16:35-43.

Epker, B. N. and Frost, H. M. (1966). Biomechanical control of bone growth and development: a histologic and tetracycline study. *J. Dent. Res.*, 45:364-371.

Eriksson, P. O. and Thornell, L. E. (1983). Histochemical and morphological muscle-fiber characteristics of the human masseter, the medial pterygoid, and the temporal muscles. *Archs. Oral Biol.*, 28:781-795.

Faerman, M., Zilberman, U., Smith, P., Kharitonov, V. and Batsevitz, V. (1994). A Neanderthal infant from the Barakai Cave, Western Caucasus. *J. hum. Evol.*, 27:405-415.

Fay, J. C. and Wu, C-I. (1999). A human population bottleneck can account for the discordance between patterns of mitochondrial versus nuclear DNA variation. *Mol. Biol. Evol.*, 16:1003-1005.

Ferembach, D. (1969). Les affinités morphologiques de l'enfant néandertalien du Pech-de-l'Aze (Dordogne). *C. r. Acad. Sci., Paris*, 268:1485-1488.

Ferembach, D. (1970). Le crane de l'enfant du Pech-de-l'Aze. In (D. Ferembach, P. Legoux, R. Fenart, R. Empereur-Buisson and E. Vlček, Eds) L'enfant du Pech-de-l'Azé. *Arch. Inst. Paléontol. Humaine*, 33:13-51.

Ferembach, D. (1976). Les restes humains de la Grotte de Dar-es-Soltane 2 (Maroc) Campagne 1975. *Bull. Mem. Soc. Anthrop. Paris*, 3:183-193.

Foucart, J. M., Girin, J.P. and Carpentier, P. (1998). Innervation of the human lateral pterygoid muscle. *Surg. Radiol. Anat.*, 20:185-189.

Franciscus, R. G. (1999). Neanderthal nasal structures and upper respiratory tract "specialization". *Proc. natl. Acad. Sci.*, 96:1805-1809.

Franciscus, R. G. and Trinkaus, E. (1995). Determinations of retromolar space presence in Pleistocene *Homo* mandibles. *J. hum. Evol.*, 28:577-595.

Frayer, D. W. (1992). The persistence of Neanderthal features in post-Neanderthal Europeans. In (G. Bräuer and F. H. Smith, Eds) *Continuity or Replacement: Controversies in Homo sapiens evolution*, pp. 179-188. Rotterdam: A. A. Balkema.

Friedman, M. H. (1988). Functions of the medial pterygoid muscle. *Clin. Anat.*, 1:213-220.

Friedman, M. H. (1995). Pterygoid muscle function in excursive jaw movements: A clinical report. *J. Prost. Dent.*, 73:329-332.

Friel, S. (1926). An investigation into the relation of function and form. *Brit. Dent. J.*, 47:353-379.

Frommer, J. (1974). Anatomic variations in the stylohyoid chain and their possible clinical significance. *Oral Surg. Oral Med. Oral Pathol.*, 38:659-667.

Gao, J. and Messner, K. (1996). Quantitative comparison of soft tissue-bone interface at chondral ligament insertions in the rabbit knee joint. *J. Anat.*, 188:367-373.

Gans, C. and Bock, W. J. (1965). IV. The functional significance of muscle architecture: a theoretical analysis. *Ergebn. Anat. Entwickl.-Gesch.*, 38:115-142.

Gans, C. and Gorniak, G. C. (1978). Concepts of muscle: an introduction to the intact animal. In (D. S. Carlson and J. A. McNamara Jr., Eds) *Muscle adaptation in the craniofacial region*, pp. 1-16. Center Human Growth and Development, University of Michigan, Craniof. Gr. Ser., No 8.

Gaspard, M. (1972). *Les muscles masticateurs superficiels des singes à l'homme: anatomie comparée et anatomo-physiologie*. Paris: Librairie Maloine SA.

Gaspard, M., Laison, F. and Mailland, M. (1973a). Organisation architecturale et texture des muscles ptérygoïdiens chez le Primates supérieurs. *J. Biol. Buccale*, 1:215-233.

Gaspard, M., Laison, F. and Mailland, M. (1973b). Organisation architecturale et texture des muscles ptérygoïdiens chez l'homme. *J. Biol. Buccale*, 1:353-366.

Gasser, R. F. (1967). The development of the facial muscles in man. *Am. J. Anat.*, 120:357-376.

Gaughran, G. R. L. (1957). Fasciae of the masticator space. *Anat. Rec.*, 129:583-589.

Geiser, M. and Trueta, J. (1958). Muscle action, bone rarefaction and bone formation: an experimental study. *J. Bone Joint Surg.*, 40B:282-311.

Genet-Varcin, E. (1982). Vestiges humains du Würmien inférieur de Combe Grenal, Comme de Domme (Dordogne). *Annls. Paléont. (Vert.-Invert.)*, 68:133-169.

German, R. Z. and Meyers, L. L. (1989). The role of time and size in ontogenetic allometry: II. an empirical study of human growth. *Growth Dev. Aging*, 53:107-115.

Giacobini, G., de Lumley, M-A., Yokoyama, Y. and Nguyen, H-V. (1984). Neanderthal child and adult remains from a Mousterian deposit in Northern Italy (Caveran Delle Fate, Finale Ligure). *J. hum. Evol.*, 13:687-707.

Goldspink, G. (1999). Changes in muscle mass and phenotype and the expression of autocrine and systemic growth factors by muscle in response to stretch and overload. *J. Anat.*, 194:323-334.

Golovanova, L. V. (1994). Otkrytie pogrebeniua na must'erskoi stoyanke v Mezmaiskoi peshchere. *Arkheologicheskie otkrytiya 1993 goda*. Moscow: Institut Arkheologii, pp. 110-111.

Golovanova, L. V. and Romanova, G. P. (1995). Novye antropologicheskie nakhodki na must'erskoi stoyanke v Mezmaiskoi peshchere (Severi-Zaoadnyi Kavjaz). *Arkheologicheskie otkrytiya 1994 goda*, pp. 160-161. Moscow: Institut Arkheologii.

Golovanova, L. V., Hoffecker, J. F., Kharitonov, V. M. and Romanova, G. P. (1999). Mezmaiskaya Cave: a Neanderthal occupation in the Northern Caucasus. *Curr. Anthrop.*, 40:77-86.

Gorjanović-Kramberger, D. (1923-1924). Novi prilozi čeljusnom zglobu diluvijalnog čovjeka iz Krapinae. *Izvjesca o Raspravama Matematicko-Prirodoslovnoga Razeda, Zagreb*, 19-20:118-145.

Goto, T. K., Langernbach, G. E. J. and Hannam, A. G. (2001). Length changes in the human masseter muscle after jaw movement. *Anat. Rec.*, 262:293-300.

Goudot, P. (1999). The mandibular canal of a Neanderthal: the La Chapelle-aux-Saints man anatomical-radiological study. *J. Cranio-Maxillof. Surg.*, 27:134-139.

Gould, S. J. (1977). *Ontogeny and phylogeny*. Cambridge: Belknap, Harvard University Press.

Grant, P. G. (1978). The effect of position on the migration of muscle. *J. Anat.*, 127:157-162.

Grant, P. G., Buschang, P. H., Drolet, D. W. and Pickerell, C. (1980). Invariance of the relative positions of structures attached to long bones during growth: cross-sectional and longitudinal studies. *Acta Anat.*, 107:26-34.

Grant, P. G., Buschang, P. H., Drolet, D. W. and Pickerell, C. (1981). The effect of changes in muscle function and bone growth on muscle migration. *Am. J. phys. Anthrop.*, 54:547-553.

Greene, D. L. (1970). Environmental influences on Pleistocene hominid dental evolution. *BioSci.*, 20:276-279.

Gremyatskij, M. A. (1949). The skull of the Neanderthal child from the cave of Teshik Tash, southern Uzbekistan (in Russian). In (M. A. Gremyatskij and M. F. Nesturkh, Eds) *Teshik Tash: The Paleolithic Man*, pp. 137-187. Moscow: Moscow State University.

Grossman, J. W. and Zuckerman, S. (1955). An x-ray study of growth changes in the base of the skull. *Am. J. phys. Anthrop.*, 13:515-519.

Habgood, P. J. (1989). An investigation into the usefulness of a cladistic approach to the study of the origin of anatomically modern humans. *Hum. Evol.*, 4:241-252.

Hägg, U. and Matsson, L. (1985). Dental maturity as an indicator of chronological age: the accuracy and precision of three methods. *Eur. J. Orthod.*, 7:25-34.

Haines, R. W. (1932). The laws of muscle and tendon growth. *J. Anat.*, 66:578-585.

Hall, B. K. (1971). Histogenesis and morphogenesis of bone. *Clin. Orthopaed. Related Res.*, 74:249-268.

Hall, B. K. (1979). Selective proliferation and accumulation of chondroprogenitor cells as the mode of action of biomechanical factors during secondary chondrogenesis. *Teratology*, 20:81-92.

Hall, B. K. (1995). Homology and embryonic development. *Evol. Bio.* 28:1-37.

Hamilton, W. J. and Mossman, H. W. (1978). *Human embryology: prenatal development of form and function* (4th ed). London: Macmillan.

Hamparian, A. M. (1973). Blood supply of the human fetal mandible. *Am. J. Anat.*, 136:67-76.

Hannam, A. G. and Wood, W. W. (1981). Medial pterygoid muscle activity during the closing and compressive phases of human mastication. *Am. J. phys. Anthrop.*, 55:359-367.

Hannam, A. G. and McMillan, A. S. (1994). Internal organization in the human jaw muscles. *Crit. Rev. Oral Bio. Med.*, 5:55-89.

Hans, M. G., Enlow, D. H. and Noachtar, R. (1995). Age-related differences in mandibular ramus growth: a histological study. *Angle Orthod.*, 65:335-340.

Harada, Y. and Ishizehi, K. (1998). Evidence for transformation of chondrocytes and site-specific resorption during the degradation of Meckel's cartilage. *Anat. Embryol.*, 197:439-450.

Hauser, G. and De Stefano, G. F. (1989). *Epigenetic variants of the human skull*. Stuttgart: E. Schweizerbart'che.

Hawks, J. and Wolpoff, M. H. (2001). Paleoanthropology and the population genetics of ancient genes. *Am. J. phys. Anthrop.*, 114:269-272.

Heim, J-L. (1974). Les hommes fossiles de La Ferrassie (Dordogne) et le problème de la définition des Néandertaliens Classiques. *L'Anthropologie*, 78:81-112, 321-378.

Heim, J-L. (1976). Les hommes fossiles de La Ferrassie. Vol. 1: Le gisement, les squelettes adultes: crâne et squelette du tronc. *Arch. Inst. Paléontol. Humaine, Mém.*, 35:1-326.

Heim, J-L. (1982). Les enfants néandertaliens de La Ferrassie: étude anthropologique et analyse ontogénique des Hommes de Néandertal. New York: Masson.

Hems, T. and Tillmann, B. (2000). Tendon entheses of the human masticatory muscles. *Anat. Embryol.*, 202:201-208.

Hennig, W. (1966). *Phylogenetic systematics*. Urbana: University of Illinois.

Herring, S. W. (1977). Differential activity in complex muscles. *Am. Zool.*, 17:954 (abstract).

Herring, S. W. (1993). Epigenetic and functional influences in skull growth. In (J. Hanken and B. K. Hall, Eds) *The skull. Vol. 1: Development*, pp. 153-206. Chicago: University of Chicago.

Herring, S. W. and Laskers, T. C. (1981). Craniofacial development in the absence of muscle contraction. *J. Craniof. Genet. Dev. Biol.*, 1:341-357.

Herring, S. W. and Wineski, L. E. (1986). Development of the masseter muscle and oral behavior in the pig. *J. Exp. Zool.*, 237:191-207.

Herring, S. W., Anapol, F. C. and Wineski, L. E. (1991). Motor-unit territories in the masseter muscle of infant pigs. *Arch. Oral Biol.*, 36:867-873.

Herring, S. W., Muhl, Z. F. and Obrez, A. (1993). Bone growth and periosteal migration control masseter muscle orientation in pigs (*Sus scrofa*). *Anat. Rec.*, 235:215-222.

Hey, J. (1999). Mitochondrial and nuclear genes present conflicting portraits of human origins. *Mol. Biol. Evol.*, 14:166-172.

Hobgood, P. J. (1989). An investigation into the usefulness of a cladistic approach to the study of the origin of anatomically modern humans. *Hum. Evol.*, 4:241-252.

Honée, G. L. J. M. (1972). The anatomy of the lateral pterygoid muscle. *Acta Morphol. Neerl.-Scand.*, 10:331-340.

Höss, M. (2000). Neanderthal population genetics. *Nature*, 404:453-454.

Hovelacque, A. and Virenque, M. (1913). Les formations aponévrotiques de la région ptérygomaxillaire chez l'Homme et chez quelques Mammifères. *J. Anat. Physiol., Paris*, 49:427-488, 618-699.

Hovers, E., Rak, Y., Lavi, R. and Kimbel, W. H. (1995). Hominid Remains from Amud Cave in the context of the Levantine Middle Paleolithic. *Paléorient*, 21:47-61.

Hovers, E., Rak, Y. and Kimbel, W. H. (1996). Neanderthals of the Levant. *Archaeology*, 49:49-50.

Hoyte, D. A. N. and Enlow, D. H. (1966). Wolff's law and the problem of muscle attachment on resorptive surfaces of bone. *Am. J. phys. Anthrop.*, 24:205-214.

Hublin, J-J. (1998). Climatic changes, paleogeography, and the evolution of the Neandertals. In (T. Akazawa, K. Aoki and O. Bar-Yosef, Eds) *Neandertals and modern humans in Western Asia*, pp. 295-310. New York: Plenum Press.

Humphrey, T. (1971). Development of oral and facial motor mechanisms in human fetuses and their relation to craniofacial growth. *J. Dent. Res.*, 50:1428-1441.

Hurov, J. R. (1986). Soft-tissue bone inferface: how do attachments of muscles, tendons, and ligaments change during growth? A light microscopic study. *J. Morphol.*, 189:313-325.

Ingervall, B. and Helkimo, E. (1978). Masticatory muscle force and facial morphology in man. *Archs. Oral Biol.*, 23:203-206.

Ishizeki, K., Saito, H., Shinagawa, T., Fujiwara, N. and Nawa, T. (1999). Histochemical and immunohistochemical analysis of the mechanism of calcification of Meckel's cartilage during mandible development in rodents. *J. Anat.*, 194:265-277.

Ishizeki, K., Takahashi, N. and Nawa, T. (2001). Formation of the sphenomandibular ligament by Meckel's cartilage in the mouse: possible involvement of epidermal growth factor as revealed by studies in vivo and in vitro. *Cell Tissue Res.*, 304:67-80.

Jabbour, R. S. and Richards, G. D. (1998). Condylar region morphology in Neandertal mandibles: issues of ontogeny, homology and interpretation. *Am. J. phys. Anthrop.*, 26 (Suppl.):127.

Jabbour, R. S, Richards, G. D. and Anderson, J. Y. (2002). Mandibular condyle traits in Neanderthals and other *Homo*: a comparative, correlative, and ontogenetic study. *Am. J. phys. Anthrop.*, 119:144-155.

Jidoi, K., Nara, T. and Dodo, Y. (2000). Bony bridging of the mylohyoid groove of the human mandible. *Anthrop. Sci.*, 108:345-370.

Johanson, D. C., Lovejoy, C. O., Kimbel, W. H., White, T. D., Ward, S. C., Bush, M. E., Latimer, B. M. and Coppens, Y. (1982). Morphology of the Pliocene partial hominid skeleton (A.L. 288-1) from the Hadar Formation, Ethiopia. *Am. J. phys. Anthrop.*, **57**:403-451.

Jones, F. W. (1941). *The principles of anatomy as seen in the hand*. London: Baillière, Tindall, and Cox.

Kally, J. (1955a). Novi podaci o mandibulama Krapinskog pračovjeka. *Iz. Hrva.t Medic. Proslosti., Zagreb*, 125-137.

Kally, J. (1955b). Lage und form des foramen mandibulare beim Krapina-Menschen. *Osterr. Z. Stomatol.*, 52:523-526.

Kally, J. (1970). Komparativne napomene o čeljustima Krapinskih praljudi s obzirom ma položaj me u hominidima. In (M. Malez, Ed) *Krapina 1899-1969*, pp. 153-164. Zagreb: Iz zav Jugoslavenske akad znanosti i umjetnosti.

Kane, A. A., Lo, L-J., Christensen, G. E., Vannier, M. W. and Marsh, J. L. (1997). Relationship between bone and muscles of mastication in hemifacial microsomia. *Plast. Reconstr. Surg.*, 99:990-997.

Kantomaa, T. (1988). The shape of the glenoid fossa affects the growth of the mandible. *Eur. J. Orthod.*, 10:249-254.

Kantomaa, T. (1989). The relation between mandibular configuration and the shape of the glenoid fossa in the human. *Eur. J. Orthod.*, 11:77-81.

Kardon, G. (1998). Muscle and tendon morphogenesis in the avian hind limb. *Development*, 125:4019-4032.

Katsaros, C. (2001). Masticatory muscle function and transverse dentofacial growth. *Swed. Dent. J.*, 51 (Suppl.):1-48.

Kaufman, S. M. and Irish, E. F. (1970). Styloid process variation: radiologic and clinical study. *Arch. Otolaryng.*, 91:460-463.

Kaul, S. S and Pathak, R. K. (1984). The mylohyoid bridge in four population samples from India, with observations on its suitability as a genetic marker. *Am. J. phys. Anthrop.*, 65:213-218.

Keith, A. (1931). *New discoveries relating to the antiquity of man.* London: Williams and Norgate.

Kilaridis, S. (1995). Masticatory muscle influence on craniofacial growth. *Acta Odont. Scand.*, 53:196-202.

van der Klaauw, C. J. (1963). Projections, deepenings and undulations of the surface of the skull in relation to the attachment of muscles. *Ergebn. Anat. Entwickl.-Gesch.*, Ser. 2, Pt. **55**:1-247.

Knese, K. H. and Biermann, H. (1958). Die Knochenbildung an Sehnenund Bandansätzen im Bereich ursprünglich condraler Apophysen. *Z. Zellforsch.*, 49:142-187.

Korfage, J. A. M. and Van Eijden, T. M.G. J. (1999). Regional differences in fibre type composition in the human temporalis muscle. *J. Anat.*, 194:355-362.

Korfage, J. A. M. and Van Eijden, T. M. G. J. (2000). Myosin isoform composition of the human medial and lateral pterygoid muscles. *J. Dent. Res.*, 79:1618-1625.

Koski, K. and Garn, S. M. (1957). Tooth eruption sequence in fossil and modern man. *Am. J. phys. Anthrop.*, 15:469-488.

Krieg, W. L. (1987). Early facial growth accelerations: a longitudinal study. *Angle Orthod.*, 57:50-62.

Krings, M., Stone, A., Schmitz, R. W., Krainitzki, H., Stoneking. M. and Pääbo, S. (1997). Neandertal DNA sequences and the origins of modern humans. *Cell*, 90:19-30.

Krings, M., Capelli, C., Tshentscher, F., Geisert, H., Meyer, S., von Haeseler, A., Grosschmidt, K., Possnert, G., Pauovic, M. and Pääbo, S. (2000). A view of Neandertal genetic diversity. *Nature genetics*, 26:144-146.

Kurihara, S., Enlow, D. H. and Rangel, R. D. (1980). Remodeling reversals in anterior parts of the human mandible and maxilla. *Angle Orthod.*, 50:98-106.

Lacroix, P. (1951). *The organization of bones.* Philadelphia: Balkiston.

Laitman, J. T., Reidenberg, J. S., Marquez, S. and Gannon, P. J. (1996). What the nose knows: new understandings of Neanderthal upper respiratory tract specializations. *Proc. natl. Acad. Sci.*, 93:10543-10545.

Lahr, M. M. (1995). Commentary on: testing hypotheses about recent human evolution from skulls. *Curr. Anthrop.*, 36:180-181.

Larnach, S. and Macintosh, N. (1971). The mandible in Eastern Australian Aborigines. *Oceanic Monograph*, No. 17.

Lasker, G. W. (1969). Human biological adaptability: the ecological approach in physical anthropology. *Science*, 166:1480-1486.

Last, R. J. (1954). The muscles of the mandible. *Proc. Roy. Soc. Med.*, 47:571-578.

Latham, R. A. and Scott, J. A. (1970). A newly postulated factor in the early growth of the human middle face and the theory of multiple assurance. *Archs. Oral Biol.*, 15:107-1100.

Leakey, M., Tobias, P. V., Martyn, J. E. and Leakey, R. E. F. (1969). An Acheulean industry with prepared core technique and the discovery of a contemporary hominid mandible at Lake Baringo, Kenya. *Proc. prehist. Soc.*, 35:48-76.

Lebel, S., Trinkaus, E., Faure, M., Fernandez, P., Guérin, C., Richter, D., Mercier, N., Valladas, H. and Wagner, G. A. (2001). Comparative morphology and paleobiology of Middle Pleistocene human remains from the Bau de l'Aubesier, Vaucluse, France. *Proc. nat. Acad. Sci.*, 98:11097-11102.

Le Double, A. F. (1906). *Traité des variations des os de la face de l'homme et leur signification au point de vue de l'anthropolgie zoologique.* Paris: Vigot Frères.

Lee, S. K., Kim, Y. S., Oh, H. S., Yang, K. H., Kim, E. C. and Chi, J. G. (2001). Prenatal development of the human mandible. *Anat. Rec.*, 263:314-325.

Legoux, P. (1961). Remarques sur certains aspects de la mandibule de l'enfant d'Ehringsdorf. *C. r. Acad. Sci., Paris*, 252:1821-1823.

Levelle, C. L. B. and Moore, W. J. (1970). Proportionate growth of the human jaws between the fourth and seventh months of intrauterine life. *Archs. Oral Biol.*, 15:453-459.

Lewis, A. B. and Garn, S. M. (1960). The relationship between tooth formation and other maturational factors. *Angle Orthod.*, 30:70-77.

Lewis, O. J. (1989). *Functional morphology of the evolving hand and foot*. Oxford: Clarendon.

Lieberman, D. E. (1995). Testing hypotheses about recent human evolution from skulls. *Curr. Anthrop.*, 36:159-197.

Lieberman, D. E. (1999). Homology and hominid phylogeny: problems and potential solutions. *Evol. Anthrop.*, 7:142-151.

Lieberman, D. E. (2000). Ontogeny, homology, and phylogeny in the hominid craniofacial skeleton: the problem of the browridge. In (P. O'Higgins and M. J. Cohn, Eds) *Development, Growth, and Evolution*, pp. 86-122. San Diego: Academic Press.

Lioubine, V. P. (1998). La grotto Moustérienne Barakaevskaïa (Nord Caucase). *L'Anthropologie*, 102:67-90.

Lioubine, V. P., Autlev, P. U., Zubov, A. A., Romanova, G. P. and Kharitonov, V. M. (1986). The discovery of the Neanderthal skeletal remains at the Barakai Site (Western Caucasus). *Voprosy Anthrop.*, **77**:60-70 (in Russian).

Logan, W. H. G. and Kronfeld, R. (1933). Development of the human jaws and surrounding structures from birth to the age of fifteen years. *J. Am. Dent. Assoc.*, 20:379-427.

Long, M. (1947). The development of the muscle-tendon attachment in the rat. *Am. J. Anat.*, 81:159-197.

Lovejoy, C. O., Cohn, M. J. and White, T. D. (1999). Morphological analysis of the mammalian postcranium: a developmental perspective. *Proc. Nat. Acad. Sci.* 96:13247-13252.

de Lumley, H., de Lumley, M-A. and Fournier, A. (1982). La mandibule de l'homme de Tautavel. *1st Congr. Internat. Paléontol. Humaine*, Vol. 1, pp. 178-221.

de Lumley, M-A. (1972). La mandíbula de Bañolas. *AMPURIAS* (Barcelona), 34:1-91.

de Lumley, M-A. (1973). Anténéandertaliens et Néandertaliens du bassin méditerranéen occidental européen. *Ed. Lab. Paleontol. Hum. Prehist., Études Quaternaires, Mém. No. 2*. Marseille: Université Provence, pp. 105-229.

Lundy, J. K. (1980). The mylohyoid bridge in the Khoisan of Southern Africa and its unsuitability as a Mongoloid genetic marker. *Am. J. phys. Anthrop.*, 53:43-48.

Madre-Dupouy, M. (1991). Principaux caractères de l'enfant néandertalien du Roc de Marsal, Dordogne (France). *L'Anthropologie*, 95:523-534.

Madre-Dupouy, M. (1992). L'enfant du Roc de Marsal: étude analytique et comparative. Cahiers de Paléoanthrop., Paris: C. N. R. S.

Mandarim-de-Lacerda, C. A. and Alves, M. U. (1992). Human mandibular prenatal growth: bivariate and multivariate growth allometry comparing different mandibular dimensions. *Anat. Embryol.*, 186:537-541.

Mann, A. E., Lampl, M. and Monge, J. M. (1990). Patterns of ontogeny in human evolution: evidence from dental development. *Yrbk. phys. Anthrop.*, 33:111-150.

Mann, A. and Vandermeersch, B. (1997). An adolescent female Neandertal mandible from Montgaudier Cave, Charente, France. *Am. J. phys. Anthrop.*, 103:507-527.

Mao, J., Stein, R. B. and Osborn, J. W. (1992). The size and distribution of fiber types in jaw muscles: a review. *J. Craniomand. Disorders*, 6:192-201.

Martin, H. (1923). *L'homme fossile de La Quina*. Paris: Librairie Octave Doin.

Martin, H. (1926). Mâchoire humaine moustérienne trouvée dans le station de La Quina. *L'Homme préhist.*, 13:3-21.

Matyas, J. R., Bodie, D., Andersen, M. and Frank, C. B. (1990). The developmental morphology of a "periosteal" ligament insertion: growth and maturation of the tibial insertion of the rabbit medial collateral ligament. *J. Orthoped. Res.*, 8:412-424.

Matyas, J. R., Anton, M. G., Shrive, N. G. and Frank, C. B. (1995). Stress governs tissue phenotype at the femoral insertion of the rabbit MCL. *J. Biomechan.*, 28:147-157.

Mayr, E. (1974). Cladistic analysis or cladistic classification? *Z. Zool. Syst. Evolut.-forsch.*, 12:94-128.

McBurney, C. B. M., Trevor, J. C. and Wells, L. H. (1953). The Haua Fteah fossil jaw. *J. Roy. Anthrop. Inst.*, 83:71.

McCown, T. D. and Keith, A. (1939). *The stone age of Mount Carmel II: the fossil human remains from the Levalloiso-Mousterian*. Oxford: Clarendon.

McDevitt, W. E. (1989). *Functional anatomy of the masticatory system*. London: Wright.

Merida-Velasco, J. A., Sanchez-Montesinos, I., Espin-Ferra, J., Garcia-Garcia, J. D. and Roldan-Schilling, V. (1993). Developmental differences in the ossification process of the human corpus and ramus mandibulae. *Anat. Rec.*, 235:319-324.

Miller, A. J. (1991). *Craniomandibular muscles: their role in function and form*. Boca Raton: CRC Press.

Minugh-Purvis, N. (1988). Patterns of craniofacial growth and development in Upper Pleistocene hominids. Ph. D. Dissertation, University of Pennsylvania.

Minugh-Purvis, N. (1998). The search for the earliest modern Europeans. In (T. Akazawa, K. Aoki and O. Bar-Yosef, Eds) *Neanderthals and modern humans in Western Asia*, pp. 339-352. New York: Plenum.

Mollier, G. (1937). Beziehungen zwischen Form und Funktion der Sehnen im Muskel-Sehenen-Knochen-System. *Morph. Jb.*, 79:161-199.

Moore, S., Richards, G. D., and Olson, M. (2003). Recent human mental foramen ontogeny: its significance for craniofacial growth theory and phylogenetics of Pleistocene *Homo*. *Am. J. phys. Anthrop.* Suppl. 36:154.

Moore, W. J. (1965). Masticatory function and skull growth. *J. Zool.*, 146:123-131.

Moore, W. J. and Lavelle, C. L. B. (1974). *Growth of the facial skeleton in the Hominoidea*. San Francisco: Academic Press.

Moorrees, C. F. A., Fanning, E. A. and Hunt, E. E. Jr. (1963a). Age variation of formation stages for ten permanent teeth. *J. Dent. Res.*, 42:1490-1502.

Moorrees, C. F. A, Fanning, E. A. and Hunt, E. E. Jr. (1963b). Formation and resorption of three deciduous teeth in children. *Am. J. phys. Anthrop.*, 21:205-213.

Mosolov, N. N. (1972). On the anatomy of human masticatory musculature. In (G-H. Schumacher, Ed) *Morphology of the maxillo-mandibular apparatus*, pp. 65-69. Leipzig: Veb Georg Thieme.

Moss, M. L. (1960). Functional analysis of human mandibular growth. *J. Pros. Dent.*, 10:1149-1159.

Moss, M. L. (1968). The primacy of functional matrices in orofacial growth. *Dent. Practit.*, 19:65-73.

Moss, M. L and Renkow, R. M. (1968). The role of the functional matrix in mandibular growth. *Angle Orthod.*, 38:95-103.

Moss, M. L. and Simons, M. R. (1968). Growth of the human mandibular angular process: a functional cranial analysis. *Am. J. phys. Anthrop.*, 28:127-138.

Moss, M. L. and Moss-Slentijin, L. (1978). The muscle-bone interface: an analysis of a morphological boundary. In (D. S. Carlson and J. A. McNamara, Jr., Eds) *Muscle adaptation in the craniofacial region*. Center Human Growth Development, University of Michigan, Craniof. Growth Ser., No. 8:1-16.

Moss, M. L. and Salentijin, V. (1970). The logarithmic growth of the human mandible. *Acta Anat.*, 77:341-360.

Moyers, R. E. (1950). An electromyographic analysis of certain muscles involved in temporomandibular movement. *Am. J. Orthod.*, 36:481-515.

Moyers, R. E. (1964). The infant swallow. *Trans. Eur. Orthod. Soc.*, 40:180-187.

Moyers, R. E., Bookstein, F. L. and Guire, K. E. (1979). The concept of pattern in craniofacial growth. *Am. J. Orthod.*, 76:136-148.

Moyers, R. E. and Carlson, D. S. (1996). Maturation of the orofacial neuromusculature. In (D. H. Enlow and M. G. Hans, Eds) *Essentials of facial growth*, pp. 233-240. Philadelphia: W. B. Saunders.

Murphy, T. R. and Grundy, E. M. (1969). The inferior alveolar neurovascular bundle at the mandibular foramen. *Dent. Pract.*, 20:41-48.

Nagar, Y. and Arensburg, B. (2000). Bilateral aplasia of the condyles of a 1,400-year-old mandible from Israel. *Am. J. phys. Anthrop.*, 111:135-139.

Nakata, S., Mizuno, M., Koyano, K., Nakayama, E., Watanabe, M. and Murakami, T. (1995). Functional masticatory evaluation in hemifacial microsomia. *Eur. J. Orthod.*, 17:273-280.

Nanda, R. S. (1955). The rates of growth of several facial components measured from cephalometric roentgenograms. *Am. J. Orthod.*, 41:653-673.

Nanda, R. S. (1969). Root resorption of deciduous teeth in Indian children. *Archs. Oral Biol.*, 14:1021-1030.

Nanda, S. K., Merow, W.W. and Sassouni, V. (1967). Repositioning of the masseter muscle and its effect on skeletal form and structure. *Angle Orthod.*, 37:304-308.

Noden, D. M. (1982). Patterns and organization of craniofacial skeletogenic and myogenic mesenchyme: a perspective. In (A. D. Dixon and B. G. Sarnat, Eds) *Factors and mechanisms influencing bone growth*, pp. 167-203. New York: Alan R. Liss.

Noden, D. M. (1986). Origins and patterning of craniofacial mesenchymal tissues. *J. Craniof. Genet. Dev. Biol.*, 2 (Suppl.):15-31.

Noden, D. M. and de Lahunta, A. (1985). *The embryology of domestic animals: developmental mechanisms and malformations*. Baltimore: Williams and Wilkins.

Nordborg, M. (1998). On the probability of Neanderthal ancestry. *Am. J. Hum. Genet.*, 63:1240-1242.

O'Dell, N. L., Todd, G. I. III and Bernard, G. R. (1970). Musculoskeletal arrangements for lateral mandibular movements in the rabbit and rat: electromyographic and other analyses. *J. Dent. Res.*, 49:1111-1117.

Öğütcen-Toller, M. and Keskin, M. (2000). Computerized 3-dimensional study of the embryonic development of the human masticatory muscles and temporomandibular joint. *J. Oral Maxillofac. Surg.*, 58:1381-1386.

Osburn, J. W. (1989). The temporomandibular ligament and the articular eminence as constraints during jaw opening. *J. Oral Rehabil.*, 16:323-333.

Osburn, J. W. (1993). A model to describe how ligaments may control symmetrical jaw opening movements in man. *J. Oral Rehabil.*, 20:585-604.

Ossenberg, N. S. (1974a). The mylohyoid bridge: an anomalous derivative of Meckel's cartilage. *Am. J. phys. Anthrop.*, 41 (Suppl.):496.

Ossenberg, N. S. (1974b). The mylohyoid bridge: an anomalous derivative of Meckel's cartilage. *J. Dent. Res.*, 53:77-82.

Ouchi, Y., Abe, S., Sun-Ki, R., Agematus, H., Watanabe, H. and Ide, Y. (1998). Attachment of the sphenomandibular ligament to bone during intrauterine embryo development for the control of mandibular movement. *Bull. Tokyo Dent. Coll.*, 39:91-94.

Ovchinnikov, I. V., Götgerström, A., Romanova, G. P., Kharitonov, V. M., Lidén, K. and Goodwin, W. (2000). Molecular analysis of Neanderthal DNA from the northern Caucasus. *Nature*, 404:490-493.

Pap, I., Tillier, A-M., Arensburg, B. and Chech, M. (1996). The Subalyuk Neanderthal remains (Hungary): a re-examination. *Annls. Hist.-Nat. Mus. Nat. Hungarici*, 88:233-270.

Parsons, F. G. (1896). An account of the myology of the Myomorpha, together with a comparison of the muscles of the various suborders of rodents. *Proc. Zool. Soc. Lond.*, 159-192.

Patte, M. (1957). *L'enfant néanderthalien du Pech-de-l'Aze*. Paris: Masson et Cie.

Patte, E. (1958). L'enfant du Pech-de-l'Azé. In (GHR von Koenigswald, Ed) *Hundert Jahre Neanderthaler [Neanderthal Centenary] 1856-1956*, pp. 270-276. Utrecht Netherlands: Kemink en Zoon NV.

Pirinen, S. (1995). Endocrine regulation of craniofacial growth. *Acta Odont. Scand.*, 53:179-185.

Piveteau, J. (1959). Les restes humains de la grotte de Regourdou (Dordogne). *C. r. Acad. Sci., Paris*, 248:40-44.

Piveteau, J. (1963-1966). La grotte de Regourdou (Dordogne): paléontologie humaine. *Annls. Paléont.*, 49:285-304; 50:155-194; 52:163-170.

Ponce de León, M. S. and Zollikofer, C. P. E. (2001). Neanderthal cranial ontogeny and its implications for late hominid diversity. *Nature*, 412:534-538.

Posselt, U. (1952). Studies in the mobility of the human mandible. *Acta Odont. Scand.*, 10 (Suppl.):1-160.

Presley, R. (1993). Preconception of adult structural pattern in the analysis of the developing skull. In (J. Hanken and B. K. Hall, Eds) *The skull. Vol. 1: Development*, pp. 347-377. Chicago: University of Chicago.

Quam, R. M. and Smith, F. H. (1998). A reassessment of the Tabun C2 mandible. In (T. Akazawa, K. Aoki, and O. Bar-Yosef, Eds) *Neandertals and modern humans in Western Asia*, pp. 405-421. New York: Plenum Press.

Raadsheer, M. C., Van Eijden, T. M. G. J., Van Ginkel, F. C. and Prahl-Anderson, B. (1999). Contribution of jaw muscle size and craniofacial morphology to human bite force magnitude. *J. Dent. Res.*, 78:31-42.

Rabkin, S. (1952). Variation in structural morphogenesis of the human face and jaws. *J. Dent. Res.*, 31:535-547.

Radovčić, J., Smith, F. H., Trinkaus, E. and Wolpoff, M. H. (1988). *The Krapina Hominids: an illustrated catalog of skeletal collection*. Zagreb: Croatian Nat. His. Mus.

Rak, Y. (1998a). The derived mandible of *Homo neanderthalensis*. *Am. J. phys. Anthrop.*, 26 (Suppl.):183.

Rak, Y. (1998b). Does any Mousterian cave present evidence of two hominid species? In (T. Akazawa, K. Aoki and O. Bar-Yosef, Eds) *Neandertals and modern humans in Western Asia*, pp. 353-366. New York: Plenum Press.

Rak, Y. and Kimbel, W. H. (1995). Diagnostic Neandertal characters in the Amud 7 infant. *Am. J. phys. Anthrop.*, 20 (Suppl.):177-178.

Rak, Y., Kimbel, W. H. and Hovers, E. (1994). A Neandertal infant from Amud Cave, Israel. *J. hum. Evol.*, 26:313-324.

Rak, Y., Kimbel, W. H. and Hovers, E. (1996). On Neanderthal autapomorphies discernible in Neandertal infants: a response to Creed-Miles *et al*. *J. hum. Evol.*, 30:155-158.

Raven, H. C. and Hill, J. E. (1950). Regional anatomy of the gorilla. In (W. K. Gregory, Ed) *The anatomy of the gorilla*, pp. 15-189. New York: Columbia University Press.

Rayne, J. and Crawford, G. N. C. (1971). The development of the muscles of mastication in the rat. *Ergebn. Anat. Entwickl.-Gesch.*, 44:1-55.

Rayne, J. and Crawford, G. N. C. (1972). The growth of the muscles of mastication in the rat. *J. Anat.*, 113:391-408.

Relethford, J. H. (1999). Models, predictions, and the fossil record of modern human origins. *Evol. Anthrop.*, 8:7-10.

Relethford, J. H. (2001). Absence of regional affinities of Neandertal DNA with living humans does not reject multiregional evolution. *Am. J. phys. Anthrop.*, 115:95-98.

Rhoads, M. L. and Franciscus, R. G. (1996). Mandibular notch crest orientation in Neanderthals and recent humans. *Am. J. phys. Anthrop.*, 22 (Suppl.):196.

Richany, S. F., Blast, T. H. and Anson, B. J. (1956). The development of the first branchial arch in man and the fate of Meckel's cartilage. *Quart. Bull. Northwest. Univ. Med. Sch.*, 30:331-355.

Richards, G. D. (in prep.). Basicranial evolution and ontogeny in *Homo sapiens*. Ph. D. Dissertation, University of California, Berkeley.

Richards, G. D. and Plourde, A. M. (1995). Reconsideration of the 'Neanderthal' Infant, Amud-7. *Am. J. phys. Anthrop.*, 20 (Suppl.):180-181.

Richards, G. D., Mardini, S., Rapal, K., Moore, S. and Olson, M. (in prep.). Ontogeny of the *sulcus colli* region in humans: implications for mandibular nerve (V_3) anesthesia.

Ricketts, R. M. (1972). A principle of arcial growth of the mandible. *Angle Orthod.*, 42:368-386.

Rieppel, O. (1993). The conceptual relationship of ontogeny, phylogeny, and classification: the taxic approach. *Evol. Bio.* 27:1-32.

Rightmire, G. P. (1995). Comment on: testing hypotheses about recent human evolution from skulls. *Curr. Anthrop.*, 36:1182-183.

Ringqvist, M. (1971). Histochemical fiber types and fiber sizes in human masticatory muscles. *Scand. J. Dent. Res.*, 79:366-368.

Ringqvist, M. (1973). Isometric bite force and its relationship to dimensions of the facial skeleton. *Acta Odont. Scand.*, 31:35-42.

Ringqvist, M. (1974). Fiber types in human masticatory muscles: relation to function. *Scand. J. Dent. Res.*, 82:333-355.

Robinson, J. T. (1953). *Telanthropus* and its phylogenetic significance. *Am. J. phys. Anthrop.*, 11:445-501.

Rosas, A. (1987). Two new mandibular fragments from Atapuerca/Ibeas (SH site): a reassessment of the affinities of the Ibeas mandibles sample. *J. hum. Evol.*, 16:417-427.

Rosas, A. (1992). Ontogenia y filogenia de la madíbula en la evolución de hominidos: aplicación de un modelo de morfogenesis a las mandíbulas fóssles de Atapuerca. P.h. D. Dissertation: Universidad Complutense, Madrid.

Rosas, A. (1995). Seventeen new mandibular specimens from the Atapuerca/Ibeas Middle Pleistocene hominid sample (1985-1992). *J. hum. Evol.*, 28:533-560.

Rosas, A. (1997). A gradient of size and shape for the Atapuerca sample and Middle Pleistocene hominid variability. *J. hum. Evol.*, 33:39-331.

Rosas, A. (2000). Ontogenetic approach to variation in Midle Pleistocene hominids: evidence from the Atapuerca-SH mandibles. *Hum. Evol.*, 15:83-98.

Rosas, A. (2001). Occurrence of Neanderthal features in mandibles from the Atapuerca-SH site. *Am. J. phys. Anthrop.*, 114:74-91.

Rosas, A., Bermudez de Castro, J. M. and Aguirre, E. (1991). Mandibules et dents d'Ibeas (Espagne) dans le contexte de l'èvolution humaine en Europe. *L'Anthropologie*, 95:89-102.

Rosas, A. Bastir, M., Martinez-Maza, C., and Bermudez de Castro, J. M. (2002). Sexual dimorphism in the Atapuerca-SH hominids: the evidence from the mandibles. *J. hum. Evol.*, 42:451-474.

Roth, V. L. (1988). The biological basis of homology. In (C. J. Humphries, Ed) *Ontogeny and Systematics*, pp. 1-26. New York: Columbia University Press.

Rowlerson, A., Mascarello, F., Veggetti, A and Carpené, E. (1983). The fibre-type composition of the first branchial arch muscles in Carnivora and Primates. *J. Mus. Res. Cell Motility*, 4:443-472.

Sanchez, F. (1999). Comparative biometrical study of the Mousterian mandible from Cueva del Boquette de Zafarraya (Málaga, Spain). *Hum. Evol.*, 14:125-138.

Sato, I., Ishikawa, H., Shimada, K., Ezure, H. and Sato, T. (1994). Morphology and analysis of the developing temporomandibular joint and masticatory muscle. *Acta Anat.*, 149:55-62.

Saunders, S., DeVito, C., Herring, A., Southern, R. and Hoppa, R. (1993). Accuracy tests of tooth formation age estimations for human skeletal remains. *Am. J. phys. Anthrop.*, 92:173-188.

Sausse, F. (1975). La mandibule Atlanthropienne de La Carrière Thomas I (Casablanca). *L'Anthropologie*, 79:81-112.

Sawyer, D. R., Allison, M. J., Elazy, R. P. and Pezzia, A. (1978). The mylohyoid bridge of Pre-Columbian Peruvians. *Am. J. phys. Anthrop.*, 48:9-16.

Sawyer, D. R., Gianfortune, V., Kiely, M. L. and Allison, M. J. (1990). Mylohyoid and jugular foramen bridging in Pre-Columbian Chileans. *Am. J. phys. Anthrop.*, 82:179-182.

Schaeffer, J. P. (1935). The ontogenetic development of the human face. In (C. T. Gilden, Jr., Ed) *The human face: A symposium*, pp. 17-37. Philadelphia: The Dental Cosmos.

Schiaffino, S., Gorza, L., Sartore, S., Saggin, L., Ausoni, S., Vianello, M., Gunderson, K. and Lomo, T. (1989). Three myosin heavy chain isoforms in type 2 skeletal muscle fibers. *J. Muscle Res. Cell Motil.*, 10:197-205.

Schoch, R. M. (1986). *Phylogeny reconstruction in paleontology*. New York: Van Nostrand Reinhold.

Schoetensack, O. (1908). *Der unterkiefer des Homo heidelbergensis aus den sanden von Mauer bei Heidelberg: Ein beitrag zur paläontologie des menschen*. Leipzig: Engelmann.

Scholz, M., Bachmann, L., Nicholson, G. J., Bachmann, J., Giddings, I., Rüschoff-Thale, B., Czarnetzki, A. and Pusch, C. M. (2000). Genomic differentiation of Neanderthals and anatomically modern man allows a fossil-DNA-based classification of morphologically indistinguishable hominid bones. *Am. J. Hum. Genet.*, 66:1927-1932.

Schour, I. and Massler, M. (1941). The Development of the Human Dentition. *J. Am. Dent. Assoc.*, 28:1153-1160.

Schumacher, G-H. (1959). Die kaumuskulatur von menschlichen Früh- und Neugeborenen. *Zeit. Anat. Enteickl.-gesch.*, 121:304-321.

Schumacher, G-H. (1961). *Funktionelle Morphlogie der Kaumuskulatur*. Jena: Fischer Verlag.

Schumacher, G-H. (1962). Struktur- und Funktionswandel der Kaumuskulatur nach der Geburt. *Fortfch Kieferorthop*, 23:135-166.

Schumacher, G-H. (1980). Comparative functional anatomy of jaw muscles. In (K. Kubota, Y. Nakamura, and G-H. Schumacher, Eds) *Jaw position and jaw movement*, pp. 76-93. Berlin: Veb Verlag Volk und Gesundheit.

Schumacher, G-H. (1989). Innervation pattern in jaw muscles of various mammalian chewing types. *Acta Morphol. Neerl.-Scand.*, 27:139-147.

Schumacher, G-H., Lau, H., Freund, E., Schultz, M., Himstedt, H. W. and Menning, A. (1976). Zur topographie der muskulären nervenausbreitungen: Kaumuskeln. m. pterygoideus medialis und lateralis verschiedener Kautypenvertreter (Schluß). *Anat. Anz.*, 139:71-87.

Schwartz, J. H. and Tattersall, I. (1995). Toward a definition of *Homo neanderthalensis* and *Homo sapiens*: 1. the nasal region. In (J. Gilbert, F. Sánchez, L. Gilbert and F. Ribot, Eds) *The hominids and their environment during the lower and middle Pleistocene of Eurasia*, pp. 299-310. Proc. Internat. Conf. Hum. Paleo., Orce 1995.

Schwartz, J. H. and Tattersall, I. (1996a). Toward distinguishing *Homo neanderthalensis* from *Homo sapiens*, and vice versa. *Anthropologie*, 34:79-88.

Schwartz, J. H. and Tattersall, I. (1996b). Significance of some previously unrecognized apomorphies in the nasal region of *Homo neanderthalensis*. *Proc. natl. Acad. Sci.*, 93:10852-10854.

Schwartz, J. H. and Tattersall, I. (2000). The human chin revisited: what is it and who has it? *J. hum. Evol.*, 38:367-409.

Schwartz, J. H., Tattersall, I. and Laitman, J. T. (1999). New thoughts on Neanderthal behavior: evidence from nasal morphology. In (H. Ullrich, Ed) *Hominid evolution: Lifestyles and survival strategies*, pp. 166-186. Gelsenkirchen/Schwelm: Edition Archaea.

Sciote, J. J. and Morris, T. J. (2000). Skeletal muscle function and fibre types: the relationship between occlusal function and the phenotype of jaw-closing muscles in human. *J. Orthod.*, 27:15-30.

Scott, J. H. (1951). Development of joints concerned with early jaw movement in the sheep. *J. Anat.*, 85:36-43.

Scott, J. H. (1954). The growth and function of the muscles of mastication in relation to the development of the facial skeleton and of the dentition. *Am. J. Orthod.*, 40:429-449.

Scott, J. H. (1957). Muscle growth and function in relation to skeletal morphology. *Am. J. phys. Anthrop.*, 15:197-234.

Scott, J. H. (1967). *Dento-facial development and growth*. Oxford: Pergamon.

Scott, J. H. and Dixon, A. D. (1972). *Anatomy for Students of Dentistry*, 3rd ed. Baltimore: Williams and Wilkins.

Sergi, S. and Ascenzi, A. (1955). La mandibola neandertaliana Circeo III. *Riv. Antropol.*, 17:337-403.

Shaughnessy, T., Fields, H., and Westbury, J. (1989). Association between craniofacial morphology and fiber-type distributions in human masseter and medial pterygoid muscles. *Internatl. J. Adult Orthod. Orthognath. Surg.*, 4:145-155.

Shellswell, G. B. and Wolpert, L. (1977). The pattern of muscle and tendon development in the chick wing. In (D. A. Ede, J. R. Hinchliffe and M. Balls, Eds) *Vertebrate limb and somite morphogenesis*, pp. 78-86. Cambridge: Cambridge University Press.

Sillman, J. H. (1948). Serial study of occlusion (Birth to Ten Years of Age). *Am. J. Orthod.*, 34:969-979.

Simon, B. and Kömives, O. (1938). Dimensional and positional variations of the ramus of the mandible. *J. Dent. Res.*, 17:125-149.

Simpson, G. G., Roe, A. and Lewontin, R. C. (1960). *Quantitative zoology*. New York: Harcourt, Brace and World.

Skerry, T. (2000). Biomechanical influences on skeletal growth and development. In (P. O'Higgins and M. J. Cohn, Eds) *Development, growth, and evolution: implications for the study of the hominid skeleton*, pp. 29-39. San Deigo: Academic Press.

Skinner, M. (1997). Age at death of Gibraltar 2. *J. hum. Evol.*, 32:469-470.

Smerdu, V., Karsch-Mizrachi, I., Campione, M., Leinwand, L. and Schiaffino, S. (1994). Type IIx myosin heavy chain transcripts are expressed in type IIb fibers of human skeletal muscle. *Am. J. Physiol.*, 267:C1723-C1728.

Smith, B. H. (1986). Dental development in *Australopithecus* and early *Homo*. *Nature*, 323:327-330.

Smith, B. H. (1991). Standards of human tooth formation and dental age assessment. In (M. A. Kelly and C. S. Larsen, Eds) *Advances in Dental Anthropology*, pp. 143-168. New York: Wiley-Liss.

Smith, B. H. (1993). The physiological age of KNM-WT 15000. In (A. Walker and R. Leakey, Eds) *The Nariokotome Homo erectus skeleton*, pp. 195-220. Cambridge: Harvard University Press.

Smith, F. H. (1976). *The Neandertal remains from Krapina: a descriptive and comparative study*. Knoxville: University of Tennessee, Report No 15.

Smith, F. H. (1978). Evolutionary significance of the mandibular foramen area in Neanderthals. *Am. J. phys. Anthrop.*, 48:523-532.

Smith, F. H., Trinkaus, E., Pettitt, P. B., Karavanić, I. and Paunović, M. (1999). Direct radiocarbon dates for Vindija G1 and Velika Pecina Late Pleistocene hominid remains. *Proc. natl. Acad. Sci.*, 96:12281-12286.

Smith, J. W. (1954). The elastic properties of the anterior cruciate ligament of the rabbit. *J. Anat.*, 88:369-380.

Sokal, R. R. and Rohlf, F. J. (1987). *Introduction to biostatistics*, 2nd ed. San Francisco: W. H. Freeman.

Sonntag, C. F. (1923). On the anatomy, physiology, and pathology of the chimpanzee. *Proc. Zool. Soc., Lond.*, 23:323-429.

Sonntag, C. F. (1924). On the anatomy, physiology, and pathology of the orang-outan. *Proc. Zool. Soc. Lond.*, 24:349-450.

Soussi-Yanicostas, N., Barbet, J. P., Laurnet-Winter, C., Barton, P. and Butler-Browne, G. S. (1990). Transition of myosin isozymes during development of human masseter muscle. *Development*, 108:239-249.

Sperber, G. H. (1981). *Craniofacial embryology*, 3rd ed. Year Book: Chicago.

Spyropoulos, M. N. (1977). The morphogenetic relationship of the temporal muscle to the coronoid process in human embryos and fetuses. *Am. J. Anat.*, 150:395-410.

Starkie, C. and Stewart, D. (1931). The intra-mandibular course of the inferior dental nerve. *J. Anat.*, 65:319-323.

Stefan, V. H and Trinkaus, E. (1998a). La Quina 9 and Neandertal mandibular variability. *Bull. Mém. Soc. Anthrop. Paris*, 10:293-324.

Stefan, V. H and Trinkaus, E. (1998b). Discrete trait and dental morphometric affinities of the Tabun 2 mandible. *J. hum. Evol.*, 34:443-468.

Steindler, A. (1955). *Kinesiology of the human body under normal and abnormal conditions*. Springfield: Thomas.

Straus, W. A. Jr. (1950). On the zoological status of *Telanthropus capensis*. *Am. J. phys. Anthrop.*, 8:495-498.

Straus, W. A. Jr. (1962). The mylohyoid groove in primates. *Biblthca. primatol.*, 1:197-216.

Strickland, N. C. (1981). Muscle development in the human fetus as exemplified by m. sartorius: A quantitative study. *J. Anat.*, 132:557-579.

Strickland, N. C. (1983). The arrangement of muscle fibers and tendons in two muscles used for growth studies. *J. Anat.*, 136:175-179.

Stringer, C. B. (1982). Towards a solution of the Neanderthal problem. *J. hum. Evol.*, 11:431-438.

Stringer, C. B., Hublin, J-J. and Vandermeersch, B. (1984). The origin of anatomically modern humans in Western Europe. In (F. H. Smith and F. Spencer, Eds) *The origins of modern humans*, pp. 51-135. New York: Liss.

Stringer, C. B. and Dean, M. C. (1997). Age at death of Gibraltar 2: a reply. *J. hum. Evol.*, 32:471-472.

Stingl, J. (1972). Contribution to study of the postnatal development of skeletal muscle. *Folia Morphol.*, 20:121-123.

Suzuki, H. (1970). The skull of the Amud Man. In (H. Suzuki and F. Takai, Eds) *The Amud man and his cave site*, pp. 123-206. Japan: University of Tokyo.

Swindler, D. R and Wood, C. D. (1973). *An atlas of primate gross anatomy: baboon, chimpanzee, and man*. Seattle: University of Washington Press.

Symons, N. B. B. (1954). The attachment of the muscles of mastication. *Brit. Dent. J.*, 96:76-81.

Szabo, J. (1935). L'homme Moustérien de La Grotte Mussolini (Hongrie): étude de la mandible. *Bull. Mem. Soc. Anthrop. Paris*, 6:23-30.

Templeton, A. R. (2002). Out of Africa again and again. *Nature*, 416:45-51.

Testut, L. (1889). Recherches anthropologiques sur le squelette quaternaire de Chancelade (Dordogne). *Bull. Soc. Anthrop. Bio. Lyon*, 8:131-246.

Thilander, B. (1995). Basic mechanisms in craniofacial growth. *Acta Odont. Scand.*, 53:144-151.

Tillier, A-M. (1982). Les enfants néandertaliens de Devil's Tower (Gibraltar). *Z. Morph. Anthrop.*, 73:125-148.

Tillier, A-M. (1983a). Le crâne d'enfant d'Engis 2: un exemple de distribution des caractéres juvéniles, primitifs et néanderthaliens. *Bull. Soc. Roy. Belge. Anthrop. Prehist.*, 94:51-75.

Tillier, A-M. (1983b). L'enfant néanderthalien du Roc de Marsal (Campagne du Bugue, Dordogne): le squelette facial. *Annls. de Paléont. (Vert.-Invert.)*, 69:137-149.

Tillier, A-M. (1984). L'enfant Homo 11 de Qafzeh (Israël) et son apport à la compréhension des modalités de la croissance des squelettes Moustériens. *Paléorient*, 10:7-48.

Tillier, A-M. (1986). Quelques aspects de l'ontogénèse du squelette cranien des néanderthaliens. In (V. V. Novotny and A. Mizerova, Eds) *Fossil man: New facts, new ideas*. Brun: *Anthropos*, 23:207-216.

Tillier, A-M. (1988). A propos de sequences phylogenetique et ontogénètique chez les néanderthaliens. In (E. Trinkaus, Ed) *L'Homme de Neandertal, Vol 3; Anatomie*, pp. 125-135. Liège: Actes Colloque Internat. (1986).

Tillier, A-M. (1989). The evolution of modern humans: evidence from young Mousterian individuals. In (P. Mellars and C. Stringer, Eds) *The human revolution: Behavioural and biological perspectives on the origin of modern humans*, pp. 286-297. Princeton: Princeton University.

Tillier, A-M. (1991). La mandible et les dents. In (O. Bar-Yosef and B. Vandermeersch, Eds) *Le squelette Moustérien de Kébara*, pp. 97-111. Cahiers Paléanthrop., Paris: C. N. R. S.

Tillier, A-M. (1992). The origins of modern humans in Southwest Asia: ontogenetic aspects. In (T. Akasawa, K. Aoki, and T. Kimura, Eds) *The evolution and dispersal of modern humans in Asia*, pp. 15-28. Tokyo: Hokusen-sha.

Tillier, A-M. (1995). Neanderthal ontogeny: a new source for critical analysis. *Anthropologie*, 33:63-68.

Tillier, A-M. (1998). Ontogenetic variation in Late Pleistocene *Homo sapiens* from the Near East: implications for methodological bias in reconstructing evolutionary biology. In (T. Akazawa, K. Aoki and O. Bar-Yosef, Eds) *Neanderthals and modern humans in Western Asia*, pp. 381-388. New York: Plenum.

Tillier, A-M., Arensburg, B. and Duday, H. (1989). La mandibule et les dents du néanderthalien de Kebara (Homo 2) Mont Carmel, Israel. *Paléorient*, 15:39-59.

Tobias, P. V. (1967). The hominid skeletal remains of Haua Fteah. In (C. B. M. McBurney, Ed) *The Haua Fteah (Cyrenaica) and the stone age of the south-east Mediterranean*, pp. 338-352. Cambridge: Cambridge University Press.

Tobias, P. V. (1991). *Olduvai Gorge, Vol. 4, Parts 1-4. The skulls, endocasts, and teeth of Homo habilis*. Cambridge: Cambridge University Press.

Toussaint, M., Otte, M., Bonjean, D., Bocherens, H., Falguères, C. and Yokoyama, Y. (1998). Les restes humains nèandertaliens immatures de la couche 4A de la grotte Scladina (Andenne, Belgique). *C. r. Acad. Sci. Paris, Sci. (terre planètes)*, 326:737-742.

Tracy, W. E and Savara, B. S. (1966). Norms of size and annual increments of five anatomical measurements of the mandible. *Archs. Oral Biol.*, 11:587-598.

Trevor, J. C. and Wells, L. H. (1967). Preliminary report on the second mandibular fragment from Haua Fteah, Cyrenaica. In (C. B. M. McBurney, Ed) *The Haua Fteah (Cyrenaica) and the stone age of the south-east Mediterranean*, pp. 336-337. Cambridge: Cambridge University Press.

Trinkaus, E. (1983). *The Shanidar Neanderthals*. New York: Academic.

Trinkaus, E. (1987). The Neanderthal face: evolutionary and functional perspectives on a recent hominid face. *J. hum. Evol.*, 16:429-443.

Trinkaus, E. (1990). Cladistics and the hominid fossil record. *Am. J. phys. Anthrop.*, 83;1-11.

Trinkaus, E. (1993). Variability in the position of the mandibular mental foramen and the identification of Neandertal apomorphies. *Riv. Antropol., Roma*, 71:259-274.

Trinkaus, E. (1995a). Near Eastern late archaic humans. *Paléorient*, 21:9-24.

Trinkaus, E. (1995b). Comment on: testing hypotheses about recent human evolution from skulls. *Curr Anthrop.*, 36:185-186.

Tuli, A., Choudhry, R., Choudhry, S., Raheja, S. and Agarwal, S. (2000). Variation in shape of the lingula in the adult human mandible. *J. Anat.*, 197:313-317.

Turner, A. A. and Chamberlain, A. (1989). Speciation, morphological change and the status of African *Homo erectus*. *J. hum. Evol.*, 18:115-130.

Türp, J. C., Alt, K. W., Vach, W. and Harbich, K. (1998). Mandibular condyles and rami are asymmetric structures. *Cranio*, 16;51-56.

Tyrrell, A. J. and Chamberlain, A. T. (1998). Non-metric trait evidence for modern human affinities and the distinctiveness of Neanderthals. *J. hum. Evol.*, 34:549-554.

Ubelaker, D. (1984). *Human skeletal remains: excavation, analysis, and interpretation*. Washington: Taraxacum.

Vandermeersch, B. (1981). *Les hommes fossiles de Qafzeh (Israël)*. Cahiers Paléontol., Paris: C. N. R. S.

Vandermeersch, B. and Tillier, A-M. (1977). Étude préliminaire d'une mandibule d'adolescent provenant des niveaux moustérians de Qafzeh, Israël. *Eretz-Israel*, 13:164-176.

Van Eijden, T. M. G. J., Koolstra, J. H. and Brugman, P. (1995). Architecture of the human pterygoid muscles. *J. Dent. Res.*, 74:1489-1495.

Van Eijden, T. M. G. J., Koolstra, J. H. and Brugman, P. (1997). Architecture of the human jaw-closing and jaw-opening muscles. *Anat. Rec.*, 248:464-474.

Van Eijden, T. M. G. J. and Turkawski, S. J. J. (2001). Morphology and physiology of masticatory muscle motor units. *Crit. Rev. Oral Biol. Med.*, 12:76-91.

Van Spronsen, P. A., Weijs, W. A., Valk, J., Prahl-Anderson, B. and van Ginkel, F. C. (1991). Relationship between jaw muscle cross-sections and craniofacial morphology in normal adults, studied with magnetic resonance imaging. *Eur. J. Orthod.*, 13:351-361.

Van Spronsen, P. A., Weijs, W. A., Valk, J., Prahl-Anderson, B. and van Ginkel, F. C. (1992). A comparison of jaw muscle cross-sections of long-faced and normal adults. *J. Dent. Res.*, 71:1279-1285.

Van Spronsen, P. A., Koolstra, J. H., van Ginkel, F. C., Weijs, W. A., Valk, J. and Prahl-Anderson, B. (1997). Relationship between the orientation and moment arms of the human jaw muscles and normal craniofacial morphology. *Eur. J. Orthod.*, 19:313-328.

Van Valen, L. M. (1982). Homology and Causes. *J. Morphol.*, 173:305-312.

Vargervik, K. (1997). Discussion: Relationship between bone and muscles of mastication in hemifacial microsomia. *Plast. Reconstr. Surg.*, 99:998-999.

Vargervik, K. and Miller, A. J. (1984). Neuromuscular patterns in hemifacial microsomia. *Am. J. Orthod.*, 86:33-42.

Varrela, J. (1992). Dimensional variation of craniofacial structures in relation to changing masticatory-functional demands. *Eur. J. Orthod.*, 14:31-36.

Vlček, E. (1993). *Fossil Menschenfunde von Weimar-Ehringsdorf*. Stuttgart: Konrad Theiss.

Vogel, K. G. (1995). Fibrocartilage in tendon: a response to compressive load. In (S. L. Gordon, S. J. Blair and L. J. Fine, Eds) *Repetitive motion disorders of the upper extremity*, pp. 205-215. Rosemont: Am. Acad. Orthopaed. Surg.

von Lenhossék, M. (1921). Das innere relief des unterkieferastes. *Arch. Anthrop.*, 18:49-59.

Wadu, S. G., Penhall, B. and Townsend, G. C. (1997). Morphological variability of the human inferior alveolar nerve. *Clin. Anat.*, 10:82-87.

Washburn, S. L. (1947). The relation of the temporal muscle to the form of the skull. *Anat. Rec.*, 99:239-248.

Watanabe, K. and Watanabe, M. (2001). Activity of jaw-closing and jaw-opening muscles and their influence on dentofacial morphological features in normal adults. *J. Oral Rehabil.*, 28:873-879.

Weidenreich, F. (1936). The mandibles of *Sinanthropus pekinensis*: a comparative study. *Palaeont. Sinica*, Ser. D, 7:1-163.

Weidenreich, F. (1938-39). On the earliest representatives of modern mankind recovered on the soil of East Asia. *Peking Nat. Hist. Bull.*, 13:161-174.

Weidenreich, F. (1945). The palaeolithic child from the Teshik-Tash Cave in Southern Uzbekistan (Central Asia). *Am. J. phys. Anthrop.*, 3:21-32.

Weijs, W. A. (1989). The functional significance of morphological variation of the human mandible and masticatory muscles. *Acta Morphol. Neerl.-Scand.*, 27:149-162.

Weijs, W. A., Brugman, P. and Klok, E. M. (1987). The growth of the skull and jaw muscles and its functional consequences in the New Zealand rabbit (*Oryctolagus cuniculus*). *J. Morphol.*, 194:143-161.

White, T. D., Suwa, G., Simpson, S. and Asfaw, B. (2000). Jaws and teeth of *Australopithecus afarensis* from Maka, Middle Awash, Ethiopia. *Am. J. phys. Anthrop.*, 111:45-68.

Wickwire, N. A., Gibbs, C. H., Jacobson, A. P. and Lundeen, H. C. (1981). Chewing patterns in normal children. *Angle Orthod.*, 51:48-60.

Wiley, E. O. (1981). *Phylogenetic systematics: the theory and practice of phylogenetic systematics*. New York: John Wiley and Sons.

Williams, P. L. and Warwick, R. (1980). *Gray's Anatomy*, 36th ed. Philadelphia: W.B. Saunders.

Wilson, S., Johns, P. and Fuller, P. M. (1984). The inferior alveolar and mylohyoid nerves: an anatomic study and relationship to local anesthesia of the anterior mandibular teeth. *J. Am. Dent. Assoc.*, 108:350-352.

Winkler, L. A. (1991). Morphology and variability of masticatory structures in the orangutan. *Int. J. Primatol.*, 12:45-65.

Wolpoff, M. H., Smith, F. H., Malez, M., Radovčić, J. and Rukavina, D. (1981). Upper Pleistocene human remains from Vindija Cave, Croatia, Yugoslavia. *Am. J. phys. Anthrop.*, 54:499-545.

Wolpoff, M. H. and Crummett, T. L. (1995). Comment on: Testing hypotheses about recent human evolution from skulls. *Curr Anthrop.*, 36:186-188.

Wolpoff, M. H. and Caspari, R. (1999). Letter to the editor. *Evol. Anthrop.*, 8:10.

Wood, B. (1991). *Koobi Fora research project, Vol. 4. Hominid cranial remains*. Oxford: Clarendon.

Woodburn, R. T. (1978). *Essentials of Human Anatomy*, 6th ed. New York: Oxford University Press.

Woodside, D. G. (1973). Some effects of activator treatment on the mandible and the midface. *Trans. Eur. Orthod. Soc.*, 443-447.

Yamada, K. and Kimmel, D. B. (1991). The effect of dietary consistency on bone mass and turnover in the growing rat mandible. *Archs. Oral Biol.*, 36:129-138.

Yamano, S. and Yamaguchi, B. (1976). On the mylohyoid canal in the human mandible. *Bull. Tokyo Nat. Sci. Mus.*, Ser. D (Anthrop.), 2:37-44.

Zollikofer, C. P. E., Ponce de León, M. S. and Martin, R. D. (1995). Neanderthal computer skulls. *Nature*, 375:283-285.

Zuckerman, S., Ashton, E. H. and Pearson, J. B. (1962). The styloid of the primate skull. *Biblthca. primatol.*, 1:217-228.

www.ingramcontent.com/pod-product-compliance
Ingram Content Group UK Ltd.
Pitfield, Milton Keynes, MK11 3LW, UK
UKHW060200240426
12048UKWH00029B/1664